In A Page
Medicine

In A Page
Medicine

Scott Kahan, MD
Class of 2002
Medical College of Pennsylvania—Hahnemann University
Philadelphia, Pennsylvania

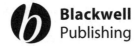

Blackwell
Publishing

Blackwell Publishing, Inc., 350 Main Street, Malden, Massachusetts 02148-5018, USA
Blackwell Science Ltd, 9600 Garsington Road, Oxford OX4 2DQ, UK
Blackwell Science Asia Pty Ltd, 550 Swanston Street, Carlton South, Victoria 3053, Australia
Blackwell Verlag GmbH, Kurfürstendamm 57, 10707 Berlin, Germany

03 04 05 06 5 4 3 2 1

ISBN: 1-405-10325-6

Library of Congress Cataloging-in-Publication Data

Kahan, Scott.
  In a page medicine / Scott Kahan.
    p. cm.
  Includes index.
  ISBN 1-40510-325-6
  1. Clinical medicine—Handbooks, manuals, etc.   I. Title.

  RC55 .K26 2003
  616—dc21
                                                          2002028220

A catalogue record for this title is available from the British Library

Acquisitions: Beverly Copland
Development: Julia Casson
Production: Debra Lally
Cover design: Gary Ragaglia
Interior design: Meral Dabcovich
Typesetter: Techbooks in York, PA
Printed and bound by Sheridan Books in Ann Arbor, MI

For further information on Blackwell Publishing, visit our website:
www.medirect.com

Table of Contents

Table of Contents

Section Four: Gastrointestinal Disease   59

Shahwali Arezo, MD
Scott Kahan, MD

Table of Contents

Section Five: Renal Disease 101
Joseph H. Brezin, MD, FACP

Section Six: Infectious Disease 111
Jose Delgado, MD

Table of Contents

Table of Contents

Table of Contents

Section Twelve: Rheumatologic & Immunologic Disease   217

Carolyn O'Connor, MD
Karen Carpency, MD

Abbreviations

α_1-AT	α-1 Antitrypsin Deficiency	CA	Cancer
5-FU	5-Fluorouracil	CABG	Coronary Artery Bypass Graft
5-HT	Serotonin	CAD	Coronary Artery Disease
A-a	Arterial-Alveolar Gradient	cANCA	Cytoplasmic Antineutrophilic Cytoplasm Antibody
AAA	Abdominal Aortic Aneurysm		
ABG	Arterial Blood Gas	CAP	Community-Acquired Pneumonia
AC	Acromioclavicular Joint	CATH	Cardiac Catheterization
ACE	Angiotensin-Converting Enzyme	CBC	Complete Blood Count
ACTH	Adrenocorticotropic Hormone	CD	Crohn's Disease
ADA	American Diabetes Association	CEA	Carcinoembryonic Antigen
ADH	Antidiuretic Hormone (Vasopressin)	CF	Cystic Fibrosis
		CHF	Congestive Heart Failure
Afib	Atrial Fibrillation	CIS	Carcinoma in situ
AFP	α-Fetoprotein	CK	Creatine Kinase
AGUS	Atypical Glands of Unknown Significance	CKD	Chronic Kidney Disease
		CLL	Chronic Lymphocytic Leukemia
AIDS	Acquired Immunodeficiency Syndrome	CMC	Carpometacarpal
		CML	Chronic Myelogenous Leukemia
AIH	Autoimmune Hepatitis	CMV	Cytomegalovirus
AIN	Acute Interstitial Nephritis	CN	Cranial Nerve
AIP	Acute Interstitial Pneumonitis	CNS	Central Nervous System
ALL	Acute Lymphoblastic Leukemia	CO	Cardiac Output
ALS	Amyotrophic Lateral Sclerosis	COPD	Chronic Obstructive Pulmonary Disease
ALT/SGPT	Alanine Aminotransferase		
AMA	Antimicrosomal Antibodies	COX	Cyclooxygenase
AMI	Acute Myocardial Infarction	CP	Chest Pain
AML	Acute Myelogenous Leukemia	CPAP	Continuous Positive Airway Pressure
ANA	Antinuclear Antibody		
AP	Anteroposterior	CPK	Creatine Phosphokinase
AR	Aortic Regurgitation	CRF	Chronic Renal Failure
ARDS	Acute Respiratory Distress Syndrome	CRP	C-Reactive Protein
		CSF	Cerebrospinal Fluid
ARF	Acute Renal Failure	CT	Computerized Tomography
AS	Ankylosing Spondylitis	CV	Cardiovascular
ASA	Aspirin	CVA	Cerebrovascular Accident
ASCUS	Atypical Squamous Cells of Unknown Significance	CVA	Costovertebral Angle
		CVD	Cerebrovascular Disease
ASD	Atrial Septal Defect	CVVH	Continuous Venovenous Hemofiltration
ASMA	Anti-smooth Muscle Antibodies		
ASO	Antistreptolysin	CWP	Coal Worker's Pneumoconiosis
AST/SGOT	Aspartate Aminotransferase	CXR	Chest X-Ray
AT	Antitrypsin	DBP	Diastolic Blood Pressure
ATN	Acute Tubular Necrosis	DDx	Differential Diagnosis
AV	Arterovenous	DFA	Direct Fluorescent Antibody
AV	Atrioventricular	DHEA-S	Dehydroepiandrosterone Sulfate
AVM	Arterovenous Malformation	DI	Diabetes Insipidus
AXR	Abdominal X-Ray	DIC	Disseminated Intravascular Coagulation
BMI	Body Mass Index		
BOOP	Bronchiolitis Obliterans Organizing Pneumonia	DIP	Distal Interphalangeal Joint
		DJD	Degenerative Joint Disease
BP	Blood Pressure	DM	Dermatomyositis
BPH	Benign Prostatic Hypertrophy	DM	Diabetes Mellitus
BSO	Bilateral Salpingo-oophorectomy	DRE	Digital Rectal Exam
BUN	Blood Urea Nitrogen	DUB	Dysfunctional Uterine Bleeding
BV	Bacterial Vaginosis	DVT	Deep Venous Thrombosis

Abbreviations

Dx	Diagnosis	HAV	Hepatitis A Virus
Dysfn	Dysfunction	Hb	Hemoglobin
EBV	Epstein-Barr Virus	HBV	Hepatitis B Virus
ECG	Electrocardiogram	HCC	Hepatocellular Carcinoma
ECHO	Echocardiogram	HCG	Human Chorionic Gonadotropin
ED	Emergency Department	HCT	Hematocrit
EEG	Electroencephalogram	HCV	Hepatitis C Virus
EF	Ejection Fraction	HD	Hodgkin's Disease
EGD	Esophagogastroduodenoscopy	HDL	High-Density Lipoprotein
EKG	Electrocardiogram	HDV	Hepatitis D Virus
ELISA	Enzyme-Linked Immunosorbent Assay	HEV	Hepatitis E Virus
		HGSIL	High-Grade Squamous Intraepithelial Lesion
EMG	Electromyogram		
EN	Erythema Nodosum	HHV	Human Herpesvirus
ERCP	Endoscopic Retrograde Cholangiopancreatography	HIV	Human Immunodeficiency Virus
		HLA	Human Leukocyte Antigen
ESR	Erythrocyte Sedimentation Rate	HP	Hypersensitivity Pneumonitis
ESRD	End-Stage Renal Disease	HPV	Human Papillomavirus
ET	Essential Thrombocytosis	HRT	Hormone Replacement Therapy
EtOH	Alcohol	HS	Hereditary Spherocytosis
F	Fever	HSP	Henoch-Schönlein Purpura
FAP	Familial Adenomatous Polyposis	HSV	Herpes Simplex Virus
FENa	Fractional Excretion of Sodium	HTLV	Human T-Cell Lymphocytic Virus
FEV_1	Forced Expiratory Volume	HTN	Hypertension
FH	Family History	HUS	Hemolytic-Uremic Syndrome
FiO_2	Fractional Inspiration of Oxygen	IABP	Intra-Aortic Balloon Pump
FNA	Fine-Needle Aspiration	IBD	Inflammatory Bowel Disease
FRC	Forced Residual Capacity	ICU	Intensive Care Unit
FSGS	Focal Sclerosing Glomerulosclerosis	IF	Intrinsic Factor
		IFG	Impaired Fasting Glucose
FSH	Follicle-Stimulating Hormone	IFN	Interferon
FUO	Fever of Unknown Origin	IgE	Immunoglobulin E
FVC	Forced Ventilatory Capacity	IgG	Immunoglobulin G
G6PD	Glucose-6-Phosphate Dehydrogenase Deficiency	IgM	Immunoglobulin M
		IL	Interleukin
GBM	Glomerular Basement Membrane	IM	Idiopathic Myelofibrosis
GBS	Guillain-Barré Syndrome	IMA	Inferior Mesenteric Artery
GCS	Glasgow Coma Scale	INH	Isoniazid
G-CSF	Granulocyte Colony-Stimulating Factor	INR	International Normalization Ratio
		IPF	Idiopathic Pulmonary Fibrosis
GERD	Gastroesophageal Reflux Disease	ITP	Idiopathic Thrombocytopenic Purpura
GFR	Glomerular Filtration Rate		
GH	Growth Hormone	IVC	Inferior Vena Cava
GI	Gastrointestinal	IVCD	Idioventricular Conduction Delay
GM-CSF	Granulocyte-Macrophage Colony-Stimulating Factor	IVF	Intravenous Fluids
		IVIG	Intravenous Immunoglobulin
GN	Glomerulonephritis	JVD	Jugular Venous Distension
GnRH	Gonadotropin-Releasing Hormone	JVP	Jugular Venous Pressure
GU	Genitourinary	LA	Left Atrium
GVH	Graft-Versus-Host disease	LAD	Left Axis Deviation
HA	Headache	LBBB	Left Bundle Branch Block
HACEK	*Haemophilus, Actinobacillus, Cardiobacterium, Eikenella, Kingella*	LBP	Low Back Pain
		LCR	Ligase Chain Reaction
		LDH	Lactate Dehydrogenase
HAP	Hospital-Acquired Pneumonia	LDL	Low-Density Lipoprotein

Abbreviations

LEEP	Loop Electrosurgical Procedure	OTC	Over-the-Counter
LES	Lower Esophageal Sphincter	PA	Pernicious Anemia
LFT	Liver Function Test	PAN	Polyarteritis Nodosum
LGSIL	Low-Grade Squamous Intraepithelial Lesion	pANCA	Perinuclear Antineutrophilic Cytoplasmic Antibody
LGV	Lymphogranuloma Venereum	PaO₂	Partial Pressure of Oxygen
LH	Luteinizing Hormone	PAP	Pulmonary Artery Pressure
Li	Lithium	PBC	Primary Biliary Cirrhosis
LLQ	Left Lower Quadrant	PCN	Penicillin
LMN	Lower Motor Neuron	PCOS	Polycystic Ovarian Syndrome
LOC	Loss of Consciousness	PCP	*Pneumocystis carinii* Pneumonia
LP	Lumbar Puncture	PCR	Polymerase Chain Reaction
LSB	Left Sternal Border	PE	Physical Examination
LUQ	Left Upper Quadrant	PE	Pulmonary Embolism
LV	Left Ventricle	PEEP	Positive End Expiratory Pressure
LVH	Left Ventricular Hypertrophy	PEFR	Peak Expiratory Flow Rate
MAC	*Mycobacterium avium* Complex	PET	Positron Emission Tomography
MAI	*Mycobacterium avium-intracellulare*	PFT	Pulmonary Function Test
MAO	Monoamine Oxidase	PICC	Peripherally-Inserted Central Catheter
MCP	Metacarpophalangeal Joint	PID	Pelvic Inflammatory Disease
MCV	Mean Corpuscular Volume	PIP	Proximal Interphalangeal Joint
M/E	Myeloid: Erythroid Precursor Ratio	PM	Polymyositis
MEN	Multiple Endocrine Neoplasia	PML	Progressive Multifocal Leukoencephalopathy
MG	Myasthenia Gravis	PMN	Polymorphonuclear Cell
MGUS	Monoclonal Gammopathy of Uncertain Significance	PND	Paroxysmal Nocturnal Dyspnea
MI	Myocardial Infarction	PNH	Paroxysmal Nocturnal Hemoglobinuria
MIBG	Metaiodobenzylguanidine Study (neuroectodermal tissue study)	PPD	Purified Protein Derivative
		PPI	Proton Pump Inhibitor
MPGN	Membranoproliferative Glomerulonephritis	PR	Pityriasis Rosea
		PSA	Prostate-Specific Antigen
MR	Mitral Regurgitation	PSC	Primary Sclerosing Cholangitis
MRA	Magnetic Resonance Angiography	PSGN	Post-Streptococcal Glomerulonephritis
MRCP	Magnetic Retrograde Cholangiopancreatography	PT	Prothrombin Time
		PTCA	Percutaneous Transluminal Coronary Angioplasty
MRI	Magnetic Resonance Imaging	PTH	Parathyroid Hormone
MS	Mitral Stenosis	PTT	Partial Thromboplastin Time
MS	Multiple Sclerosis	PTU	Propylthiouracil
MTP	Metatarsophalangeal Joint	PTX	Pneumothorax
MVP	Mitral Valve Prolapse	PUD	Peptic Ulcer Disease
N/V	Nausea/Vomiting	PV	Polycythemia Vera
NF	Neurofibromatosis	PVD	Peripheral Vascular Disease
NG	Nasogastric	PZA	Pyrazinamide
NHL	Non-Hodgkin's Lymphoma	RA	Rheumatoid Arthritis
NPO	Nulla per Os (nothing by mouth)	RA	Right Atrium
NSAID	Nonsteroidal Anti-inflammatory Drug	RAD	Right Axis Deviation
		RAS	Renal Artery Stenosis
NSCLC	Non-small Cell Lung Cancer	RBBB	Right Bundle Branch Block
NTG	Nitroglycerin	RBC	Red Blood Cell
NYHA	New York Heart Association	RF	Rheumatoid Factor
OA	Osteoarthritis	RF	Risk Factor
OCP	Oral Contraceptive Pill		

Abbreviations

RFLP	Restriction Fragment Length Polymorphism	TFT	Thyroid Function Test
RHD	Rheumatic Heart Disease	TIA	Transient Ischemic Attack
Rif	Rifampin	TIBC	Transferrin Iron-Binding Capacity
RLQ	Right Lower Quadrant	TIPS	Transjugular Intrahepatic Porto-Systemic Shunt
ROM	Range of Motion	TLC	Total Lung Capacity
RPGN	Rapidly Progressive Glomerulonephritis	TMP-SMX	Trimethoprim-Sulfamethoxazole
RPR	Rapid Plasma Reagin	TNF	Tumor Necrosis Factor
RS	Reed-Sternberg cell	TOA	Tubo-Ovarian Abscess
RTA	Renal Tubular Acidosis	TPA	Tissue Plasminogen Activator
RUQ	Right Upper Quadrant	TPR	Total Peripheral Resistance
RV	Residual Volume	TR	Tricuspid Regurgitation
RV	Right Ventricle	TRH	Thyroglobulin-Releasing Hormone
RVH	Right Ventricular Hypertrophy	TSH	Thyroid-Stimulating Hormone
S/S	Signs and Symptoms	TTE	Transthoracic Echocardiogram
S_1	First heart sound	TTP	Thrombotic Thrombocytic Purpura
S_2	Second heart sound	TURP	Transurethral Resection of the Prostate
S_3	Third heart sound		
S_4	Fourth heart sound	Tx	Treatment
SAH	Subarachnoid Hemorrhage	U/A	Urinalysis
SBE	Subacute Bacterial Endocarditis	U/S	Ultrasound
SBP	Systolic Blood Pressure	UC	Ulcerative Colitis
SCLC	Small Cell Lung Cancer	UGI	Upper Gastrointestinal Series
SGOT	See AST	UMN	Upper Motor Neuron
SI	Sacroiliac joint	URI	Upper Respiratory Infection
SIADH	Syndrome of Inappropriate Antidiuretic Hormone	UTI	Urinary Tract Infection
		V/Q	Ventilation-Perfusion Ratio
SK	Seborrheic Keratosis	VATS	Video-Assisted Thoracoscopic Surgery
SLE	Systemic Lupus Erythematosis		
SLL	Small Lymphocytic Lymphoma	VC	Vasoconstriction
SMA	Chemistry Panel	VCUG	Voiding Cystourethrogram
SMA	Superior Mesenteric Artery	VD	Vasodilation
SOB	Shortness of Breath	VDRL	Venereal Disease Research Laboratory
SSRI	Selective Serotonin Reuptake Inhibitor	VIP	Vasoactive Intestinal Peptide
STD	Sexually Transmitted Disease	VP	Ventriculo-Peritoneal
SVC	Superior Vena Cava Syndrome	Vtach	Ventricular Tachycardia
SVR	Systemic Venous Resistance	VWD	Von Willebrand's Disease
SVT	Supraventricular Tachycardia	VWF	Von Willebrand's Factor
TAH	Total Abdominal Hysterectomy	VZV	Varicella Zoster Virus
TAP	Thorax, Abdomen, Pelvis	WBC	White Blood Cell
TB	Tuberculosis	WPW	Wolff-Parkinson-White Syndrome
TCA	Tricyclic Antidepressant	WT	Weight
TEE	Transesophageal Echocardiogram		

Contributors

Shahwali Arezo, MD
Assistant Professor of Medicine
Allegheny General Hospital
Pittsburgh, Pennsylvania

J Brad Bellotte, MD
Resident, Neurosurgery
Allegheny General Hospital
Pittsburgh, Pennsylvania

Joseph Brezin, MD, FACP
Associate Professor of Medicine
MCP-Hahnemann University
Attending Nephrologist
Hahnemann University Hospital
Philadelphia, Pennsylvania

Karen Carpency, MD
Resident, Family Practice
Franklin Square Hospital
Baltimore, Maryland

Jeffrey M. Caterino, MD
Resident, Emergency Medicine/Internal Medicine
Allegheny General Hospital
Pittsburgh, Pennsylvania

Kathleen Owens DeAntonis, MD
Fellow, Academic Pediatrics
Children's Hospital of Pittsburgh
Pittsburgh, Pennsylvania

Jose A. Delgado, MD
Resident, Internal Medicine
Allegheny General Hospital
Pittsburgh, Pennsylvania

Richard F. Frisch, Jr., MD
Resident, Orthopedic Surgery
Albert Einstein Medical Center
Philadelphia, Pennsylvania

Aditi Ghatge, MD
Resident, Internal Medicine
Thomas Jefferson University
Philadelphia, Pennsylvania

Erica Linden, MD
Resident, Internal Medicine
Massachusetts General Hospital
Boston, Massachusetts

Contributors

Tejas Mehta, MD
Fellow, Cardiovascular Disease
Allegheny General Hospital
Pittsburgh, Pennsylvania

Pankaj Mohan, MD
Clinical Cardiologist
Associate Program Director For Education—Internal Medicine
Allegheny General Hospital
Pittsburgh, Pennsylvania

Carolyn Riester O'Connor, MD
Chief of Rheumatology
MCP-Hahnemann University
Philadelphia, Pennsylvania

Alexis Palley
Class of 2003
MCP-Hahnemann University
Philadelphia, Pennsylvania

John Leander Po, PhD
Class of 2003
MD-PhD Program Student
MCP-Hahnemann School of Medicine
Philadelphia, Pennsylvania

Nabeel R. Rana, MD
Resident, General Surgery
Christiana Care Health System
Newark, Delaware

Brett Sachse, MD
Resident, General Surgery
Allegheny General Hospital
Pittsburgh, Pennsylvania

Sudhakar Reddy Satti, MD
Resident, Radiology
MCP-Hahnemann University
Philadelphia, Pennsylvania

Ellen G. Smith, MD, FAAFP
Chairman and Director of Education
Department of Family Practice
Pinnacle Health System
Harrisburg, Pennsylvania

Josef Stehlik, MD
Fellow, Cardiovascular Disease
Department of Cardiology
Allegheny General Hospital
Pittsburgh, Pennsylvania

Contributors

Marcus Teshome, MD
Resident, Internal Medicine
Graduate Hospital
Philadelphia, Pennsylvania

Chanel T. Tyler, MD
Resident, Obstetrics/Gynecology
University of Massachusetts Memorial Health Center
Worcester, Massachusetts

David Wein
Class of 2004
University of Florida College of Medicine
Gainesville, Florida

Mary Helen Whited, MD
Fellow, Internal Medicine
University of Arizona
Tucson, Arizona
Mayo Clinic Scottsdale/Mayo Clinic Hospital
Scottsdale, Arizona

Ernest F. Wiggins, MD
Resident, General Surgery
Monmouth Medical Center
Long Branch, New Jersey

Scott M. Zelasko, MD
Resident, General Surgery
David Grant Medical Center
Travis Air Force Base
Fairfield, California

Consultants

Rosemary Patricia Fiore, MD, PhD
Attending Physician, Department of Medicine and Jacqueline Wilentz Breast Center
Monmouth Medical Center
Long Branch, New Jersey

Murray Gordon, MD
Associate Professor of Medicine
MCP-Hahnemann University
Senior Attending
Division of Endocrinology
Allegheny General Hospital
Pittsburgh, Pennsylvania

Alan B. Haratz, MD
Clinical Instructor of Medicine
MCP-Hahnemann University School of Medicine
Medical Director, Davita-Atlantic Artificial Kidney Center
Philadelphia, Pennsylvania

Neil Robert Holland, MD, BS
Neurologist, Herman Anayiotos, Gennaro & Gilson Neurology, P.A.
Active Staff
Monmouth Medical Center
Long Branch, New Jersey
Riverview Medical Center
Red Bank, New Jersey

Martin J. Luria, MD
Chief of Endocrinology
Medical Director, Diabetes Treatment Center
Monmouth Medical Center
Long Branch, New Jersey

James Joseph McGinty, Jr., MD
Executive Chief Resident
Department of General Surgery
Allegheny General Hospital
Pittsburgh, Pennsylvania

Carolyn Riester O'Connor, MD
Chief of Rheumatology
MCP-Hahnemann University
Philadelphia, Pennsylvania

Walter Joseph O'Donnell, MD, FACP
Clinical Director, Pulmonary/Critical Care Unit
Massachusetts General Hospital
Assistant Professor of Medicine
Harvard Medical School
Boston, Massachusetts

Consultants

Jeffrey L. Osofsky, MD, MBA
Cardiologist-Monmouth Cardiology Associates, LLP
Monmouth Medical Center
Long Branch, New Jersey

John J. Raves, MD
Senior Attending Staff
Division of General Surgery
Allegheny General Hospital
Pittsburgh, Pennsylvania

Ellen G. Smith, MD, FAAFP
Chairman and Director of Education
Department of Family Practice
Pinnacle Health System
Harrisburg, Pennsylvania

Ben Terrany, MD
Attending Physician Gastroenterology
Monmouth Medical Center
Long Branch, New Jersey

Allan Robert Tunkel, MD
Director, Internal Medicine Residency Program
Professor of Medicine
Vice-Chair for Education
MCP Hahnemann University
Co-Director, Medicine-Pediatrics Residency Program
MCP Hahnemann University–St. Christopher's Hospital for Children
Philadelphia, Pennsylvania

Reviewers

Sean Armin
Class of 2003
University of California, Los Angeles
Lost Angeles, California

Shane Kim
Class of 2002
University of Kansas School of Medicine
Kansas City, Kansas

Andrew Louie
Class of 2004
George Washington University
Washington, D.C.

Mark Mills, MD
Resident, Radiology
Baptist Memorial Hospital
Memphis, Tennessee

Christopher Quinn
Class of 2004
Michigan State University College of Osteopathic Medicine
East Lansing, Michigan

Jason Sluzevich, MD
Resident, Internal Medicine
University Hospital
Cincinnati, Ohio

Christina Thiruvathukal
Class of 2004
George Washington University
Washington, D.C.

Preface

Much of the idea for this book came from the difficulty that I experienced during medical school handling the incredible amount of medical information (and the lack of clear organization) that confronted me. So many times I became distracted by all there is to know in medicine. I found it difficult to know where to start my studies—due to the wide breadth of information available—and where to end my studies—due to the great depth of medical knowledge. What is necessary for a medical student to know?

Whereas entire books—even many volumes of books in some cases—have been written on nearly every human disease, there exists a basic nucleus of information central to any given disease. The luxury of being students is that we can forgo the esoteric clinical details in favor of concentrating on the "big picture." It is so essential, especially in medicine, to learn to walk before attempting to run. Just as baseball pitchers must prove that they can throw a fastball accurately before they can learn to throw a curve, so medical students should take the same approach to their education.

When I proposed the idea for *In A Page Medicine* to the editors at Blackwell Publishing, I envisioned a series of high-yield, "big picture" review books that would not bog readers down with too much breadth or depth of discussion. I wanted to present the most important human diseases in a manner that facilitates—even demands—that readers concentrate on the major issues. By presenting each disease on a simple one-page template, I hope that students will be able to master the nucleus of each disease without becoming seduced by the seemingly infinite amount of detail that normally surrounds it.

Along the way, we were somewhat constrained by the size of the template and the need to keep the discussion of each disease to a single page. We had to be quite succinct in our explanations and descriptions. In many cases, we sacrificed details such as drug dosages. Furthermore, we had to abbreviate liberally.

Nonetheless, the finished product appears to be highly effective. Reviews from medical students and residents have been very positive. I believe *In A Page Medicine* will prove very useful as a review for the boards, as a pocket reference during rounds, and even as a primary text to keep students focused on the big picture before advancing to more comprehensive texts. I hope readers will find this book as useful as I do.

I welcome any suggestions, questions, and advice. Please address your comments to drkahans@aol.com.

Acknowledgments

Perhaps the greatest strengths of *In A Page Medicine* is its diverse group of authors: Advanced medical students who have recently sat for the boards, residents who have experienced medicine from the viewpoints of both students and physicians, and experienced faculty physicians. My name on the cover is a technicality—this book became a reality because of the contributions of these physicians and physicians-in-training. I am so grateful to them. Special thanks go to Jeff Caterino, Walter O'Donnell, Josef Stehlik, and Ellen Smith.

I have enjoyed the opportunity to work with several physicians and professors who have been great mentors to me, especially those at MCP-Hahnemann University and Allegheny General Hospital. Their dedication to students and to their profession is appreciated by so many of the students, residents, and patients who learn from them. Although I can mention only a few here, I thank them all: Drs. Charles Puglia, Burton Landau, Jay Adler, Walter O'Donnell, Richard Shannon, Barbara Clark, Ronald Monah, Punkaj Mohan, Jim McGinty, John Raves, Donald Atkinson, Joseph Young, Paul Lebovitz, Jen Lewis, Wayne Goldman, Mark Lazarus, and Paige Rackliffe.

All my thanks to the staff at Blackwell Publishing, especially Bev Copland and Julia Casson. I hope to work with them to bring many more projects to print.

Finally, I thank my family and friends. Many of them contributed directly to this book; all of them have contributed directly to my life.

Scott Kahan

Cardiac Disease

JOSEF STEHLIK, MD
TEJAS MEHTA, MD

1. Coronary Artery Disease

Etiology

- Classically secondary to atherosclerotic plaque formation causing luminal narrowing and decreased myocardial oxygen supply
- Atherosclerotic plaque formation is a complex interaction involving lipid-laden macrophages, smooth muscle proliferation, and growth factors
- Other causes are rare, but include infection (syphilis), inflammatory disorders (rheumatic vasculitis), congenital anomalies, and coronary artery aneurysm
- Endothelial dysfunction is the earliest sign of the start of atherosclerosis

Epidemiology

- Risk factors for atherosclerosis include dyslipidemia (HDL < 40, LDL > 160), HTN, tobacco use, diabetes mellitus, male gender, family history of premature CAD (male < 55, female < 65), obesity (BMI > 30), advanced age, elevated homocysteine, and elevated lipoproteins

Differential Dx

- Acute MI
- Pericarditis
- Pulmonary embolus
- Pneumothorax
- Costochondritis
- GERD
- Esophageal spasm
- Stress/anxiety
- Aortic dissection
- Aortic stenosis
- Any cause of pleurisy
- Pancreatitis
- Biliary colic
- Zoster
- Trauma
- Metastatic malignancy

Signs/Symptoms

- Wide range of signs and symptoms depending on severity—may be asymptomatic (especially in diabetics)
- Exertional chest pain/pressure (Levine's sign = clenched fist over chest); may radiate to neck, jaw, shoulders, and arms
- Exertional shortness of breath
- Nausea
- Diaphoresis
- Fatigue
- Lightheadedness or near-syncope
- Altered blood pressure and heart rhythm

Diagnosis

- EKG changes: ST depression indicates myocardial ischemia; ST elevation indicates acute myocardial injury; Q wave denotes prior MI
- Stress testing: Used to demonstrate significant CAD
  - Exercise stress test: Preferred method; patient exercises on treadmill while being monitored with EKG, attempting to reproduce physiologic stress
  - Pharmacologic: Used when patients are unable to exercise due to PVD, joint disease, or lung disease
  - Radioisotope imaging/echocardiography: Used with stress testing to increase sensitivity/specificity and when the EKG cannot be interpreted
- Coronary angiography is the gold standard to document significant CAD and assess the need for revascularization
- Cardiac MRI may soon be used to evaluate the entire cardiovascular system; C-Reactive Protein and other markers of inflammation may be used to monitor CAD

Treatment

- Treat atherosclerosis with diet, exercise, tobacco cessation, and lipid-lowering medications (i.e., statins)
- Nitrates for symptomatic control of chest pain
- Aggressive treatment of hypertension and diabetes
- Aspirin and β-blockers
- New studies suggest ACE inhibitors and statins are very important in the treatment of CAD, as they decrease inflammation and the activity of atherosclerotic plaques
- True unstable angina (CP with EKG changes) or complicated MI (MI with CHF, Vtach, etc) should forgo stress testing and proceed to catheterization
- Interventional treatments for significant CAD
  - PTCA: angioplasty +/− stenting
  - CABG: for left main or triple-vessel disease
- Treat underlying non-atherosclerotic causes as necessary: infection, vasculitis, etc

Prognosis/Clinical Course

- Prognosis and clinical course are variable depending on severity of disease at time of detection, ranging from symptomatic control and primary prevention of CAD to PTCA/CABG to sudden cardiac arrest
- Aggressive primary and secondary prevention is crucial to lower morbidity and mortality
- 14% of patients with newly diagnosed angina pectoris progress to unstable angina, MI, or death within one year
- Cardiac rehabilitation decreases hospitalizations but does not alter mortality
- Other sequalae include CHF, valvular heart disease, and arrhythmias

2. Acute Myocardial Infarction

Etiology

- Due to an imbalance between myocardial oxygen demand and supply
- ST-segment elevation MI is most often secondary to occlusive thrombus formation on a disrupted atherosclerotic plaque (also secondary to coronary vasospasm or thrombus formation in the absence of atherosclerosis)
- Unstable angina/non-ST-segment elevation MI is most often secondary to nonocclusive narrowing due to atherosclerotic plaque

Epidemiology

Differential Dx

- Pericarditis
- Pulmonary embolus
- Pneumothorax
- Costochondritis
- GERD
- Esophageal spasm
- Stress/anxiety
- Aortic dissection
- Aortic stenosis
- Any cause of pleurisy
- Pancreatitis
- Biliary colic
- Zoster
- Trauma
- Metastatic malignancy

Signs/Symptoms

- Classic symptoms of MI include chest pain, SOB, nausea, diaphoresis, lightheadedness, and near-syncope
- Signs include hypotension, arrhythmias, and evidence of pulmonary edema
- May be asymptomatic—especially in diabetics (atypical symptoms, such as abdominal pain or isolated arm/jaw pain, are more common in diabetics and women)
- Unstable angina/non-ST-segment elevation MI
    - Chest discomfort at rest lasting for more than 20 minutes *or*
    - New-onset exertional angina *or*
    - Increased intensity of preexisting anginal symptoms

Diagnosis

- History and physical exam
- EKG should be done initially in ED, at 2 hours, and 6–12 hours later (normal EKG *does not* rule out MI)
    - Compare with old EKG, if possible
    - ST elevation signals ST-segment elevation MI
    - ST depression and/or T wave inversion signals unstable angina/non-ST elevation MI
    - Q wave denotes prior MI
- Serum cardiac enzymes act as biochemical markers of myocardial necrosis: MB isoenzyme of creatinine phosphokinase (CK-MB), troponin I, and troponin T
    - Positive enzymes indicate ST or non-ST elevation MI
    - Negative enzymes suggest unstable angina
- Patients with hemodynamic instability or recurrent pain should be evaluated/treated even if negative test results

Treatment

- Initial medical therapy
    - Continuous EKG monitoring
    - Aspirin ASAP (or clopidrogrel or ticlopidine)
    - β-Blockers: 1st dose IV, then oral (not in CHF pts)
    - Nitroglycerin for ischemic pain, CHF, and/or HTN
    - Oxygen for hypoxia (O_2 sat $<$ 92%), respiratory distress, pulmonary congestion
    - IV heparin or lovenox if no contraindications
    - Glycoprotein IIb/IIIa receptor inhibitor if angioplasty is planned, hemodynamic instability, or persistent symptoms despite therapy
    - Morphine sulfate for pain relief, pulmonary sxs
- Consider thrombolysis in ST elevation MI if $<$12 hours since onset and if no contraindications
- Interventional therapy: PTCA (angioplasty $+/-$ stenting) or CABG

Prognosis/Clinical Course

- PTCA: Preferred initial therapy (if available within 2 hrs) for ST elevation MI, persisting ischemic pain $>$12 hours, failed thrombolytic therapy, late-developing cardiogenic shock
- CABG: Indicated emergently for failed angioplasty with persistent pain or hemodynamic instability (cardiogenic shock); indicated electively for significant CAD
- Patients should proceed to stress testing (after symptom-free interval of 24–48 hours) or coronary angiography
- High risk of progression to MI and/or death during first 2 months after acute phase of unstable angina/non-ST elevation MI
- After acute treatment, every patient should undergo risk stratification

3. Congestive Heart Failure

Etiology

- A syndrome resulting from any structural or functional cardiac disorder that impairs diastolic ventricular filling or systolic ejection of blood
  - Etiology may be pericardial (pericardial constriction or tamponade), myocardial (MI, cardiomyopathy, myocarditis), endocardial (valvular disease), arrhythmic, drug-induced (i.e., chemotherapy), or alcoholic
- Systolic dysfunction: Impaired ability of ventricle to eject blood; EF <40%
- Diastolic dysfunction: Normal contractility but impaired filling of ventricle due to ↓ ventricular relaxation, ↓ elastic recoil, or ↑ stiffness; EF >40%

Differential Dx

- Non-cardiogenic pulmonary edema
- Renal insufficiency with fluid overload
- Hepatic insufficiency
- Hypoalbuminemia
- Cirrhosis
- Anemia
- Thyrotoxicosis
- Hypothyroidism
- Thiamine deficiency
- AV shunting

Epidemiology

- Prevalence: 5 million patients in the US
- Incidence: 500,000 patients per year in the US
- Two-thirds of cases are secondary to coronary artery disease
- CHF is the leading discharge diagnosis in patients > age 65
- Two-year mortality in patients with advanced heart failure (NYHA Class III or IV) on good medical therapy is 30–50%

Signs/Symptoms

- Dyspnea on exertion, orthopnea, paroxysmal nocturnal dyspnea
- Fatigue, decreased exercise tolerance
- Lower extremity edema
- Abdominal distention
- Central and peripheral embolic events
- Weight loss
- Jugular venous distention
- Laterally displaced apical impulse; S_3
- Rales
- Hepatomegaly, hepatojugular reflux, ascites, anasarca
- Some patients with significant systolic dysfunction can be asymptomatic for a prolonged period of time

Diagnosis

- Echocardiography to determine ejection fraction, chamber enlargement, and underlying heart disease
- MRI/CT
- Left and right heart catheterization
- CXR: Cardiomegaly, pulmonary edema
- EKG may be used to rule out CHF and screen for underlying heart disease
- Exercise testing with respiratory gas analysis
- NYHA Functional Classification of Heart Failure:
  - Class I: No limitations of physical activity
  - Class II: Slight limitation of physical activity—ordinary physical activity results in CHF symptoms
  - Class III: Marked limitation of physical activity with less than ordinary physical activity
  - Class IV: Inability to do any physical activity without discomfort; symptoms may be present at rest

Treatment

- Treat underlying structural heart disease and risk factors as necessary, for example:
  - Coronary artery disease/atherosclerosis
  - Hypertension
  - Valve repair/replacement
  - Congenital heart disease
- ACE inhibitors and β-blockers have been shown to decrease mortality—consider in all patients (angiotensin receptor blockers are useful for patients who experience side effects of ACE inhibitors)
- Diuretics are useful to alleviate symptoms of fluid overload, but have not been shown to decrease mortality
- Digoxin and vasodilators (nitrates, hydralazine)
- Spironolactone for NYHA Class III/IV patients
- Treat dilated cardiomyopathy if necessary
- Biventricular pacemaker

Prognosis/Clinical Course

- Prognosis varies significantly depending on etiology, left ventricular ejection fraction, NYHA functional class, and concomitant right ventricular dysfunction
- Unless there is a reversible cause, heart failure is a progressive disorder with high morbidity (limitation of physical activity and recurrent hospitalizations) and mortality
- Proper attention to end-of-life issues in end-stage heart failure patients is very important
- High-output heart failure: Anemia, AV shunts, thyrotoxicosis, and thiamine deficiency are conditions characterized by high cardiac output—in patients with impaired cardiac reserve, these may lead to heart failure as they are not able to augment the cardiac output

4. Dilated Cardiomyopathy

Etiology

- Dilatation of the cardiac chambers and impaired systolic ventricular function—usually results in congestive heart failure
- Due to HTN, CAD (ischemic cardiomyopathy), toxins (alcohol, cocaine, heroin, doxyrubicin, lead, arsenic, cobalt), sepsis, myocarditis, Chagas' disease, rheumatic fever, valvular insufficiency (MR, AR), peripartum, thyroid disease, or nutritional deficiencies (protein, thiamine, selenium)
- Ischemic cardiomyopathy is the most common form of dilated cardiomyopathy (two-thirds of all cases)

Differential Dx

- Diastolic heart failure: Impaired relaxation of the left ventricle leads to congestive symptoms even though ventricular systolic function remains normal
- Non-cardiogenic pulmonary edema
- Renal insufficiency with fluid overload
- Hepatic insufficiency
- Hypoalbuminemia

Epidemiology

Signs/Symptoms

- Dyspnea on exertion, orthopnea, paroxysmal nocturnal dyspnea
- Fatigue, decreased exercise tolerance
- Signs of "backup": JVD, leg edema, hepatomegaly, hepatojugular reflux, ascites, anasarca
- Embolic events: TIA/CVA, PE, petechiae
- Weight loss
- Laterally displaced apical impulse
- Audible S_3
- Rales
- Some patients with significant systolic dysfunction can be asymptomatic for a prolonged period of time

Diagnosis

- Echocardiography: Dilated chambers
- MRI
- Left and right heart catheterization
- CXR: Cardiomegaly, pulmonary edema
- EKG
- Exercise testing with respiratory gas analysis provides helpful prognostic information in patients who are candidates for heart transplant

Treatment

- Treat reversible, underlying disorders
- Medical therapy for acute CHF
  - Diuretics, norepinephrine, dopamine, nitroglycerine/nitroprusside
- Medical therapy for chronic CHF
  - Decrease afterload: ACE inhibitors, hydralazine, nitroglycerine
  - Diuretics
  - β-blockers: Carvedilol, metoprolol, and so on
  - Aldactone: for CHF Classes III and IV
- Surgical therapy for appropriate candidates
  - CABG
  - Valvular replacement and repair
  - Cardiac transplant or artificial heart (soon)
  - Left-, right-, or bi-ventricular assist device
  - Cardiac myoplasty and ventricular resection

Prognosis/Clinical Course

- Prognosis depends on the severity of associated congestive heart failure—see CHF

5. Restrictive Cardiomyopathy

Etiology

- A rare form of cardiomyopathy where pathologic changes of the myocardium result in restricted filling of the ventricles; this causes reduced diastolic volumes and increased filling pressures, resulting in pulmonary congestion
- May be primary (idiopathic) or secondary to other disease states, such as hypereosinophilic syndrome (Löffler's), endomyocardial fibrosis, infiltrative diseases (amyloidosis, sarcoidosis, hemochromatosis), carcinoid, scleroderma, or post heart-transplant

Differential Dx

- Constrictive pericarditis: It may be difficult to distinguish these conditions
- Right heart failure from other causes
- Aortic stenosis
- Ischemic heart disease

Epidemiology

Signs/Symptoms

- Signs and symptoms of the underlying disease process
- Symptoms of right heart failure and low output
  - Fatigue
  - Shortness of breath
  - Lower-extremity edema
  - Jugular venous distention
  - Ascites
  - Loud S_3
- Pleural effusions

Diagnosis

- Echocardiography: Restrictive diastolic ventricular dysfunction, normal ventricular size, normal or reduced systolic function, large atrial size
- MRI
- Right heart catheterization
- After diagnosis made by imaging techniques, proceed with non-invasive search for etiology (e.g., iron studies, ACE levels)
- Consider endomyocardial biopsy if the etiology is not determined by non-invasive workup

Treatment

- Treatment of CHF symptoms: Diuretics, digoxin, etc
- Avoidance of dehydration (patients are preload-dependent)
- Treatment of underlying condition if possible
  - Eosinophilic endomyocardial disease: Steroids and cytotoxic agents
  - Hemochromatosis: Phlebotomy or iron chelation therapy
  - Sarcoidosis: Steroids
- Heart transplant in suitable candidates

Prognosis/Clinical Course

- Prognosis depends on underlying disease; poor prognosis in most patients
- Fair prognosis in patients who are suitable candidates for heart transplant

6. Hypertrophic Cardiomyopathy

Etiology

- Asymmetric left ventricular hypertrophy that results in impaired diastolic ventricular filling and outflow obstruction in the left ventricle → results in pulmonary congestion
- Familial disease caused by a mutation of genes that define the sarcomere
- The genetic mutation results in various degrees of asymmetric ventricular hypertrophy
- May be at increased risk for infectious endocarditis

Differential Dx

- "Athletic heart": Seen in well-trained athletes
- Hypertensive hypertrophic cardiomyopathy: Seen in elderly patients with long-standing, poorly treated HTN
- Aortic stenosis
- Ischemic heart disease

Epidemiology

- Autosomal dominant inheritance

Signs/Symptoms

- Syncope
- Sudden cardiac death: Atrial arrhythmias lead to hemodynamic instability (loss of preload), ventricular ectopy, ventricular tachycardia, ventricular fibrillation
- Dyspnea, angina: Due to myocardial O_2 supply/demand mismatch
- Congestive heart failure: Due to diastolic dysfunction
- Sustained apical impulse, S_4, possible S_3
- Harsh systolic ejection murmur radiating to base and apex; increases in intensity with Valsalva maneuver
- Pulsus bispheriens

Diagnosis

- Echocardiography: Asymmetric hypertrophy, diastolic dysfunction, dynamic LV outflow tract obstruction
- EKG: High voltage, deeply inverted T waves in some cases, left ventricular hypertrophy
- Family history

Treatment

- Lifestyle modifications: Avoid dehydration; avoid competitive sports and strenuous activity
- Medical therapy: High-dose β-blockers, calcium-channel blockers, disopyramide
- Surgical therapy (for patients unresponsive to medical therapy): Dual-chamber pacing, surgical myectomy, septal ablation with alcohol
- Antibiotic prophylaxis for endocarditis during surgical procedures
- All first-degree relatives should undergo echocardiographic screening
- Genetic counseling should be offered to patients planning to have children

Prognosis/Clinical Course

- Incidence of sudden death varies from 1% to 8% per year
- Clinical factors conveying higher risk of sudden death include young age, male sex, history of syncope, and family history of sudden death
- Hypertrophic cardiomyopathy is the leading cause of death in competitive athletes

7. Infectious Endocarditis

Etiology

- Most cases of endocarditis involve abnormal valves: Myxomatous and degenerative changes, rheumatic valves, bicuspid aortic valves, prosthetic valves
- Left-sided endocarditis is much more common—IV drug abuse predisposes to right-sided endocarditis
- Seeding of the valve occurs during transient bacteremia
- Infectious organisms: *Streptococcus viridans* (50%), *Enterococcus* (10%), *Staphylococcus aureus* (20%), gram-negative rods (2%), HACEK, fungi (*Candida, Aspergillus*)

Differential Dx

- Septicemia without endocardial involvement (e.g., line sepsis)
- Systemic vasculitis
- Non-infectious endocarditis: Libman-Saks (in SLE), marasmic (in terminal disease)
- Acute valvular dysfunction of non-infectious etiology

Epidemiology

- 15,000 cases/year in US
- Males > Females
- Median age: 54 years (increasing)
- Mitral > aortic > tricuspid > pulmonic

Signs/Symptoms

- Fever, malaise, sweats, myalgias, arthralgias, abdominal pain, back pain, weight loss
- Heart murmur (usually new or changing)
- Vascular phenomena: Conjunctival petechiae, splinter hemorrhages, Janeway lesions (painless hemorrhagic plaques on palms and soles), major arterial emboli including stroke, septic pulmonary infarcts, mycotic aneurysms
- Immunologic phenomena: Osler's nodes (painful nodular lesions on fingers and toes), Roth's spots (pale retinal lesions surrounded by hemorrhage)
- Splenomegaly
- Signs of renal failure
- Signs of CHF and/or heart block

Diagnosis

- Duke criteria: If 2 major or 1 major and 2 minor or 5 minor criteria are present, endocarditis is considered definite
- Major criteria
  - Positive blood culture for typical organisms from two different blood cultures; persistently (>12 hours apart) positive blood cultures for typical organisms
  - Evidence of endocardial involvement: Echocardiogram showing vegetation, abscess, or new dehiscence of prosthetic valve (TEE much more accurate than TTE)
- Minor criteria
  - Predisposing heart condition or IV drug abuse
  - Fever > 38°C (100.4°F)
  - Vascular phenomena or immunologic phenomena
  - Positive blood culture not meeting major criteria
  - Positive echocardiogram not meeting major criteria
- Infectious endocarditis should always be considered in patients with fever of unknown origin

Treatment

- If suspect acute endocarditis, obtain 3 sets of blood cultures within 1 hr; then begin empiric therapy
- Adjust antibiotic according to culture and sensitivity
- 2–4 week course of antibiotics is usually needed
- For strep and staph endocarditis: β-lactam or cephalosporin (vancomycin in methicillin resistance) plus an aminoglycoside
- Indications for surgical treatment
  - CHF/hemodynamic instability due to valvular dysfunction
  - Paravalvular infection or abscess
  - Persistent bacteremia on antimicrobial therapy
  - Fungal or gram-negative bacillus endocarditis
  - *S. aureus* endocarditis of a prosthetic valve
  - Recurrent arterial emboli
  - Large vegetations (relative indication)

Prognosis/Clinical Course

- Mortality remains high—approximately 20%
- Prompt diagnosis and treatment reduces morbidity and mortality
- Some authorities recommend a screening TEE for all patients with staph bacteremia
- Patients are at risk for recurrent infection
- Prophylactic therapy with antibiotics is indicated prior to medical procedures that are likely to result in bacteremia
- CHF is the leading cause of death in patients with infectious endocarditis

8. Myocarditis

Etiology

- Infectious myocarditis: Almost any organism can cause myocarditis
  - Viral ("idiopathic") myocarditis: Coxsackie, influenza viruses, HIV, HBV, HCV, EBV, dengue
  - Bacterial: *Brucella, Clostridium,* diphtheria
  - Fungal, *Rickettsia,* spirochetes (Lyme disease), parasitic (*Trypanosoma*—Chagas' disease)
- Giant-cell myocarditis is a rare disease that causes progressive left ventricular failure and often results in dilated cardiomyopathy

Differential Dx

- Acute MI
- CHF of other causes (ischemic, valvular, HTN)
- Cardiac sarcoidosis
- Non-infectious myocarditis
  - Acute rheumatic fever
  - Toxic: Doxorubicin, anthracycline
  - Giant-cell myocarditis
  - Hypersensitivity: Immunologic reaction to a variety of drugs

Epidemiology

- Most cases of myocarditis are probably subclinical
- Viral ("idiopathic") myocarditis is the most common form of myocarditis in the US
- More frequent among younger patients (<age 45)
- Patients are usually otherwise healthy

Signs/Symptoms

- Most common presentation is new onset of CHF symptoms in a healthy young person (e.g., orthopnea, dyspnea, edema)
- Atrial and ventricular arrhythmias
- AV nodal block
- Sudden death
- Flu-like symptoms 2–3 weeks prior to the onset of CHF symptoms are common in viral myocarditis
- Patients with non-infectious myocarditis may have symptoms and signs of the primary disease

Diagnosis

- EKG: Sinus tachycardia, nonspecific ST-T changes, IVCD, AV block, atrial/ventricular arrhythmias, occasional ST elevations
- Echocardiography: Global ventricular systolic dysfunction, regional wall motion abnormalities may be present
- Troponin I may be elevated
- Coronary angiography may be used to rule out ischemic heart disease
- Antimyosin scintigraphy
- Endomyocardial biopsy (no longer routinely performed)
  - Histology shows inflammatory infiltrate with necrosis and degeneration of adjacent myocytes
  - Consider biopsy if giant-cell myocarditis or sarcoidosis is suspected

Treatment

- Viral ("idiopathic") myocarditis
  - Restriction of strenuous physical activity
  - Standard medical therapy for CHF (ACE inhibitors, diuretics, digoxin, β-blockers)
  - Standard treatment of AV conduction disturbances
  - Corticosteroids, immunosuppressives, or immunomodulators may be beneficial
- Infectious (nonviral) myocarditis
  - The above measures plus antibiotics specific to the causative organism
- Giant-cell myocarditis: Combination immunosuppressive therapy
- Heart transplant for patients in whom dilated cardiomyopathy develops

Prognosis/Clinical Course

- Viral myocarditis: Systolic function usually improves over several months; some will develop dilated cardiomyopathy
- Giant-cell myocarditis: Carries a much worse prognosis—6-month survival <50%
- Hypersensitivity myocarditis: Often results in progressive heart failure and death despite discontinuation of the offending agent
- Patients with dilated cardiomyopathy resulting from acute myocarditis represent a large group of candidates for heart transplant; given young age and lack of comorbidities, prognosis after successful transplantation is very good

9. Pericardial Disease

Etiology

- Acute pericarditis: Viral, connective tissue disease (SLE, scleroderma, RA), malignancy (lymphoma, leukemia, lung, breast), post-MI (Dressler's syndrome), post-pericardiotomy, or uremia
- Pericardial effusion/tamponade: Accumulation of fluid in the pericardium, resulting in impaired filling of the cardiac chambers; due to trauma, acute pericarditis, wall rupture, aortic dissection, cardiac surgery, or hypothyroid
- Constrictive pericarditis: Idiopathic, post-acute pericarditis, radiation-induced, or infectious (TB, parasitic, fungal)

Epidemiology

Differential Dx

- Acute pericarditis
  - Acute MI
  - Aortic dissection
  - Pleuritis
  - PE
- Pericardial effusion
  - Cardiomegaly
  - CHF due to systolic dysfunction
- Constrictive pericarditis
  - Restrictive cardiomyopathy
  - Right heart failure of a different etiology

Signs/Symptoms

- Acute pericarditis
  - Sharp, stabbing pain radiating to back
  - Relieved by leaning forward
  - May mimic anginal pain
  - Pericardial rub
  - Large effusion may cause tamponade
- Pericardial effusion/tamponade
  - Tachycardia, hypotension, dyspnea
  - Leg edema, hepatomegaly, ascites
  - Pulsus paradoxus
  - Jugular venous distension
  - Decreased cardiac sounds
- Constrictive pericarditis
  - Dyspnea, JVD, Kussmaul's sign
  - Leg edema, hepatomegaly, ascites
  - Pericardial knock

Diagnosis

- Acute pericarditis
  - EKG: PR depression, ST elevation, T waves upright initially then inverted
  - Presence of pericardial rub is diagnostic
- Pericardial effusion
  - Echocardiogram: Effusion, right atrium/ventricle collapse (if tamponade), respiration-dependent transvalvular flow variation
  - Right heart catheterization: Equalization of diastolic pressures, preserved x descent, diminished y descent
  - CXR: Cardiomegaly, globular cardiac contour
  - EKG: Low voltage
- Constrictive pericarditis
  - MRI, echocardiogram: Increased pericardial thickness
  - CXR: Pericardial calcification
  - Right heart catheterization: Increased RA pressure

Treatment

- Acute pericarditis
  - ASA or NSAIDs
  - Steroids for recurrent pain that does not respond to NSAIDs
- Pericardial effusion/tamponade
  - Therapeutic pericardiocentesis; pericardial window and stripping if recurrent
  - IV fluids
- Constrictive pericarditis
  - Pericardectomy

Prognosis/Clinical Course

- Acute pericarditis
  - Usually self-limited, unless caused by malignancy or systemic disease
- Pericardial effusion/tamponade
  - Amount of pericardial fluid needed to cause tamponade varies from as little as 50 cc (if accumulates rapidly) to several liters (if accumulates slowly)
  - Prognosis varies depending on the underlying process that led to the pericardial tamponade
  - Tamponade not relieved by pericardiocentesis is often lethal
- Constrictive pericarditis
  - Prognosis varies depending on the underlying process that led to pericardial tamponade

10. Atrial Septal Defect

Etiology

- Ostium secundum defect: 75% of all ASDs—second most common heart defect in adults (#1 is bicuspid aortic valve)
  - Defect in central portion of atrial septum; associated with MVP
- Ostium primum defect: 15% of all ASDs
  - Associated with cleft in mitral valve and significant MR
  - Defect in lower part of atrial septum and/or atrioventricular groove
- Sinus venosus: 10% of all ASDs; defect in upper part of atrial septum
  - Associated with anomalous drainage of pulmonary veins (into RA or vena cava)

Differential Dx

- Pulmonary HTN
- COPD
- Sleep apnea
- Pulmonary stenosis
- Valvular disease

Epidemiology

- Represents 1/3 of congenital heart disease in adults
- Females > males
- ASDs are often found early in life after an echocardiogram is performed for evaluation of murmur or dyspnea
- Paradoxical embolism: Flows through septal defect to left heart and arterial circulation, skipping the lungs and embolizing to the brain

Signs/Symptoms

- Signs and symptoms of all ASDs
  - Palpitations
  - Signs of right heart failure—edema, hepatomegaly, JVD, dyspnea
  - Right ventricular thrill
  - Fixed-split S_2
  - Systolic murmur (due to increased flow across pulmonary valve)
  - Cyanosis occurs with RV failure
- Ostium secundum defect is asymptomatic early; >70% symptomatic at 40 years old
- Ostium primum defect is associated with symptoms early in life
  - Syncope due to AV nodal disease
  - Additional systolic murmur from associated mitral regurgitation

Diagnosis

- EKG
  - Secundum: Right axis deviation, incomplete RBBB, may develop Afib
  - Primum: Left axis deviation, complete RBBB, 1st degree AV block
- Chest X-ray: Cardiomegaly, enlarged pulmonary artery
- Transthoracic echocardiography (TTE): Identifies exact location of most defects, except sinus venosus
- Transesophageal echocardiography (TEE): Often needed to search for sinus venosus defect
- Coronary angiography: Not needed for diagnosis of ASD, but used to search for concomitant CAD

Treatment

- Early recognition and closure are imperative for prevention of long-term sequelae—especially atrial arrythmias
- Primary goal of treatment is to prevent pulmonary hypertension and resulting right heart failure
- First option is surgical or percutaneous closure
- Pharmacologic: Primarily antiarrhythmics for Afib and diuretics for right heart failure
- Contraindications to closure include irreversible pulmonary hypertension (Eisenmenger's syndrome)

Prognosis/Clinical Course

- Left-to-right shunt occurs initially b/c RV is very compliant—flow is therefore increased through pulmonary vasculature
  - Pulmonary HTN, RV hypertrophy, and RV failure develop, so RV loses compliance
  - Reversal of flow then occurs and pulmonary obstructive disease sets in (Eisenmenger's syndrome—present in 5% of cases)
  - As a result, the prior acyanotic congenital defect becomes cyanotic
- <1% mortality with uncomplicated secundum repair—mortality ↑ if closure is delayed
- Patients who develop pulmonary HTN have ↑ mortality (whether defect is closed or not)
- After closure, must follow for right heart failure, pulmonary HTN, and arrhythmias

11. Rheumatic Heart Disease

Etiology

- Pathologic changes of various cardiac structures that result from immunologic response to streptococcal pharyngitis
- Rheumatic fever is a multisystem disorder occurring 1–5 weeks after Group A *Streptococcus* infection—usually affects heart, joints, and subcutaneous tissues
- Subsequent mitral valve disease in 75% of patients (especially MS)
- Subsequent aortic valve disease in 20% of patients
- Pulmonic or tricuspid involvement is rare

Differential Dx

- Endocarditis
- Viral infection (rubella, hepatitis B)
- Septic arthritis (*Neisseria*)
- Acute rheumatoid arthritis
- SLE
- Still's disease
- Lyme disease
- Osteomyelitis
- Sickle cell disease

Epidemiology

- Peak incidence is 5–15 years of age
- Affects males and females equally, although females have a higher risk of developing Sydenham's chorea and mitral stenosis
- 2 cases/100,000 in US; 100 cases/100,000 in developing countries
- 3% risk of RHD following untreated streptococcal pharyngitis
- Increased risk in HLA-DR 1, 2, 3, 4

Signs/Symptoms

- Fever
- Joint manifestations (75% of patients): Inflammation and pain (large joints)
- Signs of heart failure (50% clinically, 90% by echo): Dyspnea, tachycardia, mitral regurgitation, aortic regurgitation, pericarditis, varying degree of AV block
- Skin manifestations (<5%): Erythema marginatum
- Painless nodules (<5%)
- Sydenham's chorea (<5%): Rapid, purposeless movements that occur only while awake— "bag of worms" of tongue upon protrusion, squeezing/relaxing motion during handgrip, knee jerk

Diagnosis

- Throat swabs are usually negative
- Positive serum titers for anti-streptolysin, anti-DNAase B, and anti-hyaluronidase
- Elevated ESR
- Echocardiography: Assess valvular dysfunction and evidence of myocardial/pericardial involvement
- Physical exam: Duckett-Jones criteria for rheumatic fever—diagnosis requires 2 major criteria *or* 1 major and 2 minor

Major criteria	Minor criteria
– Carditis	– Previous rheumatic fever
– Polyarthritis	– Arthralgias
– Sydenham's chorea	– Fever
– Erythema marginatum	– Elevated ESR/CRP/WBC
– Subcutaneous nodules	– Prolonged PR interval

Treatment

- Antibiotics to treat initial infection: Penicillin is usually adequate
- Anti-inflammatory agents for joint symptoms
- Treat heart failure symptomatically (see discussion of CHF treatment)
- Long-term antibiotic prophylaxis should be used for any patient who develops rheumatic fever—5 years if no signs of carditis; 10 or more years if cardiac involvement
- Lifelong prophylactic antibiotics for all surgical procedures

Prognosis/Clinical Course

- Immediate mortality is 1–2%
- Untreated acute rheumatic fever lasts 3 months
- Untreated acute rheumatic fever with severe carditis extends illness to 6 months
- Most patients who develop valvular dysfunction require intervention
- Patients are at risk for reoccurrence; use prophylactic antibiotics before any surgical procedure

12. Atrial Fibrillation

Etiology

- The most common sustained arrhythmia
- Any disease that increases atrial size may predispose to Afib
- Most common causes are HTN, sick-sinus syndrome, valvular disease (MS, MR), cardiomyopathy, CAD, myocarditis, pericarditis, cardiac surgery, thyrotoxicosis, alcohol use, WPW syndrome, sepsis, pulmonary disease (asthma, COPD), idiopathic
- The major complications associated with Afib are formation of emboli (due to stagnation of blood) and heart failure

Differential Dx

- Frequent premature atrial or premature ventricular beats
- Multifocal atrial tachycardia
- Marked sinus arrhythmia
- Atrial flutter
- Atrial tachycardia with variable AV block
- Digitalis toxicity

Epidemiology

- Most common arrhythmia in clinical practice
- Incidence increases with age (5% of patients over age 65)

Signs/Symptoms

- Palpitations
- Presyncope
- Dyspnea
- Chest pain
- Irregularly irregular rhythm
- Variable intensity of S_1
- There may be a difference between the heart rate and the number of palpable pulsations over a peripheral artery (peripheral deficit)
- Patients may be asymptomatic, especially when ventricular response is controlled

Diagnosis

- EKG is diagnostic in most cases: Absent P waves; irregular, tachycardic ventricular rate
- Echocardiography is useful to evaluate possible underlying causes of Afib; TEE is used to rule out the presence of an atrial thrombus prior to initiation of antiarrhythmic therapy
- Thyroid studies to rule out underlying thyroid disease
- Holter monitor/event monitor: Especially helpful in paroxysmal Afib (see below)

Treatment

- Rate control: Initial treatment in stable patients
  - IV β-blockers, calcium-channel blockers, digoxin
- Anticoagulation: Most effective means of diminishing the risk of embolic events
  - Factors further increasing risk of embolic events: Age >60, HTN, DM, CHF, previous TIA/CVA
  - Full anticoagulation with IV heparin in hospital, then switch to oral warfarin (target INR of 2–3)
  - Contraindications: Recent surgery, gait instability, untreated GI bleed
  - ASA alone for pts <60 with no RFs for embolism
- Rhythm control (antiarrhythmic therapy)
  - Electric cardioversion or antiarrhythmic meds
- Anticoagulate 4 weeks before and after cardioversion (if TEE rules out an atrial thrombus, then not necessary to anticoagulate prior to treatment)

Prognosis/Clinical Course

- Paroxysmal Afib: Recurrent episodes of Afib, which spontaneously revert to sinus rhythm
- Persistent Afib: Patient has remained in Afib for a period of days to weeks
- Permanent Afib: Long-standing Afib
- Side effects of antiarrhythmic medications must be considered when choosing an appropriate treatment
- Anticoagulation and rate control appear to have a prognosis similar to that with treatment aimed at maintenance of sinus rhythm

13. AV Conduction Disturbances

Etiology

- Failure of appropriate conduction of atrial impulse to ventricles
- 1st degree AV block: Prolonged PR interval (>0.20 second) that remains constant; each P wave is followed by a QRS complex
- 2nd degree AV block
    - Mobitz I (Wenckebach): Progressive prolongation of PR until P wave fails to conduct—AV conduction recovers—then repeats
    - Mobitz type II: Intermittent nonconducted P waves without preceding conduction delay—PR interval remains fixed (does not prolong)
- 3rd degree AV block: Complete failure of conduction from atria → ventricles

Differential Dx

- 1st degree AV block
- 2nd degree AV block
- 3rd degree AV block
- Atrial fibrillation
- Atrial flutter with variable conduction

Epidemiology

- Most commonly found in elderly (fibrosis of conduction system), acute MI, antiarrhythmics (β-blockers, calcium-channel blockers, digoxin), vagal stimulation, paravalvular abscess, post-valve replacement (edema of conduction system), infiltrative diseases (sarcoidosis, amyloidosis), congenital complete heart block (rare)

Signs/Symptoms

- 1st degree AV block is often asymptomatic
- Palpitations
- Shortness of breath
- Dizziness, presyncope, syncope (Adams-Stokes)
- Irregular heart beat
- Jugular venous distension, cannon waves (in 3rd degree block)
- Soft S_1 in 1st degree block
- Hypotension
- Heart failure

Diagnosis

- EKG
    - 1st degree block: PR interval is prolonged (>0.2 second) and remains constant; each P wave is followed by a QRS complex
    - 2nd degree block—Mobitz type I: Progressive prolongation of PR interval until a P wave fails to conduct; RR interval progressively shortens; PP interval remains constant
    - 2nd degree block—Mobitz type II: Intermittent nonconducted P waves; PR interval remains fixed (does not prolong); PP interval remains constant
    - 3rd degree block (complete heart block): Atrial activity and ventricular activity are independent; the escape rhythm comes from either the AV junction (narrow QRS) or the ventricular pacemaker (wide QRS)
- Holter monitoring (or intermittent patient-triggered monitoring) if symptoms are transient

Treatment

- Emergent treatment of symptomatic AV block: IV atropine, IV isoprotenorol, low-dose IV dopamine, transcutaneous (external) pacing, temporary transvenous pacemaker
- Long-term treatment of AV block is a permanent pacemaker: Indicated for all cases of 3rd degree heart block, Mobitz II, and symptomatic cases of Mobitz I
- AV block in the presence of acute MI
    - Inferior wall MI is often complicated by transient AV conduction disturbance: Use temporary transvenous pacing if symptomatic and await recovery of conduction
    - Anterior wall MI: Progression to complete heart block is frequent and most patients will require permanent pacing

Prognosis/Clinical Course

- 1st degree AV block
    - Usually benign in the absence of QRS widening, but may exacerbate heart failure
    - Progressive PR prolongation in the setting of endocarditis is suggestive of a paravalvular abscess
- 2nd degree AV block
    - Mobitz type I (Wenckebach): Generally benign (no risk of progression to complete heart block)
    - Mobitz type II: Often progresses to complete heart block
- 3rd degree AV block (complete heart block) is life-threatening

14. Supraventricular Tachycardia

Etiology

- Rapid heart rhythms originating in the atria or AV junction
  - Sinus tachycardia: Not a primary cardiac arrhythmia—due to underlying causes (i.e., hypovolemia, hypotension, hyperthyroid, sepsis, LV dysfunction)
  - Multifocal atrial tachycardia (due to COPD, heart failure, or theophylline)
  - Nonparoxysmal junctional tachycardia (due to myocarditis, digitalis toxicity, inferior MI)
  - AV reentrant tachycardias, such as WPW (due to accessory pathways that allow the electrical signal to bypass the normal conduction pathway)

Differential Dx

- Atrial fibrillation
- Atrial flutter
- Sinus tachycardia
- Nonparoxysmal junctional tachycardia
- Sinus nodal reentry tachycardia
- Multifocal atrial tachycardia
- AV reentrant tachycardia (Wolff-Parkinson-White)
- Ventricular tachycardia

Epidemiology

Signs/Symptoms

- Palpitations
- Dizziness, presyncope, syncope
- Tachycardia
- Hypotension

Diagnosis

- EKG: *Narrow* QRS complex (QRS <0.10 second); identification of atrial activity helps to classify the arrhythmia
  - Sinus tachycardia: Normal P waves, normal PR interval, normal QRS
  - Multifocal atrial tachycardia: Abnormal P waves
  - Nonparoxysmal junctional tachycardia: P waves may be inverted and may occur during or after QRS
  - WPW: Short PR interval and a delta wave present at the beginning of the QRS complex
- Holter monitor/event monitor
- Electrophysiology study: To define the origin and type of SVT

Treatment

- Sinus tachycardia: Treat the underlying disorder; β-blockers may be used to slow the heart rate (i.e., in presence of myocardial ischemia)
- Multifocal atrial tachycardia: Treat the underlying pulmonary disease; calcium-channel blockers if needed
- AV reentrant tachycardias
  - Acute treatment: Vagal maneuvers, IV adenosine, IV β-blockers, IV calcium-channel blockers, electric cardioversion if severe hemodynamic compromise
  - Chronic treatment: AV nodal blocking agents, catheter ablation of the slow pathway in the AV node (curative in 95% of patients)

Prognosis/Clinical Course

- Prognosis is generally more favorable than that for ventricular tachycardias
- Wolff-Parkinson-White syndrome carries a small risk of sudden cardiac death—it is believed to result from atrial fibrillation with very fast ventricular response, leading to ventricular fibrillation
- Digitalis toxicity should be strongly considered in patients presenting in atrial tachycardia with AV block or nonparoxysmal junctional tachycardia

15. Ventricular Tachycardia

Etiology

- Ventricular tachycardia is a life-threatening arrhythmia that appears as wide QRS complexes; the most common life-threatening arrhythmia
- Defined as the onset of three or more premature ventricular beats
- The vast majority of ventricular tachycardia events are a consequence of CAD; other causes include myocardial ischemia, cardiomyopathy, myocarditis, congenital long QT syndrome, Brugada syndrome, proarrhythmic effect of certain medications (antiarrhythmics), and severe electrolyte imbalance (hypokalemia, hypomagnesemia)

Differential Dx

- Bundle branch block
- Monitor artifact
- Atrial fibrillation
- Atrial flutter
- Sinus tachycardia
- Nonparoxysmal junctional tachycardia
- Sinus nodal reentry tachycardia
- Multifocal atrial tachycardia
- AV reentrant tachycardia (Wolff-Parkinson-White)

Epidemiology

Signs/Symptoms

- Palpitations
- Shortness of breath
- Chest pain
- Dizziness, presyncope, syncope
- Tachycardia
- Hypotension
- Audible third heart sound
- Cannon waves in jugular veins
- Cardiorespiratory arrest

Diagnosis

- EKG: Wide QRS complex (QRS > 0.12 second, often >0.14 second), 100–150 bpm, AV dissociation, left axis or extreme right axis deviation, inverted T waves; may have evidence of prior MI
  - Torsades de pointes is a ventricular tachycardia in which the QRS complexes appear to be "twisting"; most commonly secondary to electrolyte imbalances, severe cardiomyopathies, or congenital long QT syndromes
- Holter monitoring
- Electrophysiology study
- Echocardiography, cardiac MRI (to detect structural heart disease)

Treatment

- If patient is stable, antiarrhythmics may be used initially: Amiodarone, procainamide, and/or lidocaine
- If patient is unstable, direct current cardioversion must be the initial treatment; antiarrhythmics may be used as well
- Automated implantable cardiovertor-defibrillator (AICD) is useful in certain patients
- Radiofrequency ablation of focus of ventricular tachycardia in selected patients

Prognosis/Clinical Course

- Prognosis varies depending on the etiology
- In patients with CAD, prognosis is very good if ventricular tachycardia is limited to the first 48 hours after acute ischemic myocardial injury
- Ventricular tachycardia lasting more than 48 hours after acute ischemic myocardial injury warrants further workup

16. Aortic Regurgitation

Etiology

- Incompetence of the aortic valve, resulting in diastolic backflow of blood into the left ventricle
- Most commonly due to rheumatic fever; other causes include congenital defects of aortic valve (bicuspid valve, ventricular septal defect), infective endocarditis, trauma (aortic dissection), collagen vascular diseases with involvement of the aortic root and aortic valve, senile degenerative valvular disease, any dilatation of aortic root (HTN, Marfan's, syphilis), connective tissue disease (rheumatoid arthritis, spondyloarthropathies)

Epidemiology

- Prevalence increases with age

Differential Dx

- Mitral stenosis
- Pulmonic regurgitation (rare)

Signs/Symptoms

- Angina
- Syncope
- Dyspnea, orthopnea, PND
- Overactivity of neck vessels
- Classic murmur: High-pitched, diastolic decrescendo murmur
- Wide pulse pressure
- de Musset's sign: Nodding of head
- Quincke's pulse: Nail bed capillary pulsation upon gentle nail pressure
- Corrigan's pulse: Sharp, rapid carotid upstroke with subsequent collapse
- Duroziez murmur: Pistol shot at the femoral artery
- Austin Flint murmur: Apical diastolic rumble

Diagnosis

- EKG is nonspecific; may show left ventricular hypertrophy
- Chest X-ray: Cardiomegaly; ascending aorta may be dilated
- Echocardiography: Evaluates aortic root dilatation and early closure of mitral valve; Doppler jet evaluation of aortic regurgitation
- Heart catheterization: Evaluates for concomitant CAD

Treatment

- Medical therapy is a short-term goal to reduce left ventricular volume and improve ejection fraction
- ACE inhibitors and vasodilators (hydralazine) are thought to decrease afterload and therefore diminish the regurgitant volume—however, only nifedipine (Ca^{++}-channel blocker) has been proven to do this
- Treat CHF as needed with diuretics, digoxin, etc
- Antibiotic prophylaxis for infective endocarditis
- β-blockers to decrease the rate of dilatation in Marfan's syndrome
- Aortic valve replacement: Indications include Class III or IV heart failure, progressive LV dilatation, decreasing ejection fraction, decreasing exercise tolerance, angina with severe aortic regurgitation, mild/moderate LV dysfunction (EF < 50%), infective endocarditis resistant to therapy
- Transplant if LV function is significantly diminished

Prognosis/Clinical Course

- Acute aortic regurgitation: Symptoms of CHF develop quickly
- Once aortic regurgitation causes decreased left ventricular function, symptoms develop within three years
- Chronic aortic regurgitation is usually asymptomatic but once symptoms begin, prognosis is poor if left untreated
- Best predictor of outcome in aortic valve replacement surgery is preoperative ejection fraction

17. Aortic Stenosis

Etiology

- Pathologic changes of aortic valve, resulting in obstruction to blood flow
- Secondary to congenital valvular disease (age < 30), bicuspid valve (age 40–60), rheumatic heart disease (age 40–60), senile degeneration (most common cause; in patients >60), peripheral pulmonary stenosis, hypercalcemia
- Rheumatic aortic stenosis never occurs alone - always associated with mitral valve disease
- Normal aortic valve area is 3–4 cm^2; mild stenosis occurs at area of 1.0–1.5; moderate stenosis 0.7–1.0; severe stenosis <0.7; critical stenosis <0.5

Differential Dx

- Mitral regurgitation
- Ventricular septal defect
- Pulmonic stenosis (rare)
- Subvalvular stenosis
- Supravalvular stenosis

Epidemiology

- 25% of all patients >65 years of age have echocardiographic evidence of aortic sclerosis (defined as thickening of the valve without obstruction of flow)
- 35% of all patients >75 years of age have echocardiographic evidence of aortic sclerosis

Signs/Symptoms

- Most cases asymptomatic; found incidentally on exam or on echo
- Angina
- Exercise-related syncope in 25% of cases (due to arrhythmia, cerebral hypoperfusion, or hypotension)
- Dyspnea, especially if LV dysfunction
- Crescendo–decrescendo systolic murmur
- Pulsus tardus et parvus: Slow, late carotid upstroke
- Nondisplaced "thrusting" apex
- May have systolic ejection click
- Audible fourth heart sound
- S_2 may be softened or muffled depending on severity of stenosis—the less audible the aortic component of S_2, the more severe the stenosis

Diagnosis

- EKG: Evidence of LVH
- Chest X-ray: Cardiomegaly, post-stenotic dilatation of aorta, calcification of aortic valve (depending on etiology)
- Echocardiography: Defines the level/severity of obstruction, calculates transvalvular gradients and valve areas, may show evidence of diastolic dysfunction
- Heart catheterization: Checks for evidence of concomitant CAD; measures gradient between left ventricle and aorta; calculates valve area

Treatment

- Antibiotic prophylaxis for all patients
- No treatment for asymptomatic patients, unless declining LV function, severe LVH, high transvalvular gradients (>80), or severely reduced valve area (<0.7)
- Medical treatment is used to stabilize the patient until surgery
- Surgical valve replacement is curative and indicated in all symptomatic patients who can tolerate surgery
- Balloon valvuloplasty may be used for those who cannot tolerate surgery and in some congenital cases (i.e., adolescents with aortic stenosis but normal cardiac output)

Prognosis/Clinical Course

- Mortality is based on presenting symptoms:
  – Angina: Median survival is 5 years
  – Syncope: Median survival is 3 years
  – If CHF is present, median survival is just 1 year
- Sudden death occurs in 10–20% of cases
- Any type of arrhythmia suggests a poor prognosis unless valve is replaced
- Overall 5-year survival is 40%
- Prognosis after surgical intervention depends on age and preoperative left ventricular function

18. Mitral Regurgitation

Etiology

- Incompetence of the mitral valve, resulting in systolic backflow of blood into the left atrium and pulmonary veins
- Due to rheumatic heart disease, mitral valve prolapse, CAD (papillary muscle rupture, LV dilatation), papillary muscle dysfunction, endocarditis, atrial myxoma, congenital
- Mitral valve prolapse: >2 mm displacement of valve into left atrium during systole, causing a mid-systolic click; progression of mitral valve prolapse to mitral regurgitation is more common in men than in women

Differential Dx

- Tricuspid regurgitation
- Aortic stenosis
- Pulmonic stenosis (rare)

Epidemiology

- Reported incidence of severe mitral regurgitation is increasing as more echocardiograms are being done to identify the lesion and as life expectancy increases
- Fewer cases of MR are secondary to rheumatic heart disease (due to the widespread use of antibiotics)

Signs/Symptoms

- May be asymptomatic for years
- Dyspnea
- Fatigue
- Palpitations related to atrial fibrillation
- Fluid retention
- Signs of right heart failure (if severe, long-standing MR): elevated JVP, edema, hepatomegaly, right-sided heave
- Pansystolic murmur best heard at the apex
- Mid-systolic click if MVP is present
- Audible third heart sound
- May or may not have evidence of atrial fibrillation

Diagnosis

- EKG: May have left atrial enlargement, bifid P wave in lead II; Afib may be present
- Chest X-ray: Left atrial enlargement, cardiomegaly, evidence of CHF
- Echocardiography: Left atrial enlargement, Doppler measurement of regurgitant jet, evaluation of valvular apparatus (TEE allows for better visualization of the valve)
- Coronary angiogram: Look for concomitant CAD

Treatment

- Afterload reduction to decrease backflow: ACE inhibitors or nitrates plus hydralazine
- Diuretics
- Digoxin for rate control in Afib or positive inotropy in CHF
- Anticoagulation for Afib or severe LV dysfunction
- Antibiotic prophylaxis for infective endocarditis
- Indications for mitral valve repair or replacement
  - Class III or IV heart failure, ejection fraction <60%, severe functional debility, LV end-systolic diameter >45, acute mitral regurgitation following MI with hemodynamic instability, MR associated with endocarditis that is resistant to therapy
- Heart transplant if left ventricular function is significantly compromised

Prognosis/Clinical Course

- Generally good prognosis unless pulmonary pressure is chronically high or if severe left ventricular dysfunction is present
- Patients with impaired left ventricular function are better served with mitral valve repair than with valve replacement
- Complications include right-sided heart failure secondary to pulmonary HTN, endocarditis, systemic emboli if Afib, or severe left ventricular dysfunction

19. Mitral Stenosis

Etiology

- Pathologic changes of mitral valve, resulting in obstruction to blood flow
- The stenotic valve causes increased left atrial pressure and consequently increased pulmonary venous pressure → this results in transudation of plasma into the lung interstitium and alveoli → this pulmonary congestion eventually leads to pulmonary HTN and right heart failure
- The increased left atrial pressure also leads to an enlarged chamber, stagnation of blood flow, and Afib, which predisposes to emboli

Differential Dx

- Severe aortic regurgitation
- Tricuspid stenosis

Epidemiology

- Almost always secondary to rheumatic heart disease, which causes scarring of the mitral valve and fusion of valve cusps; rare causes (<1%) include congenital stenosis, calcifications, and endocarditis
- Typically occurs 15–40 years after rheumatic heart disease

Signs/Symptoms

- Dyspnea is the most significant symptom (indicates pulmonary congestion)—usually precipitated by exercise, infection, pregnancy, or Afib
- Chronic cough and hemoptysis (from vessel rupture due to pulmonary HTN)
- Crackles
- Atrial fibrillation leading to systemic emboli
- Signs/symptoms of right heart failure: Pulmonary edema, pedal edema, ascites, hepatomegaly, anorexia, fatigue
- Diastolic rumble (increases in intensity with increasing stenosis) with opening snap
- Loud first heart sound

Diagnosis

- Classic triad: Diastolic rumble, opening snap, and loud first heart sound
- Echocardiogram is diagnostic: Classic "hockey stick" and calcified appearance of anterior mitral leaflet, narrowing of mitral valve orifice, left atrial enlargement
  - TEE should be used to evaluate the presence of LA thrombus if Afib is present
- EKG: Afib, LA enlargement, RV hypertrophy
- Chest X-ray: Large left atrium on lateral film, pulmonary congestion, double density of right heart border, loss of retrosternal space due to right ventricular hypertrophy
- Cardiac catheterization: May be used to assess other affected structures and to calculate mitral valve cross-sectional area, pressure gradients, and pulmonary artery pressure
- Mitral stenosis usually becomes clinically apparent when valve area is reduced to less than 2 cm^2 (normal is 4–6 cm^2)

Treatment

- Diuretics as needed for pulmonary congestion
- Digoxin to increase inotropy and as a rate-controlling agent in atrial fibrillation
- Negative chronotropes (i.e., β-blockers, calcium-channel blockers) to alleviate high heart rates
- Endocarditis prophylaxis
- Anticoagulation if Afib is present or in patients with a previous embolic event
- Surgery is indicated for symptomatic patients with moderate to severe stenosis, asymptomatic patients with pulmonary HTN, or persistent emboli despite anticoagulation
  - Balloon valvuloplasty is treatment of choice
  - Mitral valve repair (comissurotomy) for patients with symptomatic mitral stenosis who are not candidates for valvuloplasty
  - Mitral valve replacement

Prognosis/Clinical Course

- Progressive, lifelong disease—slow progression early in course with acceleration of symptoms in late stages
- If asymptomatic or minimal symptoms, >80% 10-year survival
- With significant, limiting symptoms, 0–15% 10-year survival
- Without any intervention, median survival is less than 7 years after onset of symptoms
- If severe pulmonary HTN is present, mean survival is <3 years
- Mortality for untreated patients is due to progressive heart failure (60–70%), systemic emboli (20–30%), pulmonary emboli (10%)
- Perioperative mortality is 1–2% but 10-year survival exceeds 80%

20. Tricuspid Regurgitation

Etiology

- Incompetence of the tricuspid valve, resulting in systolic backflow of blood into the right atrium
- Most commonly due to right ventricular dilatation secondary to left-sided heart conditions (valvular disease, ischemia) and/or pulmonary HTN
- Also may be caused by rheumatic heart disease, CAD, infective endocarditis, carcinoid syndrome, iatrogenic (e.g., secondary to catheter placement, transvenous pacer), connective tissue disease, congenital

Differential Dx

- Mitral regurgitation
- Aortic stenosis
- Pulmonic stenosis (rare)

Epidemiology

- Much less common than other valvular conditions
- Most frequently develops in IV drug abusers, secondary to infective endocarditis

Signs/Symptoms

- Signs of underlying condition (pulmonary HTN, left-sided cardiac disease, etc)
- Exertional dyspnea, fatigue
- Palpitations
- Edema, ascites, hepatomegaly
- Elevated jugular venous pressure, JVD
- Atrial fibrillation
- Palpable right-sided thrill/heave
- Pansystolic murmur at LSB or sub-xyphoid region
- Carvallo's sign: Increased intensity of the pansystolic murmur with inspiration
- Palpable liver

Diagnosis

- EKG: Right atrial enlargement, evidence of possible right ventricular hypertrophy
- Chest X-ray: Right atrial enlargement +/− right ventricular enlargement
- Echocardiography: Evaluates valvular apparatus and cavity size; Doppler jet evaluation of regurgitant valve and right-sided heart pressures
- Heart catheterization: Hemodynamic evaluation of right heart and pulmonary pressures as well as evaluation of concomitant CAD

Treatment

- Medical treatment for relief of symptoms of right heart failure (diuretics, etc)
- Antiarrhythmics for atrial fibrillation
- If associated with pulmonary hypertension, treat underlying cause as indicated
- Treat underlying problem (e.g., left-sided cardiac disease)
- Rare indications for valve replacement—usually only valve repair is needed
  - Repair for severe TR associated with pulmonary HTN in those undergoing mitral valve surgery
  - Repair may be indicated in cases of severe, refractory infective endocarditis
  - Valvuloplasty or replacement for severe, symptomatic TR with mean pulmonary artery pressure <60 mm Hg

Prognosis/Clinical Course

- Patients with severe tricuspid regurgitation of any cause have a poor long-term prognosis
- Prognosis is worse if associated with pulmonary hypertension
- Prognosis for isolated mild or moderate tricuspid regurgitation is good

Vascular Disease

BRETT SACHSE, MD
SCOTT KAHAN, MD

21. Atherosclerosis

Etiology

- Abnormal lipid metabolism in genetically predisposed individuals, resulting in fibrofatty intimal plaques with lipid core
- Focal area of endothelial injury → lipids and lipoproteins enter wall → macrophages are activated and take up lipids, becoming "foam" cells → smooth muscle cells migrate into intima → smooth muscle proliferation, collagen deposition, and extracellular lipid production create a plaque → lumen narrowed by plaque → ischemia → superimposed thrombus formation may completely block lumen, resulting in acute MI, stroke, etc

Differential Dx

- Familial hypercholesterolemia (defective hepatic LDL receptor)
- Vascular vasospasm
- Atheroembolism
- Vasculitis
- Hypertensive crisis
- Cholestasis
- Nephrotic syndrome
- Hypothyroidism

Epidemiology

- Male > female
- Risk factors include decreased estrogen, increased age, diabetes mellitus, hyperlipidemia, HTN, elevated homocysteine, positive family history, smoking

Signs/Symptoms

- Cardiovascular: Chest pain, dyspnea, palpitations
- Cerebrovascular: Contralateral weakness or sensory changes, changes in vision (diplopia, blindness), expressive aphasia, dysarthria, vertigo, ataxia, carotid bruit, absent pulses in neck or arms
- Peripheral vascular: Intermittent claudication, impotence, rest pain, weak femoral pulses, bruits, atrophic changes in skin (dependent rubor, hair loss, coolness of skin)
- Viscera: Epigastric postprandial pain, pain out of proportion to physical findings
- Xanthomas: Subcutaneous nodules on extensor tendons, eyelids, buttocks

Diagnosis

- Lipid panel
- Coronary involvement
  - EKG
  - Cardiac stress testing
  - Angiography of coronary vessels
- Carotid involvement
  - Duplex ultrasound of carotids
- Peripheral involvement
  - Ankle:Brachial index < 1
  - Doppler ultrasound
  - MRA or arteriogram (if revascularization is being considered)
- Urinalysis: Rule out nephrotic syndrome
- Glucose: Rule out diabetes mellitus
- TSH: Rule out hypothyroidism

Treatment

- The mainstay of treatment is the reduction of risk factors
- Diet, exercise, weight loss
- Smoking cessation
- Control of hypertension
- Lipid-lowering agents
  - Statins: Most effective agents but risk of liver damage, myositis
  - Bile acid resins (i.e., cholestyramine): Decrease absorption of cholesterol from gut
  - Niacin: Also increases HDL
- Daily aspirin

Prognosis/Clinical Course

- Cardiovascular complications: Angina pectoris, CAD, MI, sudden death
- Cerebrovascular: Stroke, transient ischemic attack
- Peripheral vascular disease: Leg ulcers, limb loss
- Viscera: Intestinal ischemia, bowel infarction
- Lipid-level goals
  - LDL < 160 in normal patients
  - LDL < 130 in patients with risk factors for heart disease
  - LDL < 100 in patients with known coronary artery disease or diabetes
  - HDL > 35

22. Hypertension

Etiology

- Blood pressure >140/90 on two separate occasions
- May be due to decreased luminal size (atherosclerotic) and/or increased arterial muscle tone
- BP = cardiac output $\times$ total peripheral resistance
  - CO is determined by blood volume, heart rate, and inotropy
  - TPR is determined by the degree of smooth muscle vasoconstriction (vasoconstrictors include angiotensin II, thromboxane A_2, catecholamines; vasodilators include prostaglandins and nitric oxide)

Epidemiology

- Males > females
- Blacks > whites
- Age > 50, diabetes mellitus, obesity, and positive family history predispose to development of HTN

Differential Dx

- Essential/idiopathic HTN
- Secondary hypertension
  - Renal: Renal artery stenosis, intrinsic renal disease
  - Endocrine: Primary aldosteronism, Cushing's syndrome, pheochromocytoma, hyperthyroidism
  - Drugs: OCP, NSAIDs, phenylephrine
  - Coarctation of aorta
- Pregnancy-induced HTN
- Anxiety
- "White coat HTN"
- Measurement error

Signs/Symptoms

- Asymptomatic early
- Headache
- Nausea/vomiting
- Blurred vision
- Retinal fundoscopic findings: Copper wiring, AV nicking, flame hemorrhages
- Fourth heart sound
- Signs of secondary hypertension may be present (see the Secondary Hyptertension entry)
- Signs of acute organ injury secondary to hypertensive emergency:
  - Encephalopathy
  - Cardiac decompensation
  - Kidney dysfunction
  - Retinal hemorrhages, exudates, papilledema

Diagnosis

- Basic studies: CBC, chemistries, urinalysis, BUN/creatinine, EKG, lipid panel, uric acid
- Consider a secondary cause of hypertension if:
  - Age of onset <20 or >50
  - BP > 180/100
  - Hypertension refractory to several medications
  - Presence of end-organ damage
  - Signs/symptoms of secondary hypertension (e.g., renal bruit, signs of hyperthyroidism)
- Hypertensive emergency: Severe HTN with evidence of acute organ injury; treat as medical emergency—hospitalize (to ICU) and immediately reduce BP with nitroprusside or nitroglycerine
- Hypertensive urgency: Severe HTN without evidence of acute organ injury—possible hospitalization; decrease BP over 24 hours

Treatment

- Lifestyle modification: Weight loss, diet, exercise, low-salt diet (about half of hypertensives will respond to salt restriction)
- Diuretics: Especially effective in blacks, CHF, elderly; contraindicated in osteoporosis, gout
- β-blockers: ↓ cardiac output, ↓ renin, vasodilation; use in CAD patients, CHF; contraindicated in asthma, COPD, diabetes (masks hypoglycemia)
- ACE inhibitors: CHF, post-MI, diabetes, chronic renal insufficiency; contraindicated in pregnancy
- Angiotensin II receptor antagonists in patients who suffer side effects of ACE inhibitors
- Calcium-channel blockers: ↓ smooth muscle contraction, resulting in vasodilation; use in angina, SVT; contraindicated in 2nd or 3rd degree heart block
- Alpha-1 blocker: Patients with BPH
- Direct vasodilators (hydralazine, nitroprusside)

Prognosis/Clinical Course

- Untreated: Shortened lifespan of 10–20 years
- Complications of untreated HTN
  - CV: Atherosclerosis, LV hypertrophy and ensuing ischemic injury, LV diastolic dysfunction, CHF, aortic aneurysm, aortic dissection
  - Cerebrovascular: CVA/TIA
  - Renal: Nephrosclerosis, renal insufficiency

23. Secondary Hypertension

Etiology

- Chronic kidney disease (CKD): Due to fluid retention and renin effects
- Pheochromocytoma: Due to excess catecholamines
- Renal artery stenosis (atherosclerotic or fibromuscular dysplasia): Due to activation of renin-angiotensin-aldosterone axis, resulting in systemic vasoconstriction (angiotensin II) and volume expansion (aldosterone)
- Mineralocorticoid excess (primary hyperaldosteronism, Cushing's syndrome): Excess aldosterone production results in sodium reabsorption and volume expansion

Epidemiology

- CKD may affect >10 million in US—HTN will develop in most
- RAS may account for 1–2% of all hypertensives; 30% of patients with multivessel coronary disease have RAS (not all of whom have HTN)
- Primary hyperaldosteronism may be underdiagnosed (1–2%)
- Pheochromocytomas account for < 0.3% but should not be missed (10% hereditary—MEN II, neurofibromatosis, von Hippel-Lindau)

Differential Dx

- Essential HTN
- Chronic kidney disease
- Renal artery stenosis
- Pheochromocytoma
- Hyperaldosteronism
- Conn's syndrome
- Cushing's syndrome
- Liddle's syndrome
- Coarctation of the aorta
- Hyperthyroidism
- Obesity/Syndrome X
- Obstructive sleep apnea
- Drugs (cocaine, amphetamines, OCP, alcohol, steroids, sympathomimetics)

Signs/Symptoms

- Severe hypertension with a negative family history, sudden elevation of BP, and/or onset before age 20 or after 50
- Signs and symptoms of end-organ damage (see the Hypertension entry)
- RAS: Presence of long flank bruit suggests fibromuscular dysplasia (in young women more than in men); localized epigastric bruit suggests atherosclerotic RAS
- Hypokalemia spontaneously or after low-dose diuretic suggests mineralocorticoid excess or Liddle's syndrome
- Pheochromocytoma: Episodic HTN in up to 50%; hyperadrenergic triad of headache, diaphoresis, and palpitations
- Buffalo hump, striae, and associated findings of Cushing's syndrome

Diagnosis

- The basic workup for HTN remains an H & P, urinalysis, basic biochemical profile, and assessment of cardiac target organ damage (EKG/echocardiogram)
- Focused studies are reserved for patients with suggestive clinical features or those with severe or refractory HTN
  - CKD screening by serum creatinine and urinalysis
  - RAS screening by MRA and captopril renal scintigraphy; definitive test is renal angiography
  - Primary hyperaldosteronism by demonstrating high serum or urinary aldosterone levels with suppressed plasma renin activity, followed by MRI of the adrenals
  - Pheo: Elevated urinary metanephrines/catecholamines followed by CT, MRI, MIBG scan, or selective venography for catecholamine levels to localize the tumor (10% extra-abdominal, 10% malignant, 10% bilateral adrenal, 10% abdominal but extra-adrenal)

Treatment

- CKD: Medication (i.e. ACE inhibitors) to completely normalize BP is essential to limit progression of kidney disease
- RAS: Angioplasty and stenting to widen the stenotic renal artery
- Pheochromocytomas and aldosterone-producing adrenal adenomas: Surgical resection
  - Preoperative α- and β-adrenergic blockade in pheochromocytoma resection
- Spironolactone in adrenal hyperplasia
- Amiloride in Liddle's syndrome

Prognosis/Clinical Course

- Good prognosis in most cases if the correct diagnosis is made
- See individual entries for further details

24. Abdominal Aortic Aneurysm

Etiology

- The abdominal aorta is the most common site for aortic aneurysms; >90% occur below the renal arteries
- Atherosclerosis, HTN, connective tissue disease (Takayasu's), Marfan's syndrome, and family tendency all predispose to development of AAA
- Bacteria account for 5% of AAAs (staph, syphilis, and *Salmonella*)
- Untreated AAA may result in rupture of the aneurysm—the larger the aneurysm, the greater the chance of rupture
- Embolism formation occurs rarely due to stagnation of blood

Differential Dx

- Aortic dissection
- Ischemic bowel
- Perforated ulcer
- Nephrolithiasis
- Appendicitis
- Acute MI
- GERD
- Musculoskeletal pain
- Pancreatitis
- Cholecystitis
- Zoster
- Trauma
- GI malignancies
- Stress/anxiety
- Any cause of pleurisy

Epidemiology

- Most common in men >60 years old with atherosclerosis and smokers

Signs/Symptoms

- Usually asymptomatic
- Pulsatile mass at the midline of the abdomen
- Abdominal bruit
- Back or abdominal pain when they leak, rupture, or rapidly expand
- Hypotension may occur with rupture

Diagnosis

- CT, MRI, or ultrasound all may be used to diagnose aneurysm and monitor size
  - CT is most accurate (i.e., for surgical landmarks)
  - AAA is often found incidentally on CT or ultrasound
- Angiography may be used but it is less reliable since it shows only the lumen of the aneurysm; it may not show the entire aneurysm sac

Treatment

- Initial treatment for small, stable aneurysms is aimed at reduction of blood pressure and cholesterol, and at smoking cessation
- A leaking or ruptured aneurysm is a medical emergency, due to the amount of internal hemorrhage that may ensue
- Surgery is the definitive treatment
- Indications for surgery
  - Symptomatic and/or ruptured aneurysm
  - Size > 4–5 cm
  - Infectious or traumatic aneurysm
  - Rapidly enlarging (>0.5 cm/year)
- Poor surgical candidates may be eligible for percutaneous prosthetic graft

Prognosis/Clinical Course

- Continue to follow patients for control of hypertension and possible reoccurrence of aneurysm
- Patients with untreated AAA run the risk of having the aneurysm rupture
  - Risk of rupture if the aneurysm is 5 cm is 5% per year
  - Rate of rupture rises for aneurysms greater than 5 cm
- A ruptured AAA has 50% mortality
- Elective repair carries 5% mortality

25. Aortic Dissection

Etiology

- Underlying cystic medial necrosis of aorta may result in a tear of the intima of the aorta, resulting in separation of the layers of the aortic wall
- Predisposing factors include HTN, atherosclerosis, Marfan's, male gender, pregnancy (3rd trimester), iatrogenic, trauma, coarctation of the aorta
- Type A is a tear of the ascending aorta $+/-$ transverse or descending aorta
- Type B involves only the descending aorta
- Dissection may also involve the abdominal aorta (may result in renal and/or mesenteric artery occlusion) or coronary arteries (may cause MI)

Epidemiology

- 80–90% of patients >60 years old
- Males >> females

Differential Dx

- Acute MI
- Pericarditis
- Pulmonary embolus
- Pneumothorax
- Coarctation of the aorta
- Ruptured aortic aneurysm
- Costochondritis
- GERD
- Esophageal spasm/rupture
- Stress/anxiety
- Aortic stenosis
- Any cause of pleurisy
- Pancreatitis
- Biliary colic
- Zoster
- Trauma
- Metastatic malignancy

Signs/Symptoms

- Acute dissection often has a sudden onset of severe pain, usually in the back or chest
- May have concomitant nausea, diaphoresis, dyspnea, or neurologic symptoms (syncope, paresthesias)
- May cause hypertension or hypotension (if tamponade or hemorrhage occurs)
- Proximal dissection: Diminished upper-limb pulses and blood pressure, aortic regurgitation, tamponade, hypotension, syncope, CHF, AMI
- Distal dissection: Diminished lower-limb pulses and blood pressure, oliguria, mesenteric ischemia

Diagnosis

- Clinical: Unequal/absent peripheral pulses/blood pressure
- CXR: >90% will show changes associated with dissection—widened mediastinum, pleural effusion, and cardiomegaly (pericardial effusion)
- EKG: Rule out MI; if EKG suggests an acute coronary syndrome, aortic dissection cannot be ruled out because the dissection may involve the coronary arteries
- TTE: Evaluate for pericardial effusion, aortic regurgitation, and possibly ascending aorta dissection
- TEE: More sensitive and specific than TTE; cannot see proximal aortic arch well
- CT can assess entire aorta and pericardium but not suitable for unstable patients; MRI has a limited role
- Aortography: For surgical landmarking

Treatment

- Treat underlying conditions—especially HTN
- Acute Type A dissection requires emergency surgery
- Type B dissections usually require only medical therapy unless complicated by limb ischemia, renal compromise, or aortic rupture
- Medical therapy with antihypertensives (nitrates, β-blockers) is aimed at decreasing blood pressure and diminishing myocardial contractility
- Acute decompensation requires supportive therapy including bed rest, β-blockers to keep SBP < 120, and surgery as needed

Prognosis/Clinical Course

- Type A dissection: Carries a 60% mortality in the first month if nonsurgical treatment is attempted; less than 10% perioperative mortality for elective repairs
- Type B dissection: Mortality <10% after 1 month without surgery
- Postoperative complications (5–10%): Paraplegia, MI, renal insufficiency, mesenteric ischemia, impotence

26. Peripheral Vascular Disease

Etiology

- Atherosclerotic obstructive disease of the arteries of the lower extremities (and, less often, of the upper extremities)
- Risk factors include hyperlipidemia, diabetes mellitus, smoking, and hypertension

Differential Dx

- Lumbar spinal stenosis: "Pseudoclaudication" (usually bilateral pain and paresthesias in lower extremities with walking and standing—symptoms abate with sitting or bending forward)
- Thrombangiitis obliterans (Buerger disease)
- Popliteal artery entrapment

Epidemiology

- Approximately 10 million patients in the US
- Diabetic peripheral vascular disease accounts for >60% of leg amputations in the United States

Signs/Symptoms

- Intermittent claudication is the characteristic symptom of PVD
  - Lower-extremity discomfort (pain, tightness, cramping) with exercise
  - May be unilateral or bilateral
  - Presents at a relatively constant walking distance
  - Symptoms disappear upon resting
  - In severe arterial obstruction, symptoms may continue even at rest
- Decreased or absent peripheral pulses
- Arterial bruits
- Pallor of feet upon exercise or elevation
- Muscle atrophy, hair loss, thickened toenails, skin fissures, shiny skin
- Ulceration, gangrene

Diagnosis

- Diagnosis is usually made clinically
- Fontaine classification
  - Stage I: Asymptomatic
  - Stage II: Intermittent claudication
  - Stage III: Rest and nocturnal pain
  - Stage IV: Necrosis, gangrene
- Noninvasive testing
  - Ankle:brachial index <1 (normal >1) and/or significant drop with exercise
  - Duplex ultrasound
  - Magnetic resonance angiography
- Peripheral angiography is a highly accurate, though invasive method of testing; used only if surgical intervention is planned

Treatment

- Correct risk factors: Smoking cessation, glucose and/or lipid control, weight reduction, foot care
- A walking program should be prescribed; regular exercise increases claudication interval
- Pharmacologic therapy
  - Antiplatelet agents (ASA, clopidrogrel)
  - Vasoactive agents (pentoxifylline, cilostazol)
- Revascularization
  - Percutaneous transluminal angioplasty with or without stent is effective for iliac disease only
  - Surgical revascularization (bypass) is indicated in 25% of patients with claudication who develop lifestyle-limiting symptoms; proper preoperative evaluation is mandatory (cardiac, cerebral risk factors)

Prognosis/Clinical Course

- Peripheral vascular disease is a marker of atherosclerotic disease—affected patients have a high incidence of coronary artery disease and cerebrovascular disease
- Five-year mortality of patients with intermittent claudications is 30%; mortality increases to more than 75% in patients with ischemia at rest (risk to life is greater than risk to limb)
- 75% of patients with claudication improve with conservative therapy
- Complications include acute arterial occlusion, arterial aneurysm, and gangrene requiring amputation

27. Shock

Etiology

- Inadequate perfusion of tissues
- Hemorrhagic shock: Depletion of intravascular volume, usually due to bleeding
- Cardiogenic shock: Insult to the myocardium results in decreased ability of the heart to pump blood
- Septic (infectious) shock: Toxins released by bacteria cause decreased vascular resistance and a shift of fluid to the extracellular space
- Neurogenic shock: Head/CNS injury causes a disruption of BP/perfusion

Differential Dx

- Low-output heart failure
- Cardiac tamponade
- Tension pneumothorax
- Massive pulmonary embolus
- Adrenal crisis
- Anaphylaxis
- Hypovolemia
- Sepsis

Epidemiology

- Most common in trauma patients, MI patients, and infectious patients

Signs/Symptoms

- Early signs
  - Orthostatic hypotension
  - Mild tachycardia
  - Diaphoresis
  - Vasoconstriction, resulting in a narrowing of the pulse pressure
- Late signs
  - Hypotension
  - Tachycardia
  - Altered mental status, seizures
- Signs and symptoms of underlying disease may be apparent
  - Fever in infection
  - Chest pain, signs of heart failure in MI
  - Dehydration, pallor, in hemorrhagic shock

Diagnosis

- The diagnosis of shock is often made clinically
  - A narrowed pulse pressure is one of the first signs
  - Decreased urine output and increased osmolality
  - Decreased mental status
  - Decreased blood pressure
  - Tachycardia
- Anion gap lactic acidosis due to tissue hypoxia
- Very few things look like shock—if shock is suspected, treat it emergently

Treatment

- Airway, Breathing, Circulation
- First step of treatment: Reestablish adequate tissue perfusion—do not wait to figure out why the patient is in shock
  - IV fluids: Initial treatment for all forms of shock, except cardiogenic—do not fluid-overload a patient with left ventricular dysfunction
  - Diuretics, vasodilators if in heart failure
  - Pressors, afterload reduction for left-sided failure
- Determine the specific type of shock and the appropriate treatment
  - Antibiotics/pressors for septic shock
  - Blood transfusion and surgery to stop bleeding for hemorrhagic shock
  - IV fluids and pressors for neurogenic shock
  - Diuretic/vasodilator/pressors for cardiogenic shock

Prognosis/Clinical Course

- Shock is a life-threatening problem
- The outcome varies depending on the type of shock and comorbidities
- Disseminated intravascular coagulation may ensue

28. Deep Venous Thrombosis

Etiology

- Thrombus formation in the deep veins of the leg/pelvis
- The major complication occurs when a thrombus breaks off and embolizes to the pulmonary arteries
- Virchow's triad indicates increased risk of thrombus formation
  - Stasis/immobilization (postsurgery, car/plane rides)
  - Hypercoagulability (cancers, protein C deficiency, nephrotic syndrome, high estrogen states—pregnancy, OCP use, obesity)
  - Endothelial trauma (infection, IV catheters, bone fractures)

Differential Dx

- Baker's cysts (popliteal fossa cysts)
- Musculoskeletal pain
- Impaired lymphatic return/lymphatic congestion
- Venous flow difficulties without thrombosis
- Cellulitis

Epidemiology

- DVTs are mostly seen in postoperative patients, bedridden patients, pregnancy, OCP use, obesity, pelvic or lower-extremity fractures, varicose veins, CHF, and any hypercoagulable state
- The incidence of DVTs in untreated surgical patients is 25%

Signs/Symptoms

- Unilateral limb swelling and warmth
- Pain/tightness
- Edema
- Fever may be present
- Increased venous markings distal to the DVT
- Homan's sign: Pain in calf with forced dorsi-flexion of foot
- Signs and symptoms of a secondary pulmonary embolism may be the only clinical evidence of DVT
  - Dyspnea
  - Chest pain
  - Tachycardia, tachypnea
  - Hemoptysis
  - Hypoxia

Diagnosis

- Age, type and duration of operation, and previous DVT history determine risk and preventive strategy
- Doppler ultrasound is usually diagnostic
- Other tests include venography and MRI

Treatment

- Preventive techniques include ambulation, sequential compression devices, heparin, or subcutaneous low-molecular-weight heparin
- If DVT is detected
  - First episode: Full anticoagulation (INR of 2–3) for 4–6 months
  - Second episode: Anticoagulation for 12 months
  - Third episode: Lifelong anticoagulation
- Inferior vena cava filter should be placed if patient has a contraindication to or failed with anticoagulation, severe pulmonary insufficiency, free-floating iliac thrombus—filter does not prevent DVTs, but merely prevents large emboli from entering the pulmonary artery
- Analgesia, compression, elevation of leg, and warm compresses for symptomatic relief

Prognosis/Clinical Course

- Prognosis is usually good
- Patients with a patent foramen ovale or septal wall defects are at risk for arterial occlusion—embolus bypasses lungs, travels from right heart to left heart, and enters the systemic circulation (rare)
  - Stroke, mesenteric infarction, and other acute vascular events may result
- Trousseau's sign (migratory thrombophlebitis): Venous thromboses that spontaneously appear, disappear, and reappear elsewhere; due to malignancy (especially GI malignancies)

Pulmonary Disease

JEFFREY M.CATERINO, MD

29. Acute Respiratory Distress Syndrome

Etiology

- ARDS is the most severe type of acute lung injury
- Caused by direct lung injury in response to a pathophysiologic stimulus—generalized lung inflammation ensues, causing ↑ pulmonary vascular permeability, interstitial edema, alveolar consolidation, and atelectasis
- Direct lung injuries include: Pneumonia, aspiration of gastric contents, pulmonary contusion, fat emboli syndrome, drowning, toxic inhalation
- Indirect injuries: Sepsis, trauma, shock, transfusion, pancreatitis, drugs

Differential Dx

- CHF
- Pneumonia
- Pulmonary embolism
- "Acute lung injury": A less severe form of ARDS in which the PaO_2/FiO_2 ratio is between 200–300
- Interstitial lung disease (i.e., sarcoid, IPF, occupational)
- Diffuse alveolar hemorrhage
- Hypersensitivity pneumonitis
- Cancer (lymphoma or leukemia)

Epidemiology

- Incidence: 18–75 cases per 100,000 population per year
- Occurs in patients who have conditions listed above
- 40% of patients with sepsis develop ARDS
- Predictors of poor outcome include sepsis and old age

Signs/Symptoms

- Abrupt onset of pulmonary infiltrates, severe hypoxemia, and extreme V/Q mismatch
- Tachypnea
- Dyspnea
- Diffuse crackles
- Rhonchi
- Rapid respiratory failure, usually requiring mechanical ventilation
- Severe hypoxemia, which responds poorly to O_2
- High peak airway pressures

Diagnosis

- Three criteria must be present for diagnosis:
  - Chest X-ray findings: Bilateral diffuse alveolar infiltrates
  - Blood gas or pulse oximeter showing hypoxemia (PaO_2/FiO_2 ratio <200)
  - Absence of cardiogenic pulmonary edema (either pulmonary capillary wedge pressure <18 or no clinical evidence of increased left atrial pressure)
- Arterial blood gas: Hypoxemia with large A-a gradient; initial respiratory alkalosis followed by hypercarbia (in severe disease) due to alveolar hypoventilation
- Swan-Ganz catheter: Pulmonary capillary wedge pressure <18; normal-to-high cardiac output

Treatment

- Primarily supportive care
- Treat the underlying cause
- Proper ventilator management is essential
  - Permissive hypercapnia: Small tidal volumes (6–8 cc/kg) are preferable to prevent overstretching of healthy alveoli (ventilator-associated lung injury)—even at the expense of hypoventilation and increased CO_2
  - Avoid oxygen toxicity: Oxygenation is best maintained with ↑ levels of PEEP, rather than high inspired O_2 concentrations (FiO_2)
- Glucocorticoids
  - If started between days 7 and 14, may prevent the development of irreversible fibrosis
  - If used at disease onset, they have been shown to *increase* mortality

Prognosis/Clinical Course

- Acute inflammatory phase: ARDS develops over 4–48 hours and can last for weeks; rapid onset of respiratory failure with inflammation, increased capillary permeability, and diffuse alveolar damage; mechanical ventilation is required
- Chronic phase: Acute symptoms either resolve or progress to the fibroproliferative phase; fibrotic lung injury occurs as lung is repaired, resulting in persistent hypoxemia, ↓ pulmonary compliance, and pulmonary HTN; survivors usually have nearly normal pulmonary function by 6–12 months; severe disease will have persistent pulmonary dysfunction
- Mortality rate is 40–60% but is decreasing due to better ventilator strategies and supportive care

30. Asthma

Etiology

- A disease of chronic airway inflammation, characterized by three elements
  - Chronic airway inflammation
  - Bronchial hyperreactivity
  - Reversible airway obstruction
- Extrinsic asthma: Hypersensitivity to an allergen (e.g., pollen, dust mites)
- Intrinsic asthma: Airway reactivity to a non-immune trigger (e.g., aspirin, NSAIDs, β-blockers, sulfites, irritant dusts, pollutants, cold, exercise, infection, stress)

Epidemiology

- Affects 5–10% of the population
- Half of cases have onset before age 10, but can develop at any age
- Males > females
- Often a family history of asthma or atopic diseases
- Mortality has been increasing, perhaps due to overreliance on bronchodilator drugs

Differential Dx

- Pulmonary edema
- Heart failure
- MI/CAD
- Pneumonia
- Bronchiolitis
- Acute bronchitis
- COPD
- Hypersensitivity pneumonitis
- Upper airway obstruction (tumor, croup, edema)
- Vocal cord dysfunction
- Pneumothorax
- Atelectasis
- Pulmonary emboli
- Angioedema
- Anxiety attacks

Signs/Symptoms

- Cough— #1 cause of cough (#2 and #3 are GERD and postnasal drip)
- Shortness of breath
- Chest tightness
- Expiratory wheeze/prolonged expirations
- Sputum production (mucorrhea)
- Overinflation with air, mucus, and debris
- Nocturnal awakenings
- Sleep disturbance
- Tachycardia/tachypnea during episodes
- Severe acute exacerbations: Accessory muscle use, unable to speak full sentences, decreased air movement, hyperinflation (increased AP diameter of thorax), altered mental status (secondary to hypoxia), pulsus paradoxus (fall in SBP by 10+ mm Hg during inspiration)

Diagnosis

- Demonstration of reversible airway dysfunction
  - 15% increase in FEV_1 after β-agonist inhaler
  - Bronchoconstriction in response to a methacholine or cold air challenge
- Pulmonary function tests: $\downarrow FEV_1$, $\uparrow TLC$, and $\uparrow RV$; improved FEV_1 with bronchodilator therapy
- PEFR: Easy to measure; used to follow course/severity of disease; 400–600 is normal; 100–300 moderate exacerbation; <100 severe exacerbation
- CXR: Hyperinflation, atelectasis
- ABG: Respiratory alkalosis in mild exacerbations; as the patient tires from hyperventilation in severe attacks, the impending respiratory failure causes pCO_2 to progress to normal and then above normal; hypoxemia and metabolic acidosis are signs of severe disease (due to poor oxygenation and V/Q mismatch)
- Sputum culture: $\uparrow$ eosinophils, possible secondary infection

Treatment

- Avoid triggers!
- Supplemental O_2 in acute attack
- $β_2$-agonists for bronchodilation
  - Short-acting (albuterol)—for acute rescue
  - Long-acting (salmeterol)—for nocturnal use, exercise, and persistent asthma
- Inhaled corticosteroids for chronic therapy: Should be used if patient is using bronchodilators more than twice per week
- Anticholinergics (ipratropium): Weak bronchodilators
- Mast cell stabilizers (cromolyn) in children
- Leukotriene inhibitors (i.e., montelukast)
- Systemic steroids (prednisone), nebulized β-agonists, and occasionally theophylline for acute, severe exacerbations

Prognosis/Clinical Course

- Episodic course with acute exacerbations separated by symptom-free periods
- Symptoms precipitated by exercise, cold air, URIs, stress, irritants, etc
- Severity of attack and response to treatment is followed by measuring PEFRs
- Status asthmaticus: Prolonged, severe attack that does not respond to initial therapy; may lead to respiratory failure and death
- *Mild, intermittent* asthma: Symptoms <2/wk; PEFR > 80% of normal
- *Mild, persistent*: sxs >2/wk; PEFR > 80%
- *Moderate persistent*: Daily sxs; PEFR 60–80%
- *Severe, persistent*: Frequent sxs and exacerbations; limited activity; PEFR <60%

31. Chronic Obstructive Pulmonary Disease

Etiology

- Progressive, irreversible airway obstruction, usually due to smoking
  - Chronic bronchitis: Productive cough for at least 3 months during 2 or more successive years
  - Emphysema: Enlargement of air spaces and destruction of parenchyma, causing closure of small airways and loss of lung elasticity
- Lung dysfunction results from airflow limitation (loss of elastic recoil, ↑ collapsibility/narrowing of small airways) and impaired gas exchange (V/Q mismatch, alveolar destruction, ↑ dead space causing hypercarbia)

Differential Dx

- CHF
- Asthma
- Pneumonia
- Bronchiolitis
- Pulmonary embolism
- Bronchiectasis
- Upper airway obstruction
- Restrictive lung diseases
- Pneumothorax
- GERD

Epidemiology

- Risk factors: Cigarette smoking (accounts for >90% of cases), air pollution, occupational inhalation, α_1-AT deficiency)
- Just 15% of smokers get COPD—genetic predisposition important
- 4th leading cause of death in US—incidence and mortality increasing
- 6th most common cause of death worldwide—increasing to 3rd due to increased cigarette use and air pollution

Signs/Symptoms

- Patients usually have a combination of bronchitis and emphysematous sxs
- Chronic bronchitis symptoms (blue bloaters)
  - Productive cough   – Rhonchi/wheezes
  - Exertional dyspnea   – Cyanosis/hypoxemia
  - Fatigue   – Obesity
  - Right heart failure   – Late CO_2 retention
- Emphysematous symptoms (pink puffers)
  - Severe dyspnea   – Minimal cough
  - ↑ work of breathing   – Weight loss
  - Prolonged expiration   – ↓ Air movement
  - Flattened diaphragm   – Barrel chest
  - Pursed-lip breathing   – "Tripod" sitting
  - Hyperresonance   – Normal pCO_2
  - Accessory muscle use
  - Minimal hypoxemia

Diagnosis

- PFTs: Gold standard for diagnosis; PFTs must show an obstructive pattern for diagnosis of COPD
  - ↓ FEV_1/FVC (<70% predicted): Best indicator of obstruction
  - ↑ Lung volumes (FRC, RV, RV/TLC ratio): Due to airway obstruction, resulting in air trapping and hyperinflation
  - ↓ diffusing capacity: Especially in emphysema
- CXR: Flattened diaphragms, hyperinflation, bullae and increased lucency in lung; small heart (radiographic appearance does not correlate with degree of lung dysfunction)
- ABG: Hypoxemia (due to V/Q mismatch), hypercarbia
- CBC: Polycythemia secondary to chronic hypoxemia
- CT scan: centrilobular emphysema, bullae

Treatment

- Stop smoking—the only way to slow progression
- Bronchodilators: Anticholinergics are the preferred agents; long-acting β-agonists decrease infections and improve symptoms
- Oxygen: Continual/nighttime O_2 improves mortality and quality of life in pts with chronic hypoxemia
- Antibiotics: Beneficial in exacerbations but not as prophylaxis
- Corticosteroids: Role of inhaled steroids is unclear—few have even a small improvement; systemic steroids are useful in acute exacerbations
- Theophylline: Causes improvement in 20%
- Noninvasive positive pressure ventilation (biPAP): Decreases need for mechanical vent in exacerbations
- Lung volume reduction surgery and lung transplant may benefit selected patients with end-stage disease

Prognosis/Clinical Course

- Chronic course with acute exacerbations
- Progression slowed by smoking cessation
- Acute exacerbations
  - ↑ sxs, ↓ lung function, ↑ sputum, fever
  - May be a bacterial (*Streptococcus pneumoniae, Haemophilus influenzae, Moraxella*) or viral infection
  - Responds to antibiotics (doxycycline, azithromycin, bactrim), steroids, and ventilatory support
- Poor prognosis with end-stage disease (pCO_2 > 60 mm Hg, poor exercise tolerance)
- Usually diagnosed in 6th decade as abnormal accelerated decline in FEV_1 for age (↓ 50–75 cc/year vs. 30 cc/year in non-COPD)
- Pulmonary HTN, cor pulmonale may result

32. Chronic Cough

Etiology

- Defined as a cough that lasts >3 weeks
- Due to stimulation of cough receptors in the nose, auditory canal, pharynx, larynx, trachea, bronchi, and pleura
- If chest X-ray is normal, >90% result from one or more of the following:
  - Smoking
  - Asthma
  - Chronic bronchitis
  - ACE inhibitors (allow bradykinin to accumulate in lungs)
  - Postnasal drip
  - GERD

Epidemiology

- Occurs in as many as one in four adults
- Incidence increases directly with the number of cigarettes smoked
- As many as 60% of cases have more than one cause of cough
- 5th most common outpatient complaint—accounts for 30 million office visits annually

Differential Dx

- Viral URI
- CHF
- Hypersensitivity pneumonitis
- Bronchiectasis
- Occupational exposure
- Tuberculosis
- Lung/esophageal cancer
- Cystic fibrosis
- Interstitial lung disease
- Airway foreign body
- Recurrent aspiration
- Psychogenic
- Intrathoracic mass (tumor, aortic aneurysm)
- Medications (aspirin, ACE inhibitor, β-blocker)

Signs/Symptoms

- Nonproductive cough
- Symptoms related to specific causes
  - Upper respiratory infection
  - Throat discomfort (post nasal drip)
  - Nasal congestion and facial pain (post nasal drip, sinusitis)
  - Increased symptoms with a specific trigger or worsening symptoms at night, in cold air, or with exercise (asthma)
  - Productive cough (chronic bronchitis, bronchiectasis)
  - Dyspepsia, belching (GERD)
- Chronic cough may be an atypical presentation of common diseases (GERD, asthma, etc)

Diagnosis

- Screen for serious causes: Chronic infection, lung cancer (weight loss, hemoptysis, fever/chills), and so on—X ray and CT if patient has concerning symptoms
- D/C smoking, causative meds, and occupational exposures
- Screening X-ray is required unless patient is young nonsmoker
- Step 1: Treat empirically for post nasal drip with antihistamine and decongestant; add nasal steroids if symptoms persist; if ineffective, obtain CT of sinuses for sinusitis
- Step 2: Evaluate for asthma with a trial of bronchodilators or a methacholine challenge test; treat asthma if found
- Step 3: Obtain chest X-ray and CT scan of the chest
- Step 4: If imaging is normal, treat empirically for GERD with PPI and antireflux measures; proceed with EGD or esophageal pH monitoring if no improvement with the PPI
- Step 5: Bronchoscopy to identify less common causes

Treatment

- Nonspecific agents (do not take the place of specific therapies): Antitussives, expectorants, mucolytics
- Postnasal drip: Antihistamine (e.g., diphenhydramine) plus decongestant (e.g., pseudoephedrine); add nasal steroid if no improvement in 1 week; add antibiotics if sinusitis is present
- Cough-variant asthma: Remove allergens; treat with inhaled bronchodilators, inhaled steroids, leukotriene antagonists, and mast cell stabilizers as needed
- GERD: Proton pump inhibitor for 1–2 months; antireflux measures
- Chronic bronchitis/bronchiectasis: Smoking cessation, inhaled ipratropium and β-agonist, antibiotics, chest physiotherapy, postural drainage, expectorants
- Postviral: Antihistamine plus decongestant; add β-agonist and inhaled or systemic steroids as needed

Prognosis/Clinical Course

- >90% have resolution of symptoms if the suggested algorithm is followed
- The key to success is to rule out serious causes initially and then proceed through the algorithm
- Continue following the algorithm if only partial improvement occurs—many patients have more than one cause
- Newer, nonsedating antihistamines are not as effective as the older varieties

33. Bronchiectasis

Etiology

- Abnormal, irreversible dilatation of medium-sized airways
- Inflammatory insult (usually infectious) results in injury and fibrosis to dilated and distorted airways
- The dilated and distorted airways cannot properly clear secretions
- This predisposes patient to recurrent infection, inflammation, and further damage
- May be localized secondary to a single insult (i.e., lobar pneumonia) or diffusely spread throughout the lungs

Epidemiology

- Females > males
- Ages 20–60
- Increased in nonsmokers and white women

Differential Dx

- Pneumonia
- COPD
- Interstitial lung disease
- Chronic aspiration
- BOOP
- Asthma
- Inciting lesions
  - Infection (pneumonia, TB, measles, pertussis)
  - Inflammation (aspiration, inhalation injury)
  - Congenital (α_1-antitrypsin deficiency, cystic fibrosis, ciliary dyskinesia)
  - Scarring (COPD, pulmonary fibrosis)
  - Obstruction (neoplasm, foreign body)

Signs/Symptoms

- Classic triad
  - Persistent productive cough
  - Copious purulent sputum
  - Hemoptysis: May be mild, due to inflamed airways, or massive, due to hypertrophied bronchial arteries
- Recurrent pneumonia
- Dyspnea
- Crackles, rhonchi, wheezing
- Fever
- Pleuritic chest pain
- Weight loss
- May develop clubbing, pulmonary HTN, and cor pulmonale

Diagnosis

- CT is the gold standard
  - Dilated airways, "tram tracks" (dilated airways parallel to each other due to collapse of intervening alveoli), dilated "signet ring" bronchioles (a dilated bronchus—the ring—with a visible associated pulmonary artery—the stone)
- CXR: May be normal—sensitivity is just 50%
  - Cystic areas with fluid levels; peribronchial thickening; "tram tracks"; atelectasis
- Sputum: Many neutrophils; microorganisms representing either colonization or infection, especially *Pseudomonas*
- Bronchoscopy: Used if a foreign body or neoplasm suspected
- PFTs: Restrictive or mixed restrictive–obstructive pattern
- Sweat chloride test for cystic fibrosis; assessment for ciliary dyskinesia; serum immunoglobulins; rheumatoid factor

Treatment

- Treat the underlying cause
- Improve clearance of secretions
  - Inhaled bronchodilators
  - Postural drainage
  - Chest physiotherapy and handheld flutter valves
- Control infection
  - Vaccinations
  - Chronic prophylactic antibiotics: Either oral medications or inhaled aminoglycosides
  - Antibiotics for acute exacerbations, including anti-pseudomonal coverage
- Surgical resection in (rare) cases of localized disease
- Lung transplant as a last resort

Prognosis/Clinical Course

- Incidence has been decreasing in recent years as antibiotics have improved; however, nodular bronchiectasis due to atypical mycobacteria is increasing
- Chronic course; progression depends on the primary cause and adequacy of management
- Course is marked by recurrent infections and acute exacerbations
- Lung function may be stable or may show a slow, steady decline despite adequate management
- Bronchiectasis is an end-stage lesion of a variety of pulmonary processes—respiratory failure may ensue if the inciting event cannot be revsersed

34. Cystic Fibrosis

Etiology

- Caused by a defect in the cystic fibrosis transmembrane receptor (CFTR) protein—it results in defective ion transport in the exocrine glands
- In the lungs, abnormal Na and Cl transport causes thick, poorly cleared mucus, resulting in chronic bacterial colonization and recurrent infections
- Chronic inflammation impairs lung function, eventually resulting in respiratory failure
- Thickened secretions in the pancreas result in retention of pancreatic enzymes with eventual destruction of the pancreas and steatorrhea

Differential Dx

- Asthma
- Pneumonia
- Bronchiectasis
- GI disease
  - Chronic diarrhea
  - Food allergy
  - Gastroenteritis
  - Pancreatic insufficiency
  - Liver disease

Epidemiology

- Autosomal recessive genetic disorder
- >800 different mutations exist, each with differing phenotypes
- As many as 1 case per 3000 births (depending on ethnic group)
- Whites >> blacks > Asians
- Most common severe recessive genetic disease among whites in US
- Most common mutation (66%) is the ΔF508 deletion

Signs/Symptoms

- Pulmonary
  - Chronic cough   - Clubbing
  - Purulent sputum   - Nasal polyps
  - Wheezing, SOB   - Hemoptysis
  - Chronic sinusitis
  - Recurrent infections/pneumonias
  - Pneumothorax
- Pulmonary exacerbations: ↑ Cough and sputum, fever, wt loss, ↓ pulmonary fn
- Gastrointestinal
  - Pancreatic insufficiency (90%)
  - Protein/fat malabsorbtion
  - Diabetes mellitus (10%)
  - Obstruction/intussusception
  - Biliary stasis   - Constipation
- Sterility in 95% of males (abnl secretions in vas deferens) and 20% of females

Diagnosis

- Requires clinical symptoms (pulmonary or GI) plus diagnostic sweat chloride test (>80 mEq/L in adults)
- DNA analysis: Not used for primary diagnosis (detects less than 20% of mutations); has prognostic value after diagnosis is made; useful if diagnosis is in doubt
- PFTs: Obstructive pattern (↓ FVC, ↑ lung volumes)
- CXR: Hyperinflation, peribronchial cuffing, bronchiectasis, upper lobe > lower lobe involvement, hilar lymphadenopathy
- Sputum culture and sensitivity
- ABG: Hypoxemia, metabolic alkalosis
- Electrolytes: Hypochloremic, hyponatremic metabolic alkalosis; hyperglycemia if diabetic
- Stool analysis: Increased fecal fat due to malabsorption
- Semen analysis: Azoospermia

Treatment

- Antibiotics
  - Chronic: Inhaled tobramycin— ↑ lung function, ↓ exacerbations
  - Exacerbation: Two-drug antipseudomonal therapy treats exacerbation and prevents resistance
- Mobilization of secretions: Chest physiotherapy; inhaled bronchodilators; rhDNAase (Pulmozyme)—thins and mobilizes secretions, ↓ exacerbations by 1/3
- Nutritional therapy: ↑ fat diet, vitamin supplements, ↑ caloric requirements from work of breathing
- Control of airway inflammation: Vaccinations and steroids (chronic, prophylactic inhaled steroids; systemic steroids during exacerbations)
- Gene therapy may provide definitive cure
- Lung transplant in severe dysfunction (FEV_1< 30%) has relatively good results (60% 2-year survival)

Prognosis/Clinical Course

- Presents in adulthood in 4% of cases
- Childhood presentation: Meconium ileus, multiple respiratory tract infections, cachexia
- Adult presentation includes chronic sinus/respiratory infections
- Median survival is now >30 years
- Chronic course with acute exacerbations
- Most common infectious agents include:
  - Children: *Staphylococcus aureus, Haemophilus influenzae*
  - Adults: Resistant *Pseudomonas, Burkholdia cepacia* (highly resistant bacterium), *Aspergillus*
- Respiratory failure causes death in the majority of cases

35. Pneumonia

Etiology

- Lower respiratory tract infection of the lung parenchyma, resulting in inflammation, alveolar exudates, and consolidation
- Community-acquired pneumonia (CAP): In nonhospitalized patients
- Hospital-acquired pneumonia (HAP): Onset 2–3 days after admission
- Ventilator-associated pneumonia: Develops >48 hours after intubation
- Often distinguished by presentation into "typical" or "atypical," but clinical picture alone is not sufficient for diagnosis or treatment

Epidemiology

- 3–4 million cases/yr in US; 500,000 hospitalizations; 45,000 deaths
- 6th leading cause of death—it is the most deadly infection
- Incidence increases in the winter months
- Mortality of CAP patients who need to be hospitalized is 14%; <1% mortality in those not hospitalized
- HAP is the leading cause of nosocomial death—20–50% mortality

Differential Dx

- URI
- Bronchitis
- PE
- Vasculitis
- Asthma
- CHF
- Lung cancer
- Sarcoid
- Occupational exposure
- CAP: *Streptococcus pneumoniae* (most common), *Mycoplasma, Chlamydia pneumoniae,* HiB, *Staphylococcus aureus, Moraxella, Legionella,* gram-negative enterics, viruses, fungi, PCP, TB
- HAP: Gram-negative enterics, *Staphylococcus*
- Vent-associated: *S. aureus* and gram-negative enterics (especially *Pseudomonas*)

Signs/Symptoms

- "Typical" pneumonia is characterized by acute or subacute onset of fever, dyspnea, and productive cough
- Constitutional signs: Rigors, sweats, chills, chest discomfort, fatigue, myalgia, anorexia, HA, abdominal pain, N/V
- Physical examination
  - Tachypnea
  - Dull to percussion
  - Tachycardia
  - Egophony
  - Hypoxemia
  - Rhonchi
- "Atypical" pneumonia occurs with *Mycoplasma, Legionella, Chlamydia:*
  - More gradual onset
  - Dry cough
  - Headache, malaise
  - Minimal lung signs

Diagnosis

- Pulse oximetry
- CXR: Ranges from diffuse patchy infiltrates to lobar consolidation; may be bilateral or unilateral; pleural effusion or cavitation
- Sputum Gram stain and culture: IDSA recommends Gram stain in CAP patients and culture in all admitted patients; however, poor sensitivity/specificity
- Blood cultures: Positive in 10%; recommended by IDSA for all hospitalized patients
- Serologies for *Legionella, Mycoplasma,* and *Chlamydia;* poor sensitivity/specificity; requires follow-up titers
- *Legionella* urinary antigen (50% sensitive, 90% specific)
- HIV testing in young patients with repeated pneumonia
- Hospital-acquired pneumonia: Bronchoscopy with lavage may help identify organism and guide management (blood/sputum cultures are often not diagnostic)

Treatment

- CAP (outpatient): Macrolide (i.e., erythromycin, azithromycin), doxycycline, or quinolone
- CAP (hospitalized): [Macrolide plus 3rd generation cephalosporin] or a 2nd generation quinolone
- CAP (ICU): [Macrolide or 2nd generation quinolone] plus [3rd generation cephalosporin or β-lactam/β-lactamase inhibitor]
- Suspected aspiration: 2nd generation quinolone plus [clindamycin or β-lactam/β-lactamase inhibitor]
- CAP with structural lung disease: Antipseudomonal PCN/cephalosporin plus antipseudomonal quinolone
- HAP (mild and early-onset): 3rd generation cephalosporin or a β-lactam/β-lactamase inhibitor
- HAP (severe, late-onset, ICU, or vent-associated): [2nd generation quinolone or aminoglycoside] plus [antipseudomonal PCN/cephalosporin, imipenem, or aztreonam]; add vancomycin if staph is a concern

Prognosis/Clinical Course

- Vaccines available for *S. pneumoniae,* influenza
- Treat CAP for 14 days; HAP for 14–21 days
- Pneumonia severity index (PSI): A scoring system used to determine the risk of mortality
- Risk Class I: Age < 50 and absence of neoplasm, liver disease, CHF, CVA, and/or renal disease—discharge on oral antibiotics
- Risk Classes II–V use a point system based on age, sex, coexisting disease (neoplastic, liver, heart, renal), abnormal vitals, abnormal exam, abnormal labs, and pleural effusion
  - Class II: Mortality <1%; discharge
  - Class III: Mortality 1–3%; discharge or short hospital stay
  - Class IV: Mortality 9%; hospitalize
  - Class V: Mortality 30%; hospitalize

36. Lung Abscess/Aspiration

Etiology

- Aspiration pneumonia: Abnormal entry of material from stomach/airway into the lungs—three discrete syndromes:
  - Chemical pneumonitis (Mendelson's syndrome): Aspiration of gastric acid without bacterial infection
  - Pneumonia: Due to oral anaerobes $+/-$ aerobes
  - Airway obstruction by a foreign body
- Lung abscess: Most result from aspiration pneumonia and are caused by oral anaerobes; also due to PE with infarction, chest trauma, obstruction

Differential Dx

- Other cavitary lung diseases
  - TB
  - Fungal infection
  - Cancer
  - Pulmonary embolism with infarction
  - Vasculitis
  - Wegener's granulomatosis
  - Acute necrotizing pneumonia
  - Lymphoma
  - Bronchiectasis

Epidemiology

- Risk factors for aspiration: ↓ Level of consciousness, dysphagia, dental disease, GERD, intubation, tube feedings, alcoholism
- Aspiration is usually polymicrobial; consists of oropharyngeal anaerobes and aerobes
- Aspiration causes almost all cases of anaerobic pneumonia

Signs/Symptoms

- Chemical pneumonitis
  - Acute dyspnea
  - Tachycardia
  - Low-grade fever
  - Hypoxemia
  - Crackles
  - Tachypnea
  - Hypotension
  - Abrupt onset
  - May have rapid onset of respiratory distress and hypoxia
- Anaerobic pneumonia/lung abscess
  - Insidious onset over days, weeks, or months
  - Fever, malaise
  - Cough with purulent sputum
  - Poor oral hygiene
  - Dysphagia, weight loss
  - Night sweats

Diagnosis

- Chemical pneumonitis
  - Presence of a predisposing condition
  - CXR: Lobar infiltrates (lower > upper lung zones)
- Lung abscess
  - CXR: Cavity with an air-fluid level, surrounded by consolidation; especially found in dependent lung zones—superior lower lobe or posterior upper lobes; may see infiltrate or effusion
  - CT: Defines the abscess cavity
  - Sputum Gram stain and culture: Usually mixed flora; also stain for mycobacteria and fungi; very difficult to culture anaerobes
  - Bronchoscopy: Use if the lesion does not resolve as expected or if cancer or a foreign body are possible
  - Blood cultures are rarely positive
  - Leukocytosis

Treatment

- Chemical pneumonitis
  - Supportive care with O_2, mechanical ventilation
  - Hold antibiotics unless evidence of infection
  - There is no evidence that bacteria have any role, but patients are often give antibiotics as it is difficult to rule out secondary infection
- Aspiration/anaerobic pneumonia and lung abscesses
  - Treat anaerobes with clindamycin, a β-lactam/β-lactamase inhibitor, or imipenem
  - Add gram-negative coverage in nosocomial infxns
  - Treat abscess for at least 3 weeks (often months)
  - Drainage does not seem to improve the course of lung abscesses
  - Surgical resection or percutaneous drainage if nonresolving, persistent fevers, ↑ WBC, empyema, enlarging cavity, or suspected cancer

Prognosis/Clinical Course

- Chemical pneumonitis
  - 15% of cases develop ARDS
  - 60% have rapid improvement over 2–3 days
  - 25% rapidly improve, but then develop increased infiltrates, which likely represent secondary bacterial infection
- Lung abscess
  - Develops 7–14 days after initial aspiration
  - Clinical response to antibiotics in 3–4 days
  - In those who fail to respond, consider an associated condition (such as foreign body or neoplasm), a different infectious agent (i.e., fungus), or the presence of a noninfectious cavitary lung disease
  - 20% overall mortality

37. Tuberculosis

Etiology

- Airborne droplet transmission of *Mycobacterium tuberculosis* bacillus
- Organisms replicate within the alveoli
- The emergence of multidrug-resistant organisms is primarily due to failure to complete the required long courses of therapy
- Some positive PPDs are due to previous inoculation with BCG vaccine outside of the US
- Most cases of active disease involve reactivation of a previous infection

Differential Dx

- Bacterial pneumonia
- Lung cancer
- Sarcoidosis
- HIV
- CHF
- Fungal infection
- Lung abscess
- Lymphoma
- Vasculitis

Epidemiology

- 15 million people in the US are infected; 16,000 active cases per year
- Prevalence increased during the 1980s, but has been declining since 1992
- 1/3 of the world's population is infected; fewer have active disease
- Groups who require screening PPDs: HIV, close contacts of active TB cases, IV drug users, DM, silicosis, immunosuppression, cancer cases, ESRD, health care workers, low-income and immigrant groups

Signs/Symptoms

- Fever
- Night sweats
- Weight loss
- Fatigue
- Cough
- Hemoptysis
- Pleuritic chest pain
- Dyspnea is uncommon
- Pleural effusion
- Extrapulmonary involvement: Lymph nodes, bones, joints, genitourinary, CNS, abdomen, pericardium, pleura; symptoms of organ dysfunction may be present

Diagnosis

- CXR
  - Primary TB: Lower lung infiltrates; adenopathy
  - Latent TB: Nodules and fibrosis in upper lung
  - Reactivation TB: Upper lung infiltrates, cavitation
  - Miliary TB: Disseminated small nodules
  - Gohn complex: Granuloma with bacilli in center plus calcified lymph node
- Sputum (need three samples): Shows acid-fast bacilli
- Tuberculin skin test (PPD): Most common screening test
  - 15 mm of induration is positive if no risk factors
  - 10 mm of induration is positive for patients at risk
  - 5 mm is positive for patients with HIV, recent exposure, or suggestive CXR
- HIV testing should be done in all new TB patients
- Biopsy (node, liver, or bone marrow) to confirm diagnosis in extrapulmonary TB

Treatment

- Report cases to public health authorities
- Respiratory isolation
- Active TB: Isoniazid (INH) and rifampin (Rif) for 6 months plus pyrazinamide (PZA) for 2 months
  - Add ethambutol in areas of INH resistance (most of the US) pending culture
  - Multidrug-resistant TB is known
- Extrapulmonary TB: Same treatment as active TB
- Latent TB should be treated due to possibility of active transformation—especially in high-risk groups
  - INH for 9 months or Rif for 4 months
  - Rif/PZA for 2 months (caution in liver disease)
  - Treat latent infection unless previously treated
- BCG vaccine is unreliable—disregard previous BCG exposure in evaluation of patients

Prognosis/Clinical Course

- Primary TB: Usually asymptomatic or a self-limited; noninfectious; leads to latent TB
- Active TB: Clinical symptoms, positive sputum, or CXR consistent with TB; 65% 5-year mortality if untreated; easily curable
- Latent TB infection: Positive PPD but no clinical, CXR, or culture proof of active infection; TB may reactivate when the immune system is weakened
- Disseminated TB: Inadequate host defenses (i.e., HIV) allow systemic spread (diffuse, multiple, small nodes of infection) with multiorgan symptoms
- 90% of cases remain latent; never become active
- Treatment cures >95%

38. HIV-Related Lung Disease

Etiology

- The immunosuppression caused by HIV causes a variety of pulmonary manifestations, both infectious and noninfectious
- Bacterial infections often begin prior to the development of overt AIDS; their frequency increases as the patient's CD4 count drops
- For all infectious etiologies, the presentation in HIV may differ widely from the common presentations in immunocompetent individuals
- Noninfectious causes of HIV-induced lung disease can mimic infection and should be considered in the differential diagnosis

Differential Dx

- Bacteria: *S. pneumoniae, H. influenzae, S. aureus, Pseudomonas, Rhodococcus*
- Mycobacteria
- Pneumocystis (PCP)
- Fungal: *Histoplasma, Aspergillus, Coccidioides, Cryptococcus*
- Cancer: Kaposi's sarcoma, lymphoma, lung cancer
- Sinusitis, bronchitis
- Lymphocytic interstitial pneumonia
- Nonspecific interstitial pneumonitis
- BOOP
- 1° pulmonary HTN

Epidemiology

- 70% of patients with HIV have at least one pulmonary manifestation
- CD4 count provides an indicator as to likely pathogenic organisms
  - >400   Bacterial, tuberculosis
  - 200–400   Recurrent pneumonia, nontuberculous mycobacteria
  - <200   PCP, Kaposi's sarcoma, disseminated TB
  - <100   MAC, fungal, CMV, toxoplasmosis

Signs/Symptoms

- PCP: Dyspnea, dry cough, fever; most common cause of respiratory failure in AIDS patients—ARDS-like picture
- Bacterial pneumonia: Fever/chills, cough
- TB: Cough, hemoptysis, fever; miliary and extrapulmonary involvement is more common with HIV
- MAC and CMV: Severe disseminated infection that may spread to lungs; rarely causes clinical disease
- Fungal infection depends on geography: *Histoplasma, Aspergillus, Coccidioides*
- Kaposi's sarcoma: Cough, dyspnea, fever, oral/skin lesions, hemtopysis

Diagnosis

- Obtain CD4 count to narrow differential diagnosis
- CXR
  - Pneumothorax: suggests PCP
  - Opacities: Bacteria, PCP, TB, Kaposi's sarcoma, fungi, CMV
  - Diffuse nodules: Kaposi's sarcoma, TB, fungi
  - Mediastinal nodes: TB, MAC, Kaposi's sarcoma, lymphoma, fungi
  - Cavitation: TB, PCP, *Pseudomonas, Rhodococcus,* fungi, CMV
- CT: May aid in diagnosis if chest X-ray is normal
- Sputum: PCP staining; culture for AFB, fungus, bacteria
- Serology: *Histoplasma* or *Cryptococcus* antigen
- Blood cultures: For bacteria and fungus
- Serum LDH: ↑ in > 90% of PCP patients
- Bronchoscopy: Used if diagnosis is in doubt; good for PCP, TB, fungal, and viral cases

Treatment

- PCP: TMP-SMX × 2–3 weeks is the drug-of-choice; systemic steroids are indicated with moderate to severe disease (PaO$_2$ <70); lifelong prophylaxis in those with previous PCP or CD4 < 200 (TMP-SMX, dapsone, or pentamidine)
- Bacterial pneumonia: Normal empiric pneumonia coverage; consider *Pseudomonas* coverage if CD4 < 50
- Disseminated fungal infection: IV amphotericin B or itraconazole for *Aspergillus* and *Histoplasma;* fluconazole for *Cryptococcus;* prophylaxis with fluconazole/itraconazole
- Lymphocytic interstitial pneumonitis or nonspecific interstitial pneumonitis: Excellent response to systemic steroids

Prognosis/Clinical Course

- Prognosis depends on etiologic agent
- PCP usually responds to therapy and improves within a few days; high mortality if it progresses or respiratory failure ensues (80% mortality)
- Bacterial infections: Higher rate of complications and death (more empyema, effusions, and so on) than in the general population; more likely to relapse
- Lymphoid interstitial pneumonitis and nonspecific interstitial pneumonitis have a benign course
- Pulmonary HTN: High one-year mortality, mostly due to cor pulmonale

39. Interstitial Lung Diseases

Etiology

- A group of disorders characterized by inflammation and fibrosis of the alveolar walls, perialveolar tissue, and other interstitial structures
- More than 200 causes; four major categories include:
  - Pneumoconioses
  - Hypersensitivity pneumonitis (HP)
  - Drug-induced: antibiotics (PCN), amiodarone, β-blockers, radiation, chemotherapeutics, antirheumatics (i.e., gold)
  - Idiopathic disorders: ARDS, sarcoid, aspiration, SLE, RA, BOOP, IPF, interstitial pneumonia, alveolar proteinosis, amyloidosis, lymphoma

Differential Dx

- CHF
- COPD
- Asthma
- Infection
- Pneumoconioses
- HP
- Pulmonary embolism
- Pulmonary HTN
- Vasculitis

Epidemiology

- Age of presentation and incidence depend on causative factors and exposures
- Pneumoconioses present later in life after a long history of exposure
- Hypersensitivity pneumonitis presents after an exposure
- Smoking may increase the risk of pulmonary effects

Signs/Symptoms

- All types have similar symptoms, restrictive pulmonary function, and interstitial X-ray features
- Progressive dyspnea
- Tachypnea
- Nonproductive cough
- Fine crackles
- Fatigue
- Weight loss
- Findings of associated disease (drug toxicity, connective tissue disorder)
- Digital clubbing
- Signs of pulmonary hypertension and cor pulmonale (increased P_2 heart sound, RV heave, tricuspid regurgitation, peripheral edema, JVD)

Diagnosis

- History: Elicit occupational exposures, familial diseases, drug exposures, and time course of symptoms
- CXR: Reticular or reticulonodular infiltrates; ↓ lung volumes; honeycombing occurs late; may be normal
- CT: More sensitive than CXR
- PFTs: Restrictive pattern (↓ TLC, ↓ FRC, ↓ RV); ↓ diffusion
- ABG: May show hypoxemia and respiratory alkalosis
- Bronchoscopy with lavage and biopsy: Identifies the type of inflammatory cells, specific antigens/infectious etiologies; biopsy may give a definitive diagnosis, especially for infection, cancer, sarcoid
- Thoracoscopic or open lung biopsy is the gold standard—indicated if bronchoscopic biopsy is not diagnostic
- Labs: Serum precipitating antibodies (HP), angiotensin-converting enzyme (sarcoid), ANA, RF, U/A

Treatment

- Remove the offending agent and/or stop smoking
- Oxygen if patient is hypoxemic ($PaO_2 < 55$ mm Hg)
- Treatment is etiology-dependent
  - Finding a cause is important because treatment and prognosis vary markedly
  - Systemic steroids are often beneficial, especially in patients with idiopathic interstitial pneumonias, connective tissue disease, pneumoconioses, sarcoid, and HP
  - Other immunosuppressive agents may be indicated, such as methotrexate or cyclosporine
- Lung transplant should be considered in appropriate, end-stage patients
- See related entries for disease-specific therapies

Prognosis/Clinical Course

- Symptom onset
  - Acute: HP, infection, eosinophilic pneumonia, acute interstitial pneumonia
  - Subacute: Drug-induced, RA, SLE
  - Insidious onset: IPF, pneumoconioses, drug-induced, sarcoidosis
- Chronic, progressive course unless offending agent is removed or appropriately treated
- Prognosis varies widely depending on etiology and time of diagnosis; IPF is the most serious (2–5 year median survival)
- Lung cancer risk is increased by silicosis, asbestosis, and IPF

40. Hypersensitivity Pneumonitis

Etiology

- Immune-mediated inflammation of parenchyma, alveolar walls, and terminal airways; chronic fibrosis occurs with repeated exposure
- Also known as extrinsic allergic alveolitis, it is a non-atopic, non-asthmatic, immune-related reaction to an inhaled allergen
  - Animal/plant proteins: *Actinomycetes* (hay, grain, ventilation systems); *Aspergillus* (hay, grain); wood dust; cheese workers; mammals, birds
  - Low-molecular-weight chemicals (Toluene, isocyanates)
  - Drugs (gold, amiodarone, NSAIDs, nitrofurantoin)

Epidemiology

- Exposure is usually occupational or hobby-related
- Farmer's lung, bird fancier's lung, and chemical worker's lung are the most common causes in the United States
- Smoking actually decreases the risk
- Prevalence is unknown due to underreporting of occupational illness
- Farmer's lung: Occurs in 1% of those exposed; 2 million exposed/year

Differential Dx

- Asthma
- Occupational asthma
- CHF
- Pneumonia
- COPD
- Other interstitial lung diseases: Drug-induced, pneumoconioses, IPF, sarcoidosis, collagen vascular disease
- Eosinophilic pneumonia
- Industrial bronchitis: Chronic bronchitis from occupational exposure
- Irritant gas inhalation

Signs/Symptoms

- Acute
  - Fever/chills
  - Nonproductive cough
  - Dry bibasilar crackles
  - Absence of wheezing
  - Dyspnea
- Subacute
  - Progressive cough and dyspnea
  - Fatigue
  - Weight loss
  - Diffuse dry crackles
  - May progress to cyanosis
- Chronic: All subacute symptoms plus
  - Presence of pulmonary fibrosis
  - Hypoxemia and clubbing
  - Increased dyspnea
  - Eventual respiratory failure

Diagnosis

- No pathognomonic tests exist; diagnosis is based on history, exam, CXR, antigen exposure, and presence of antibody to the specific antigen
- Serology for serum precipitins: Antibodies against suspected protein antigens
- CXR: Normal or may have patchy nodular infiltrates; with repeated exposure, a diffuse reticulonodular pattern $+/-$ fibrosis develops; apical sparing; honeycombing
- CT: Global lung involvement with patchy reticulonodular infiltrates; no adenopathy
- PFTs: Restrictive with $\downarrow$ diffusion capacity; may develop mixed restrictive-obstructive pattern in chronic disease
- ABG: Hypoxemia
- Bronchoalveolar lavage: Lymphocytic predominance
- Lung biopsy: Supports the diagnosis but is not diagnostic
- May have $\uparrow$ ESR, CRP, immunoglobulins, RF, eosinophilia

Treatment

- As in other allergic diseases, the key to treatment is to avoid antigen exposure
- Bronchodilators
  - β-agonists (albuterol) $+/-$
  - Anticholinergics (ipratropium)
- Acute and subacute disease
  - Systemic corticosteroids will decrease inflammation and provide symptomatic relief
  - No need for long-term therapy if antigen exposure is avoided
- Chronic disease
  - 1–2 month trial of systemic corticosteroids may reduce symptoms
  - Steroids will not reverse fibrosis
  - Steroids have no effect on long-term prognosis

Prognosis/Clinical Course

- Course may be acute, subacute, or chronic
- The temporal relationship to an occupational exposure may provide a clue to the diagnosis
- The patient may have asthma-like symptoms if IgE is triggered
- Acute form develops 6–12 hours after exposure and resolves over 24–72 hours
- Chronic form results from prolonged, recurrent, low-level exposure; eventually leads to fibrosis if antigen exposure is not avoided
- Fibrotic changes, once they occur, are irreversible

41. Pneumoconioses

Etiology

- Inflammation and fibrosis caused by occupational inhalation and accumulation of mineral dust in the lungs—results in progressive lung fibrosis; may continue even in the absence of continued exposure
- Nonallergic in nature (distinguishes it from hypersensitivity pneumonitis)
- Causes: Coal, asbestos (construction/shipyard workers, mechanics), silica (mining, sand blasting), talc, cement, metals (beryllium, antimony, tin, silver, bronze)

Epidemiology

- Numbers vary—at least 2.4 million workers have been exposed (it is estimated that more than 100,000 have clinical disease)
- Asbestos: Greatly increases the risk of bronchogenic carcinoma and malignant mesothelioma, especially in smokers
- Coal worker's pneumoconiosis (CWP) is seen in 12% of all coal miners and 50% of anthracite miners

Differential Dx

- Occupational asthma
- Asthma
- Chronic infection
- Pulmonary edema/CHF
- Pulmonary hemorrhage
- Pulmonary vasculitis
- COPD/chronic bronchitis
- Interstitial lung diseases
  - Hypersensitivity pneumonitis
  - Interstitial pulmonary fibrosis
  - BOOP
  - Sarcoidosis
  - Collagen vascular
  - Drugs
  - Radiation

Signs/Symptoms

- Initially few symptoms
- Gradual, progressive dyspnea
- Nonproductive cough
- Hypoxemia
- Tachypnea
- Crackles
- Clubbing
- Decreased lung volumes
- At end stage, right-sided heart failure and cor pulmonale ensue

Diagnosis

- History of exposure is most important aspect of workup
- PFTs: Restrictive pattern with diminished lung volumes with or without decreased diffusing capacity
- Imaging (CXR and CT scan)
  - Asbestosis: CXR has irregular linear opacities, pleural thickening, and calcified pleural plaques; may have pleural effusions, ground glass infiltrate, honeycombing; CT shows subpleural curvilinear lines parallel to the pleural surface; fibrosis eventually seen
  - Coal: CXR shows a diffuse reticulonodular pattern, with very small nodules; calcification is uncommon; may eventually develop large areas of fibrosis
  - Silicosis: CXR shows perihilar lymph node calcifications with many small nodules in upper lobes
  - Large, confluent densities appear late in each disease
- Lung biopsy often reveals the etiologic agent (rarely done)

Treatment

- No specific therapies are available
- Avoid further exposure
- Stop smoking
- Test for coexisting TB in silicosis
- O_2 if oxygenation is impaired

Prognosis/Clinical Course

- May eventually develop progressive massive fibrosis—large, confluent densities and significant pulmonary impairment
- Asbestos: Pleural plaques seen with exposure; a fraction of patients develop clinical disease (asbestosis—a diffuse interstitial fibrosis); most require 10 years of exposure to develop clinical impairment; strong association with lung cancer and cancerous mesotheliomas; death from respiratory failure or lung cancer
- Silicosis: Associated with TB superinfection
- Coal: Collections of coal dust (macules) form in upper lobes; 10% result in massive fibrosis
- Beryllium: Produces either pneumonitis or a chronic interstitial pneumonia with sarcoid-like granulomas throughout the body

42. Idiopathic Pulmonary Fibrosis

Etiology

- IPF is an interstitial lung disease in which an unknown stimulus produces repeated episodes of patchy acute lung injury of the bronchioles and alveoli; interstitial pulmonary inflammation (alveolitis) at these sites results in progressive fibrosis
- IPF is a form of idiopathic interstitial pneumonia (others include BOOP, nonspecific interstitial pneumonitis, desquamative interstitial pneumonia [DIP], and acute interstitial pneumonia [AIP]); these disorders are distinguished by histologic criteria and have differing histories and responses to treatment

Epidemiology

- Mean age at diagnosis—60
- Strong association with smoking
- 10–20 cases/100,000 population
- Increased incidence in the US

Differential Dx

- Interstitial pneumonia (DIP, AIP, nonspecific interstitial pneumonitis)
- BOOP
- CHF
- Asthma or COPD
- Pneumoconioses
- Hypersensitivity pneumonitis
- Collagen vascular disease
- Sarcoidosis
- Recurrent aspiration
- Radiation pneumonitis
- Drug toxicity
- Eosinophilic pneumonia
- Alveolar proteinosis
- Infection

Signs/Symptoms

- Progressive exertional dyspnea
- Chronic, dry cough
- Tachypnea
- Bibasilar fine crackles
- Constitutional symptoms (fatigue, weight loss) occasionally
- Digital clubbing
- Signs of pulmonary hypertension and cor pulmonale in late stages (increased P_2 heart sound, RV heave, tricuspid regurgitation, peripheral edema, JVD)

Diagnosis

- Often diagnosed clinically, but invasive diagnostics (such as biopsy) should be used if diagnosis in doubt; three criteria required for diagnosis:
  - Exclusion of other interstitial lung diseases
  - Symptoms, CXR, and PFTs consistent with IPF
  - Biopsy or CT scan consistent with IPF
- CXR: Reticulonodular pattern with interstitial (linear) markings in lung bases; ↓ lung volume; honeycombing (ring-shaped opacities representing dilation of airspaces)
- PFTs: Restrictive pattern (↓ TLC, VC, FRC, RV) with diffusion abnormalities
- CT: Patchy linear opacities, honeycombing, and subpleural cyst formation (especially at bases)
- ABG: Hypoxemia, respiratory alkalosis
- Bronchoscopy: Diagnoses IPF in a few cases; useful in establishing an alternative diagnosis
- Thoracoscopic lung biopsy: Required in unclear cases

Treatment

- Stop smoking
- Vaccinate against pneumococcus and influenza
- Supplemental O_2 as needed
- Systemic corticosteroids for immunosuppression
  - Trial course—continue only if there is a clinical response (only 20% respond)
  - May add azathioprine or cyclophosphamide
  - In true IPF, no definitive evidence of improved symptoms or survival from immunosuppressives
  - Immunosuppressives may be effective in other types of idiopathic interstitial pneumonia
- Lung transplant is the only curative treatment—recommended early in appropriate patients
- Gamma-interferon is under investigation

Prognosis/Clinical Course

- Most patients have a chronic, progressive course with rare remissions
- Median survival is less than 5 years
- Stable or improving course within the first year carries a good prognosis
- Occasional acute exacerbations with decompensation
- Increased incidence of pulmonary embolism
- Increased incidence of secondary bronchogenic carcinoma
- No proven response to therapy in true IPF
- Death is often caused by progressive pulmonary fibrosis leading to cor pulmonale and respiratory failure; may also be due to cardiac disease, PE, cancer, or opportunistic infection

43. BOOP

Etiology

- Bronchiolitis obliterans organizing pneumonia (BOOP): Inflammation and fibrosis obstruct bronchioles and alveolar air spaces with plugs of granulation tissue (organizing pneumonia); usually idiopathic
- Secondary BOOP may be caused by infection, transplants, ARDS, toxic inhalation, collagen vascular disease, or aspiration
- Bronchiolitis obliterans (BO): Bronchiolar inflammation and obstruction, without extension of lesions into the alveoli; usually occurs in organ transplants and collagen vascular disease

Differential Dx

- ARDS
- COPD
- TB
- Drug reactions
- Infections
- Chronic eosinophilic pneumonia
- Interstitial lung disease
- Other idiopathic pneumonias (IPF, AIP)
- Pulmonary alveolar proteinosis
- Pulmonary infarction
- Lung neoplasm

Epidemiology

- Idiopathic BOOP: 7 cases per 100,000 hospital admissions
- Occurs in 5th and 6th decades
- Males = females
- No relation to tobacco use

Signs/Symptoms

- Flu-like prodrome
- Insidious onset of nonproductive cough
- Dyspnea
- Fever
- Malaise
- Weight loss
- Fatigue
- Inspiratory crackles
- Wheezing is rare

Diagnosis

- BOOP is a pathologic diagnosis
  - CXR: Bilateral patchy alveolar infiltrates
  - CT: Patchy consolidation and ground glass infiltrates, bronchial wall thickening and dilation
  - PFTs: Restrictive, decreased diffusing capacity, hypoxia
  - Lung biopsy: Recommended for definitive diagnosis, shows granulation tissue within small airways and inflammation of alveoli—differentiates BOOP from other interstitial lung disease
  - ABG: Hypoxemia
  - Elevated ESR
- Important distinctions
  - 1° versus 2° BOOP
  - BOOP versus BO (mixed restrictive/obstructive picture; immune-mediated; seen in transplant patients)

Treatment

- BOOP responds well to oral systemic steroids—full recovery is achieved in 2/3 of patients
- Antibiotics have no role in treatment
- Cyclophosphamide is rarely needed but may be used if steroids fail or for recurrent relapses

Prognosis/Clinical Course

- Excellent prognosis
- Rarely improves without therapy
- 2/3 of patients recover completely with steroid treatment—lung function and CXR normalize
- Response to therapy may occur as soon as 2 weeks or may take months
- Relapses are common; most patients will also respond to systemic steroids
- Nonresponse or repeated relapses may necessitate chronic steroids or the addition of other immunosuppressives

44. Sarcoidosis

Etiology

- A systemic, granulomatous, inflammatory disorder of unknown cause
- Pathogenesis is unclear; possibly involves an exaggerated immune response to an unknown antigen, resulting in T cell activation; involved organs demonstrate accumulated T cells, multinucleated giant cells, and histiocytes in characteristic noncaseating granulomas
- No specific etiologic agent has been identified
- 90% have lung involvement; 50% have extrathoracic involvement
- 2/3 of cases resolve spontaneously; 1/3 have chronic waxing and waning of symptoms

Epidemiology

- Females > males
- Affects all ages; greatest incidence is among ages 20–40
- Affects many more blacks than whites (most characteristic patient is an African American woman in her thirties)
- Prevalence: 10–40 cases per 100,000 in the US
- Smoking is *not* a risk factor

Differential Dx

- HIV
- Tuberculosis
- Lung neoplasm
- Lymphoma
- Berylliosis
- Brucellosis
- Histoplasmosis or other fungal infections
- Interstitial lung disease
- Pulmonary fibrosis
- Hypersensitivity pneumonitis
- Pneumoconioses
- BOOP
- Wegener's granulomatosis
- Lung vasculitis

Signs/Symptoms

- Pulmonary: Cough, dyspnea, chest discomfort, hemoptysis
- Constitutional: Fever, weight loss, fatigue
- Polyarthritis
- Ocular: Uveitis in 25%
- Neurologic: Cranial nerve palsies, aseptic meningitis, pituitary disease, neuropathy, seizures
- Cardiac: Cardiomyopathy, arrythmias
- Dermatologic: Erythema nodosum
- Lymphadenopathy, splenomegaly (20%)
- Hepatic: ↑ LFTs and cholestasis in 20%
- Hypercalcemia
- Acute syndromes: Löfgren's (erythema nodosum, adenopathy, tenosynovitis) and Heerfordt's (fever, uveitis, parotiditis)

Diagnosis

- A diagnosis of exclusion; based on clinical and X-ray findings plus biopsy showing noncaseating granulomas
- Biopsy: Noncaseating granulomas; may obtain sample from lymph node, transbronchial biopsy, skin lesion, salivary glands, or liver
- CXR: Often shows bilateral hilar lymphadenopathy
- CT: Nonspecific alveolitis; diffuse nodular adenopathy
- PFTs: Normal or restrictive pattern with poor diffusion
- ABG: Increased A-a gradient, hypoxemia
- Serum ACE is elevated in 50–80% of cases (nonspecific)
- Elevated serum and urine calcium
- EKG: Conduction abnormalities
- Gallium scanning is nonspecific
- Slit lamp exam annually for ocular disease
- Monitor disease progression: Follow symptoms and PFTs

Treatment

- Observation is recommended for 6 months if limited to the lungs as the majority of cases will spontaneously remit; difficult to determine which patients require treatment, which is important because of severe side effects of steroids
- Treat if severe or progressive pulmonary disease or if extrapulmonary involvement (cardiac, ocular, CNS, constitutional, hypercalcemia, arthritis, liver, renal)
- Systemic steroids are the mainstay of treatment
- 25–40% relapse—treat relapses with steroids
- Methotrexate in refractory cases or to decrease steroid requirements—other immunosuppressives have limited benefits
- Bronchodilators as needed for symptomatic relief
- Ophthalmic steroids for ocular sarcoid
- NSAIDs for erythema nodosum
- Lung transplant in severe disease; however, may recur

Prognosis/Clinical Course

- Staged based on radiographic pulmonary involvement; stages are not a continuum—patients present at any stage and do not progress through stages
- Stage 0 (8% of patients): Systemic disease but normal CXR and PFTs
- Stage 1 (50%): Bilateral hilar adenopathy; normal lung parenchyma; PFTs are normal or near-normal; 75% remit within 2 years
- Stage 2 (29%): Hilar adenopathy, diffuse interstitial disease, nodules; restrictive PFTs with ↓ diffusing capacity; 50% remit
- Stage 3 (12%): Diffuse interstitial disease without adenopathy; 20% remit
- Stage 4: *Irreversible* lung fibrosis, ↓ lung volume, bronchiectasis, restrictive PFTs with ↓ diffusing capacity

45. Hemoptysis

Etiology

- Expectoration of blood (gross blood or streaking) from below the vocal cords
- Must rule out GI bleeding (hematemesis) or nasopharyngeal bleeding (hemoptysis is bright red and alkaline, whereas GI tract blood is generally acidic and may be black)
- Massive hemoptysis is variously defined as more than 100–500 cc of blood in a 24-hour period
- Up to 30% of cases will have no identifiable etiology of the hemoptysis

Epidemiology

- Bronchitis (50% of cases) and cancer (10–20% of cases) are the most common causes
- Vasculitis, TB, and alveolar hemorrhage in 10% of cases; these must be strongly considered in the differential diagnosis because early treatment is critical

Differential Dx

- Infection: Bronchitis, TB, pneumonia, lung abscess, aspergillus
- Lung cancer
- PE
- Vasculitis
- SLE/RA
- Goodpasture's syndrome
- Wegener's granulomatosis
- Bronchial adenoma
- Pulmonary edema
- Bronchiectasis
- Foreign body or trauma
- Instrumentation: Lung biopsy, bronchoscopy
- Drugs: Anticoagulants, ASA, cocaine, solvents, amiodarone
- Cardiac: MS, CHF
- Coagulopathy

Signs/Symptoms

- Either streaking or frank blood
- Crackles
- Associated symptoms related to the underlying cause—for example:
  - Sputum in bronchitis
  - Fever in pneumonia
  - Weight loss in cancer
  - Coexistent renal disease in Goodpasture's syndrome or Wegener's granulomatosis
  - Pleuritic chest pain in PE
  - Purulent sputum in bronchiectasis

Diagnosis

- Initial workup includes a CXR, acid-fast bacilli stain, sputum cytology and Gram stain/culture, PT/PTT, CBC, SMA-7, and U/A
- Consider respiratory isolation until TB is ruled out
- CXR is 1st test; may localize bleeding or identify disease
- CT scan may show an area of focal bleeding
- Minor hemoptysis
  - Bronchoscopy is required if any risk factor for cancer is present: Age > 40, abnormal X-ray, hemoptysis > 1 wk, tobacco use (>40 pack-years), anemia, weight loss
- Major hemoptysis
  - Active bleeding requires immediate bronchoscopy
  - Stable patients may undergo chest CT if there is no active bleeding; bronchoscopy should follow
  - Bronchoscopy is both diagnostic and therapeutic; may localize bleeding and allows for balloon tamponade or vasoconstrictor injection at the site of bleeding

Treatment

- Minor hemoptysis: treat the specific etiology
- Massive hemoptysis
  - Maintain airway, O_2, stabilize hemodynamics
  - Bed rest, cough suppression
  - Place bleeding side in dependent position to prevent blood from draining into opposite lung
  - Intubation as needed for airway control; a double-lumen tube will preserve oxygenation if bleeding is persistent—may separate bleeding lung from nonbleeding lung
  - Control of bleeding:
    1. Bronchoscopic balloon tamponade
    2. Arteriography and embolization in persistent bleeding
    3. Emergent thoracic surgery if embolization is not available and bleeding persists

Prognosis/Clinical Course

- Mortality depends on the cause, volume of bleeding, rate of bleeding, and presence of underlying pulmonary disease
- Massive hemoptysis is a medical emergency (up to 30% mortality); death usually results from asphyxiation due to alveolar flooding and hypoxemia; less commonly, death results from exsanguination
- Less than 5% of cases of hemoptysis are massive
- Significant risk of recurrent hemorrhage in massive hemoptysis, even if bleeding has ceased

46. Goodpasture's Syndrome

Etiology

- A progressive autoimmune disease of the lungs and kidneys caused by autoantibodies to Type IV collagen of the basement membrane of glomeruli and alveoli
- The resulting inflammatory response causes lung capillary leakage, alveolar hemorrhage, and rapidly proliferative glomerulonephritis
- Patients may have renal disease only, in which case the process is called anti-GBM disease; Goodpasture's syndrome, by definition, has both pulmonary and renal involvement

Differential Dx

- Wegener's granulomatosis
- Microscopic polyangiitis
- HSP
- Churg-Strauss syndrome
- Behcet's syndrome
- Drugs (penicillamine, cocaine)
- Connective tissue disease: SLE, RA, sarcoidosis
- CHF
- Coagulopathy
- Mitral stenosis
- Necrotizing lung infection

Epidemiology

- Onset is usually in the 30s and 40s, but may affect patients of all ages
- Elderly patients are more likely to present with nephritis alone
- Recent respiratory infection may precipitate the disease in susceptible patients
- Very unusual to develop pulmonary symptoms in nonsmokers
- Strong association with HLA-DR2

Signs/Symptoms

- Hemoptysis
- Dyspnea
- Cough
- Tachypnea
- Cyanosis
- Inspiratory crackles
- Severe distress requiring mechanical ventilation
- The absence of hemoptysis does not exclude the presence of pulmonary hemorrhage
- Renal failure
- Hematuria

Diagnosis

- Serum: Positive for anti-GBM antibody
- Chest X-ray: Bilateral alveolar infiltrates
- ABG: Hypoxemia
- Biopsy: Both kidney and lung show linear IgG deposits in basement membrane on immunofluorescence
- Urine: Hematuria, red cell casts, non-nephrotic proteinuria
- CBC: Iron deficiency anemia due to chronic subclinical hemorrhage
- Chemistries: Elevated creatinine, progressive renal failure
- pANCA: Positive in low titers in 20% of cases
- Obtain serologies to exclude connective tissue diseases (ANA, rheumatoid factor)

Treatment

- The goal of treatment is to remove the circulating antibodies as quickly as possible
- Therapy consists of two parts
  - Plasmapheresis
  - Immunosuppressives—systemic steroids (prednisone) plus cyclophosphamide
- Continue prednisone for 1–2 years; change cyclophosphamide to azathioprine after 4 months and continue for 2 years
- Patients presenting with end-stage renal disease are extremely unlikely to recover renal function
  - Treat only with immunosuppressives as needed to control pulmonary hemorrhage
  - Without treatment, antibodies will naturally fall to undetectable levels in 1 year—renal transplant is then an option

Prognosis/Clinical Course

- Symptoms can develop subacutely over days to weeks or rapidly over hours
- Untreated disease leads to rapid respiratory and renal failure and death—generally good response to steroids and plasmapheresis
- Pulmonary hemorrhage ranges from subclinical to massive and life-threatening
- RPGN may lead to permanent renal failure
- Patients with end-stage renal disease at presentation (serum creatinine >6) rarely recover renal function—require dialysis and transplant
- Therapy usually removes the autoantibodies
  - Near-complete resolution of lung dysfn
  - Variable return of renal function
- Relapses are unusual

47. Pulmonary Hypertension

Etiology

- Defined as mean pulm artery pressure >25 mm Hg (normal 12–16) at rest
- Pulmonary vasculature normally has low resistance to blood flow b/c large x-sectional area—increased resistance to flow results from elevated vasomotor tone, endothelial fibrosis and hypertrophy, or thrombosis
- 1° Pulm HTN: No identifiable cause but pts may have increased systemic vasoconstrictors (endothelin-1, thromboxane A_2) and ↓ vasodilators
- 2° Pulm HTN due to ↑ pulm blood flow, ↑ vascular resistance (PE, hypoxic VC), ↓ pulmonary vein drainage (CHF), ↓ x-section area (interstitial disease)

Differential Dx

- Collagen vascular disease
- Left-to-right shunt
- HIV
- Appetite suppressants, cocaine, amphetamines
- Left-sided heart disease
- Chronic PE
- Sickle cell disease
- Sarcoidosis
- COPD
- Interstitial disease
- Sleep apnea
- High altitude

Epidemiology

- Secondary pulmonary hypertension is much more common and underdiagnosed
- Cor pulmonale (right ventricle dysfunction due to pulmonary hypertension) is the third most common cardiac disorder in patients > age 50.

Signs/Symptoms

- Dyspnea
- Fatigue
- Chest pain (secondary to RV ischemia)
- Syncope/near-syncope
- Lung exam is nonspecific
- Hemoptysis (due to rupture of distended pulmonary vessels)
- Hoarseness (recurrent laryngeal nerve compression by enlarged pulmonary artery)
- Raynaud's phenomenon in 10%
- Cor pulmonale (↑ jugular pulse, RV heave, right-sided S_3 and S_4, eventual LV failure due to RV impingement into the LV, tricuspid and pulmonic regurgitation, hepatomegaly, peripheral edema)

Diagnosis

- CXR: ↑ hilum indicates congestion of pulmonary arteries; disease-specific findings
- EKG: RAD, RVH, RV strain (anterior lead ST depression and T wave inversion)
- Echo: Best test to estimate pulmonary artery pressures; may show RV enlargement, decreased LV size, bulging of the septum, or tricuspid regurgitation
- PFTs: Normal to mildly restrictive; may have decreased diffusing capacity or show underlying disease
- V/Q scan: Rules out chronic emboli as a cause
- ABG: Hypoxemia due to V/Q mismatch; hypocapnia
- Cardiac catheterization: Rules out cardiac causes and shunt; directly measures pulmonary artery pressures
- CT scan: Rules out interstitial disease
- Send serologies for connective tissue diseases and HIV
- Lung biopsy is not needed for diagnosis

Treatment

- Treat underlying disorders
- If NYHA class II–IV heart failure, perform invasive testing of response to vasodilators
- If vasodilator response, calcium-channel blockers may improve symptoms
- Epoprostenol (prostacyclin): An endogenous vasodilator and platelet inhibitor; decreases mortality and symptoms in severe primary disease
- Warfarin: Used in severe cases (mean PAP > 45) to prevent in situ intrapulmonary thrombosis
- Digoxin and diuretics for symptomatic relief
- Lung transplant: Used in primary disease if epoprostenol fails; has a 45% 5-year survival
- Surgery: Atrial septostomy may be palliative as a bridge to transplant

Prognosis/Clinical Course

- Primary pulmonary hypertension
  - Usually diagnosed late due to absence of early symptoms
  - Mean survival is 3 years from diagnosis
  - Survival predicted by RA pressure, cardiac output, 6-minute walk test, and vasodilator responsiveness at diagnosis
  - Later in the disease, cardiac output is decreased and the response to vasodilators diminishes
  - Death from RV failure or arrhythmia
- Secondary pulmonary hypertension
  - The underlying disease is usually far advanced when pulmonary symptoms begin

48. Pulmonary Embolism

Etiology

- PE occurs when clots from the deep venous system break off and travel to the lungs; most emboli arise from ileofemoral thrombosis but may also come from pelvic or upper extremity veins
- Risk factors: Lower-extremity venous disease, cancer, CHF, recent surgery, immobilization, family history, pregnancy, paraplegia, previous DVT, OCP use, trauma, hypercoagulable state (Factor V Leiden, antiphospholipid antibody, protein C and S deficiency)
- Nonthrombotic PE: Fat embolus, air embolus, or amniotic fluid embolism

Epidemiology

- 600,000 cases per year
- >50% of PEs are undiagnosed
- 90% arise from a lower extremity DVT
- 50% of patients presenting with DVT have concomitant PE
- Virchow's triad indicates increased risk of thrombus formation: endothelial trauma, stasis, and hypercoagulability

Differential Dx

- Acute coronary syndrome
- CHF
- Aortic dissection
- Pericarditis/tamponade
- Pneumonia
- Bronchitis
- COPD exacerbation
- Asthma
- Pleural effusion
- Pneumothorax
- Musculoskeletal chest pain
- Anxiety attack
- Rib fracture
- GERD

Signs/Symptoms

- Dyspnea
- Pleuritic chest pain
- Tachypnea
- Tachycardia
- Anxiety
- Cough
- Crackles
- Fever
- Hemoptysis (due to pulmonary infarction) in 30% of cases
- Signs of lower extremity DVT: Edema, calf tenderness, Homan's sign (pain with plantar flexion)
- Syncope in 10% of cases
- Massive PE: Hypotension; signs of acute right heart dysfunction

Diagnosis

- Pulmonary angiogram is the gold standard but is used only if the diagnosis is uncertain
- V/Q scan: Normal scan rules out PE; high-probability scan is diagnostic for PE; most patients require further testing
- Helical (spiral) CT: Sensitive for proximal PE; sensitivity and specificity for distal PE are under investigation
- D-Dimer: Nonspecific; only the ELISA test has sufficient sensitivity to rule out PE and only in low-risk patients
- Lower extremity venous duplex scanning: Diagnostic if positive but negative study does not rule out PE; used if the initial test (V/Q or CT) is nondiagnostic
- ABG: Increased A-a gradient (may be normal)
- CXR: Usually normal; may show pleural effusion, wedge-shaped infiltrate (Hampton's hump)
- EKG: Normal or tachycardia; may see $S_1Q_3T_3$ or RV strain
- Consider hypercoagulable workup

Treatment

- Oxygen
- Anticoagulation: Start IV heparin or LMWH (less bleeding, improved mortality) when PE is clinically suspected; coumadin therapy should follow for at least 6 months and may need to be continued indefinitely depending on the underlying cause
- IVC filter: Consider if anticoagulants are contraindicated, recurrent embolism despite anticoagulation, massive PE, or poor baseline cardiac or pulmonary status
- If hypotensive: IV fluids, norepinephrine, consider thrombolysis or surgery
- Systemic thrombolytic therapy: Consider in massive PE with hypotension or refractory hypoxemia
- Pulmonary embolectomy: Occasionally used in refractory hypotension and proven pulmonary emboli

Prognosis/Clinical Course

- Clinical symptoms depend on the size of the embolus, which may range from insignificant to a large saddle embolus that obstructs the main pulmonary arteries; an embolus causing >50% occlusion of the pulmonary vascular bed can cause acute RV failure
- The patient's initial cardiopulmonary status is an important predictor of outcome
- Further clinical course and likelihood of recurrence depend on the cause of the clot
- Chronic, recurrent emboli may result in pulmonary hypertension with eventual respiratory failure and cor pulmonale
- Hypercoagulable states increase the risk of recurrence
- Mortality is 2–10% in treated patients and 20–30% in untreated patients

49. Pneumothorax

Etiology

- The introduction of air into the pleural space, causing lung collapse
- Results in pain, V/Q mismatch, and hypoxemia
- Traumatic pneumothorax (PTX): Due to penetrating or nonpenetrating chest trauma, including iatrogenic causes (i.e., central line placement)
- Spontaneous PTX: 1° PTX is due to rupture of apical pleural blebs in patients with no underlying lung disease (70%); 2° PTX occurs in patients with lung disease (especially COPD, asthma, CF, infection, cancer, interstitial disease)

Differential Dx

- COPD exacerbation
- Asthma
- Pulmonary embolus
- Myocardial infarction
- Pericarditis
- Aortic dissection
- Musculoskeletal chest pain
- Pleuritis

Epidemiology

- 20,000 spontaneous pneumothoraxes per year in the US—usually smokers (20:1)
- 1° spontaneous: Tall, thin, smoker, age 20–40; male >> female
- 2° spontaneous: Age > 40; male > female; COPD increases risk 10×
- Only 10–20% occur with exertion, most occur at rest

Signs/Symptoms

- Acute, pleuritic chest pain
- Dyspnea or tachypnea
- Tachycardia
- ↓ Breath sounds on the affected side
- Hyperresonance to percussion
- Decreased tactile fremitus
- May have respiratory distress or respiratory failure especially in those with underlying lung disease
- Symptoms worsen with increased size of the PTX
- Tension PTX: Hypotension, absent breath sounds, distended neck veins, tracheal deviation to opposite side, diaphoresis, cyanosis, cardiovascular collapse

Diagnosis

- CXR
  - Presence of a thin, radiolucent pleural line
  - Absence of vascular lung markings peripheral to the radiolucent line
  - Tracheal deviation to opposite side of pneumothorax
- CT: Very sensitive but used only if CXR inconclusive
- EKG: Tachycardia, nonspecific ST changes, T wave inversion
- ABG: Hypoxemia due to V/Q mismatch; normal pCO_2
- Tension PTX: Occurs when air enters the pleural space during each breath but the air is unable to be released during expiration; results in a significant increase in intrapleural pressure and impedes venous return to the heart, producing cardiovascular collapse; a clinical diagnosis

Treatment

- 100% oxygen increases the rate of air reabsorption—2% of intrapleural air is normally reabsorbed daily but O_2 therapy increases reabsorption fourfold
- Acute treatment options: Observation, catheter aspiration, chest tube if large PTX or catheter fails
- Recurrence prevention: Pleurodesis, VATS, thoracotomy
- 2° spontaneous PTX: Dangerous due to decreased pulmonary reserve in patients with lung disease; use chest tube +/− pleurodesis
- Traumatic PTX: Most need a chest tube unless very small
- Tension PTX: Requires *immediate* needle decompression and chest tube—do not wait for CXR

Prognosis/Clinical Course

- 1° PTX is rarely fatal
- Patients with 2° PTX may do poorly (up to 15% mortality)
- Recurrence is a common problem—30–50% of spontaneous pneumothoraxes will recur
- Smoking cessation decreases recurrence rates
- Consider recurrence prevention therapy after the first or second pneumothorax
- Consider surgery in persistent air leaks >48 hours
- Traumatic pneumothorax may develop slowly over hours to days after trauma; initial CXR may not show the pneumothorax

50. Pleural Effusion

Etiology

- Excess fluid in the pleural space; due to either excess pleural fluid formation or decreased fluid removal by the pleural lymphatics
  - Transudate: Systemic factors influence the amount of pleural fluid—the pleural surface itself is normal
  - Exudate: Arises from pleural inflammation causing increased capillary permeability or from obstruction of the lymphatic drainage
- Empyema: A grossly purulent pleural effusion
- Hemothorax: Blood in the pleural space

Epidemiology

- Greater prevalence later in life as concurrent illnesses increase
- 1.3 million cases per year in the US
  - 500,000 from CHF
  - 300,000 from bacteria
  - 200,000 from malignancy
  - 150,000 from pulmonary embolism
  - 100,000 from viral disease
  - 50,000 from cirrhosis

Signs/Symptoms

- Dyspnea
- Nonproductive cough
- Pleuritic chest pain
- Hypoxemia
- Fever
- Decreased breath sounds
- Egophony
- Dullness to percussion
- Decreased tactile fremitus
- Pleural rub
- Signs/symptoms of the primary disease process

Differential Dx

- Transudative
  - CHF
  - Nephrosis/↓ albumin
  - PE
  - Hypothyroidism
  - SVC syndrome
  - Sarcoidosis
  - Peritoneal dialysis
  - Cirrhosis
  - Trauma
- Exudative
  - Pneumonia   – PE
  - Malignancy   – TB
  - Asbestos   – Pericarditis
  - Hemothorax   – CABG
  - Chylothorax   – SLE
  - Pancreatitis   – RA
  - Uremia
  - Drugs (amiodarone)

Diagnosis

- Etiology can often be inferred from comorbid illnesses
- CXR: Blunted costophrenic angle (requires >175 cc of fluid)
- CT: More sensitive for effusion; rules out other processes
- Pleural fluid analysis: LDH, albumin, protein, cell count, Gram stain/Cx, glucose, cytology, amylase, pH, TB markers
- First, determine transudate versus exudate—exudate if
  - Pleural fluid to serum protein ratio >0.5 *or*
  - Pleural fluid to serum LDH ratio >0.6 *or*
  - Pleural fluid LDH > 2/3 serum normal limit
- Types of exudate
  - ↑ WBC: Parapneumonic, rheumatologic, pancreatitis, malignancy
  - ↓ Glucose: Malignancy, infection, rheumatologic
  - ↑ Amylase: Esophageal rupture, pancreatitis, malignancy
  - ↑ Triglycerides (>110): Chylothorax
- Pleural biopsy if cause of exudate is questionable

Treatment

- Transudative: Treat underlying cause (drain with thoracentesis if symptomatic)
- Malignant effusion: Repeated thoracentesis for symptomatic relief; pleurodesis (obliterate pleural space with talc or doxycycline) or indwelling catheter for frequent recurrences
- Parapneumonic: Treat with systemic antibiotics, thoracentesis if large (>10 mm)
  - Chest tube prevents the development of loculated, complex effusions that may require surgical intervention—insert chest tube if gross pus, positive Gram stain/culture, loculations, glucose <40, or pH < 7.0–7.2
  - May need ultrasound or CT-guided drainage
- Hemothorax: Insert chest tube; thoracotomy if necessary

Prognosis/Clinical Course

- All effusions that are unexplained or do not respond as expected to treatment should be tapped and analyzed
- Symptoms depend on the effusion size and comorbid conditions
- Course of the effusion depends on the cause
  - Malignant effusions rapidly recur and often require a sclerosing agent
  - Infectious effusions resolve with treatment of the infection
  - Transudative effusions resolve as the primary disease is corrected
  - Complicated parapneumonic effusions require urgent chest tube drainage; delay may allow formation of loculations, which require intrapleural streptokinase or surgery

51. Solitary Pulmonary Nodule

Etiology

- A circumscribed nodular density within the lung parenchyma <3 cm in size (anything bigger is considered a mass)
- Often an incidental finding on X-ray or CT; may represent a benign, asymptomatic process or a life-threatening malignancy
- Optimal workup is aimed at identifying dangerous lesions while avoiding invasive testing in cases of benign lesions
- The likelihood of malignancy is based on patient and lesion characteristics; the presence of even 1 risk factor for cancer prompts aggressive workup

Epidemiology

- Risk factors for malignancy: > 2 cm diameter, age > 40, spiculated margins, noncalcified, smoker
- 25% of lung cancers present as a single nodule

Differential Dx

- Infectious granuloma: TB, histoplasmosis, coccidiodomycosis
- Primary lung cancer
- Metastatic cancer
- Bronchial adenoma
- Lymphoma
- Benign lung neoplasms (e.g., hamartoma, lipoma)
- AVM
- Intrapulmonary lymph node
- Wegener's disease
- Rheumatoid nodule
- Amyloidosis
- Pulmonary infarction
- Mucoid impaction
- Bronchogenic cyst

Signs/Symptoms

- Asymptomatic by definition

Diagnosis

- Chest X-ray: <5 cm lesion; compare with old X-ray
- CT: More sensitive for determining nodule characteristics, size, other lesions, and calcification pattern
- Bronchoscopy (rarely diagnostic) or percutaneous fine-needle biopsy may be tried to obtain tissue
- Thoracotomy if biopsy findings are nonspecific or normal (biopsy is not sensitive enough to rule out cancer)
- Sputum cytology may give a diagnosis in central lesions
- One possible workup algorhythm
  - Review prior CXR—if no change in 2 years, no further workup
  - In patients with no risk factors for malignancy—repeat CT/CXR in 4–6 weeks, at 3 months, then every 6 months for 2 years; proceed to resection if any growth occurs
  - Intermediate/high-risk patients: Get a baseline CT, then perform either needle biopsy or thoracotomy for resection

Treatment

- If no risk factors, observation is acceptable; if lesion changes at all, aggressive workup is indicated
- Resection is indicated if the lesion is noncalcified, fast growing, of suspicious morphology, or of large size *and* the patient is a good operative candidate; otherwise, biopsy via fine needle or bronchoscopy should be attempted first (does not rule out cancer)
- Resection techniques:
  - Video-assisted thoracoscopic surgery (VATS): As good as open thoracotomy for peripheral lesions; can be extended to open thoracotomy if necessary
  - Minithoracotomy
  - Thoracotomy: Allows mediastinal and lymph node exploration
- There should be a low threshold for surgery—a malignant lesion could be deadly and surgery is relatively benign in good surgical candidates

Prognosis/Clinical Course

- Malignant versus benign nodules
- Age
  - Under 35   2% are malignant
  - 35–45   15–30% are malignant
  - Over 45   >50% are malignant
- Size
  - <1 cm   90% are benign
  - >2 cm   70% are malignant
- Stability: Lesions that are present and unchanged retrospectively for 2 years are likely benign
- Calcification: Calcifications are more likely benign—especially if they are dense, have a central core, or have a punctate or laminated pattern
- 50% 5-year survival for cancers presenting as single nodule (versus 10% survival in all cancers)

52. Lung Cancer

Etiology

- Cancer of the respiratory epithelium (bronchogenic)
- Non-small cell (NSCLC): 70% of lung cancers; spreads to regional nodes
  - Squamous (30%): Central mass in upper lobes; slow growth; late mets
  - Adenocarcinoma (30%): Peripheral mass; slow growth; early mets
  - Large cell (10%): Peripheral mass; early mets; often cavitary
- Small cell/"oat cell" (SCLC): Rapid growth and very early, widespread mets (70% have metastases at time of diagnosis); 100% in smokers
- Rare types: Carcinoid, bronchoalveolar (nonsmokers)

Epidemiology

- Leading cause of cancer death in US—2nd most common US cancer
- 170,000 new cases and 150,000 deaths yearly; 15% 5-year survival
- Peak incidence 50 to 70 years of age; increasing among women
- 90% due to smoking; other RFs include radon, asbestos, pollutants
- Number of pack-years is the major determinant of risk
- Mutations found in *ras* and *myc* oncogenes and *p53* suppressor genes

Differential Dx

- Tuberculosis
- Fungal infection
- Pneumonia
- Lymphoma
- Metastatic cancer
- AVM
- Sarcoidosis
- Bronchogenic cyst
- Pneumoconiosis
- Intrapulmonary lymph node
- Pulmonary-renal syndromes (Wegener's granulomatosis)
- Connective tissue disease
- Benign tumors: Lipoma, hamartoma, fibroma, leiomyoma, hemangioma

Signs/Symptoms

- Pulmonary: Cough, hemoptysis, dyspnea, CP, postobstructive pneumonia, effusion
- SVC syndrome: Face and neck edema due to obstruction of superior vena cava
- Pancoast syndrome: Apical tumor may lead to Horner's syndrome or shoulder/arm pain due to brachial plexus or chest wall involvement
- Horner's syn: Miosis, ptosis, anhidrosis
- Hoarseness: Due to compression of recurrent laryngeal nerve
- Extrathoracic: Anorexia, cachexia, fever, adenopathy, night sweats, sxs of mets
- Paraneoplastic syndrome (15%): SIADH, Eaton-Lambert syndrome, Trousseau's syndrome (hypercoagulability), ectopic PTH → hypercalcemia

Diagnosis

- Must establish a tissue diagnosis, extent of disease, and overall health to guide management
- CXR: Mass +/− hilar adenopathy; may see pleural effusion, atelectasis, mediastinal adenopathy
  - Squamous, large cell, and small cell have a central mass
  - Adeno has a peripheral mass
- Chest CT: Better visualizes the mass; may see lymphatic, mediastinal, or pleural spread
- Tissue diagnosis is essential
  - Sputum cytology *or*
  - Biopsy via bronchoscopy, thoracoscopy, or CT-guided fine needle aspiration
- Staging workup to determine extent of disease: CBC, chemistries, electrolytes, LFTs, amylase/lipase, CXR, CT of thorax/abdomen/pelvis, PFTs, mediastinoscopy

Treatment

- Non-small cell
  - Stages I, II, and IIIA are resectable; adjuvant chemotherapy increases survival
  - Stage IIIB: Resection with preoperative chemotherapy is investigational
  - Stage IV: No curative options; radiation treatment is palliative; survival of 6 months
  - Radiation to symptomatic sites for palliation
- Small cell: Responds very well to chemotherapy
  - Limited disease: Radiation plus 4 cycles of chemotherapy; complete response in 50%; median survival 18 months; 20% 5-year survival
  - Extensive disease: Chemotherapy; radiation does not improve survival; complete response in 25%; median survival 9 months; no 5-year survivors
- Smoking cessation decreases risk of recurrence

Prognosis/Clinical Course

- NSCLC uses TNM staging (Tumor size, Nodes involved, Metastases)
  - Stage I: Tumor with 0 nodes
  - Stage II: Tumor with positive local nodes
  - Stage III: Mediastinal nodes or extensive local tumor invasion
  - Stage IV: Distant metastases
- SCLC does not use TNM system; defined as limited (confined to hemithorax) or extensive
- SCLC: Most respond to chemotherapy (80–90%), but > 90% relapse, so 5-year survival is just 5%
- NSCLC: Resection is effective in Stage I or II disease but few present at this early stage

53. Sleep Apnea

Etiology

- A syndrome of repetitive periods of apnea (>10 seconds without air flow) or hypopnea during sleep; results in frequent desaturations and poor sleep
- May be obstructive, central, or mixed (symptoms are similar regardless)
  - Obstructive: Upper airway soft tissue impedes airflow; risk factors include narrow airways (obesity, macroglossia), alcohol, sedatives, URI, hypothyroidism, smoking, vocal cord dysfunction, bulbar disease
  - Central: Absent signal to breathe from the CNS respiratory center; apnea without respiratory effort

Epidemiology

- Occurs in 2% of women and 4% of men
- Most common in obese, middle-aged men
- Obstructive apnea is more common than central apnea
- Central apnea is more common at the extremes of age
- There is often snoring for many years prior to the onset of actual obstruction; thus snoring alone is not a reason for a full workup

Differential Dx

- Primary alveolar hypoventilation ("Ondine's curse"): Inadequate ventilation with hypoxemia despite normal airflow, normal pulmonary system, and normal respiratory drive
- Obesity-Hypoventilation syndrome (Pickwickian syndrome): Hypoventilation due to blunted central drive plus increased mechanical load of the chest wall
- Narcolepsy: Daytime sleep attacks
- Hypothyroidism

Signs/Symptoms

- Loud snoring
- Restlessness/thrashing movements during sleep
- Breath cessations or respiratory efforts without airflow while sleeping
- Obesity
- Narrowed oropharynx
- Daytime somnolence
- Daytime fatigue
- Morning sluggishness
- Cognitive impairment
- Headaches
- Impotence
- Personality changes
- The patient's bed partner often provides the most useful information

Diagnosis

- Overnight polysomnography: Monitors physiology during sleep; includes EEG, EMG, EKG, oximetry, airflow, and respiratory effort; shows apneic episodes and provides a definitive diagnosis; a positive test has 10 apneic episodes per hour lasting at least 10 seconds each
- Overnight pulse oximetry is a useful screening test
  - Highly sensitive in patients with a high pretest probability of the disease—sufficient to establish the diagnosis in these patients
  - If it is normal, it excludes the diagnosis in patients with a low pretest probability of the disease
- CBC: Erythrocytosis
- Check thyroid function to rule out hypothyroidism
- Workup is appropriate when nocturnal problems contribute to secondary daytime behavioral and physiologic problems

Treatment

- For patients with increased upper airway muscle tone: Avoid alcohol and sedatives
- For patients with increased upper airway lumen size
  - Weight reduction may be curative
  - Oral dental prosthesis
  - Nasal septoplasty if deviated septum is present
  - Uvulopalatopharyngoplasty in selected patients
- Nighttime nasal continuous positive airway pressure (CPAP) is the treatment of choice; 100% effective but may be very uncomfortable
- Bypass occlusion: Consider tracheostomy in patients with life-threatening complications and failure of other therapies
- Oxygen may worsen apnea; prescribe carefully
- Medications: Tricyclics may decrease episodes, improving daytime symptoms

Prognosis/Clinical Course

- Repetitive hypoxia may ultimately result in cardiac arrhythmias, pulmonary HTN, cor pulmonale
- Other sequelae
  - CHF (especially in patients with preexisting left ventricular dysfunction)
  - Systemic hypertension
  - Erythrocytosis
- The disease usually follows a chronic, progressive course due to continued weight gain
- There is a good response to therapy, especially nasal CPAP
- Sleep apnea *does* cause increased mortality
- Sleep apnea syndrome is one of the leading causes of daytime sleepiness

Gastrointestinal Disease

SHAHWALI AREZO, MD
SCOTT KAHAN, MD

54. Achalasia

Etiology

- Motor dysfunction of esophageal smooth muscle peristalsis and abnormal lower esophageal sphincter tone (increased LES resting pressure and failure of LES to relax in response to swallowing)
- Pathogenesis poorly understood—may be due to degenerative changes in neural innervation: Fibrosis of Auerbach's plexus? Degeneration of vagus fibers and dorsal nucleus?
- Results in obstruction and proximal dilatation
- Differentiate from diffuse esophageal spasm

Epidemiology

- 1 case per 100,000 population in US
- Usually manifests between 20 and 40 years of age but may be seen in infancy and early childhood
- Similar incidence between genders

Differential Dx

- Cancer
- Diffuse esophageal spasm
- Chagas' disease (*Trypanosoma cruzi* infection resulting in achalasia, megacolon, and cardiomyopathy)
- Scleroderma
- Primary muscle dysfunction (i.e., myotonic dystrophy)
- Metabolic disorders that affect muscle function (hypothyroidism)

Signs/Symptoms

- Progressive dysphagia is the most common symptom
- Vomiting of food a few hours after eating
- Weight loss
- Nocturnal cough due to aspiration
- Chest pain/heartburn
- Aspiration and respiratory symptoms secondary to esophageal retention, regurgitation, and overflow into trachea
- Recurrent aspiration pneumonia
- Bloating
- Inability to burp

Diagnosis

- X-ray: Dilated esophagus; "bird beak" narrowing at LES, widening of mediastinum, air–fluid level in the esophagus
- Manometry
  - LES: High resting pressure and incomplete relaxation with swallowing
  - Body: Failure of peristalsis; low-amplitude, abnormal, or absent contractions after swallowing
- Endoscopy with biopsy
  - Rule out neoplasia
  - Hypertrophied muscular wall (from trying to force contents through a "tight" LES)
  - Myenteric ganglia usually absent from the body of the esophagus

Treatment

- Treatment is palliative
- Medical treatment may give short-term improvement of symptoms: Nitrates and calcium-channel blockers
- Forced dilatation of LES with pneumatic bag is generally the treatment of choice
  - Effective in 70–90% of patients
  - 2–5% risk of perforation; 0.2% mortality rate
- Botulinum toxin injection: Effective in more than half of patients but needs to be repeated every few months; used only if dilatation cannot be performed
- Surgical option is laparoscopic or open esophagomyotomy (Heller procedure)
  - Direct section of LES
  - Often better results than pneumatic dilatation
  - 3–4% complication rate; high risk for postoperative reflux

Prognosis/Clinical Course

- Achalasia is the most treatable disorder of esophageal motility
- Surgery is the option for patients who fail pneumatic dilatation or who fear the risk of perforation with pneumatic dilatation
- 10× increased risk of esophageal carcinoma

55. Mallory-Weiss Syndrome

Etiology

- Longitudinal, partial-thickness tear at the level of the gastroesophageal junction; tear may extend into the stomach
- Follows a prolonged period of severe vomiting and retching; may result from inadequate LES relaxation during vomiting
- Bleeding is generally mild and self-limited, although massive bleeding is possible
- Distinguish from Boerhaave's syndrome (a complete-thickness tear and rupture of the esophagus) and bleeding esophageal varices—all common in alcoholics

Differential Dx

- Esophageal/gastric varices
- Boerhaave's syndrome
- Angiodysplasia
- Duodenal or gastric ulcer
- Diffuse erosive gastritis
- Gastric carcinoma
- Esophageal carcinoma
- Dieulafoy's lesion

Epidemiology

- Often seen in alcoholics
- Esophageal lacerations account for 5–10% of upper GI bleeds—most common causes of upper GI bleeding are peptic ulcers, gastritis, and mucosal tears

Signs/Symptoms

- Hematemesis following vomiting, straining, or coughing
- If significant bleeding occurs, it is more likely due to bleeding varices than Mallory-Weiss syndrome
- Bright red blood is characteristic (hematemesis of dark blood is common with esophageal varices)
- Chest pain is possible, but uncommon—chest pain is more characteristic of Boerhaave's syndrome
- Also seen in Boerhaave's syndrome is crepitus due to pneumomediastinum

Diagnosis

- Classic history: Post-retching hematemesis
- Endoscopy is diagnostic
  - Identify tear
  - Rule out other causes of bleeding
  - May also be therapeutic (see below)

Treatment

- In any GI bleeding, must monitor vitals and volume status and maintain hemodynamic stability
- Generally self-limiting—supportive treatment is often sufficient
  - Volume replacement
  - Gastric lavage
  - Vasoconstrictive medication
- Bleeding can be controlled during endoscopy by direct electrocoagulation or epinephrine injection
- Exploratory laparotomy if bleeding persists or rupture occurs
- Immediate surgery in the case of rupture (Boerhaave's syndrome)

Prognosis/Clinical Course

- Bleeding resolves spontaneously in most cases with minimal residual effects; however, infection may lead to ulcer formation
- Surgery is required in <5% of cases
- Recurrence after surgical correction is rare

56. Hiatal Hernia

Etiology

- Characterized by widening of the esophageal hiatus of the diaphragm
  - Sliding (95% of cases): An upward dislocation of the gastroe-sophageal junction; most likely due to age-related stretching of the esophageal hiatus
  - Paraesophageal: "Rolling" of the gastric fundus upward along a normally positioned cardia; most likely due to congenital hiatal defect
- In elderly, may be due to gradual stretching of esophageal hiatus
- Affected infants and children may have a congenital diaphragmatic defect

Differential Dx

- Myocardial ischemia or infarction
- GERD
- Peptic ulcer disease
- Chemical or infectious esophagitis
- Esophageal spasm
- Achalasia
- Aortic dissection
- Costochondritis

Epidemiology

- Hiatal hernias are very common, although few are symptomatic
- Affect 1–20% of adults; increasing incidence with age
- Median age for sliding hernia: 45; paraesophageal: 60
- Sliding hiatal hernia is much more common than paraesophageal hernia
- Paraesophageal hernia is more common in females (4:1)

Signs/Symptoms

- Sliding hernia
  - Displaced LES causes symptoms of GERD (heartburn and regurgitation)
  - Dysphagia, secondary to mucosal edema, stricture, or pinching of the herniated stomach by the diaphragm
- Paraesophageal hernia
  - Dysphagia and postprandial fullness due to compression of the esophagus
  - Heartburn and regurgitation
  - Hematemesis, due to ulceration of the herniated fundus
  - Dyspnea, if the stomach becomes intrathoracic
  - Aspiration and recurrent pneumonia

Diagnosis

- Upright radiograph shows an air–fluid level behind the cardiac shadow—usually caused by paraesophageal hernia
- Upper GI barium study diagnoses paraesophageal hernia in virtually every case, but is not as sensitive in detecting sliding hernia because this type can spontaneously become reduced
- Esophagoscopy is very useful in diagnosing and classifying either type of hernia

Treatment

- Treatment of sliding hernias is aimed at alleviating the symptoms of the associated reflux disease (see the Gastroesophageal Reflux Disease entry)
- Treatment of paraesophageal hernias is always operative, regardless of the severity of symptoms—because of the relatively common, life-threatening complications, patients should undergo elective repair upon diagnosis
- In infants, large intrathoracic hernia sacs may compress the lungs and mandate emergency surgical repair

Prognosis/Clinical Course

- Severe complications include strangulation, obstruction, bleeding, and perforation—these are surgical emergencies
- Sliding hernias rarely require treatment; <10% of patients have reflux symptoms; prognosis and complications depend on the duration of symptoms
- Complications are common with paraesophageal hernias—they occur in 25% of patients and include infarction, bleeding, and perforation
- Emergency repair of paraesophageal hernia carries a nearly 20% operative mortality; this rate is reduced to less than 1% with elective surgical repair

57. Esophagitis

Etiology

- Inflammation of the esophageal mucosa following injury or infection
- Most common cause is gastric reflux (see the Gastroesophageal Reflux Disease entry)
- Infectious esophagitis especially due to *Candida,* HSV, CMV, and HIV
- Chemical esophagitis occurs following ingestion (accidental or intentional) of mucosal irritants (alcohol, cigarette smoke, very hot fluids), alkali (e.g., bleach) or acids, or medications

Epidemiology

- Found in 5% of adults in US and Western countries
- Common worldwide, with the highest prevalence in China and Iran
- Higher incidence in pregnancy (due to reflux) and scleroderma patients
- Infectious cases most commonly seen in debilitated or immuno-compromised patients

Differential Dx

- Myocardial ischemia or infarction
- GERD
- Peptic ulcer disease
- Reflux from hiatal hernia
- Esophageal spasm
- Aortic dissection
- Gastritis
- Achalasia
- Costochondritis
- Scleroderma

Signs/Symptoms

- Heartburn (specific for reflux)
- Dysphagia, generally for solids
- Odynophagia
- Anemia if associated with chronic bleeding
- Severity of symptoms is not necessarily correlated with the degree of histopathology

Diagnosis

- History of caustic ingestion, immunosuppression (in cases of infectious esophagitis), or relationship of symptoms to food intake and supine position (reflux)
- Diagnostic studies for reflux—see GERD entry
- Endoscopy is diagnostic
- Findings in all cases of esophagitis include severe acute inflammation, superficial ulceration, and fibrosis
- Specific findings in nonreflux esophagitis
    - *Candida:* Grayish pseudomembranes with hyphae
    - HSV: Small, isolated ulcers and multinucleated cells with nuclear inclusions
    - CMV: Large ulcerations, nuclear inclusions in capillary endothelium
    - HIV: Diffuse inflammatory esophagitis
    - Chemical: Ranges from erythema to diffuse necrosis
- Cytology may be used to identify infectious causes

Treatment

- Reflux esophagitis: Treat underlying GERD
- Infectious esophagitis: Use appropriate antimicrobials
    - *Candida:* Nystatin, ketoconazole, fluconazole, or low-dose amphotericin B
    - HSV: Vidarabine or acyclovir
    - CMV: Gancyclovir
    - AIDS esophagitis requires steroid therapy
- Esophageal burns: Broad-spectrum antibiotics and steroids

Prognosis/Clinical Course

- Although most cases of esophagitis are well controlled with medical management, complications are seen with severe or prolonged cases (due to chronic inflammation and ulceration)
    - Stricture formation from chronic inflammation and fibrosis
    - Esophageal ulceration with possible hemorrhage
    - Reflux laryngitis
    - Pulmonary aspiration
    - Barrett's esophagus

58. Esophageal Varices

Etiology

- Due to prolonged or severe cases of portal HTN—collateral porto-caval bypass channels become engorged and portal blood flow is diverted through the coronary veins of the stomach into the esophageal venous plexus and eventually into the caval circulation
- Dilated esophageal varices may rupture and bleed due to increased tension in the veins or after erosions from gastritis
- Esophageal varices themselves do not cause problems, but potential rupture and hemorrhage represent a life-threatening complication

Differential Dx

- Duodenal/gastric ulcer
- Diffuse erosive gastritis
- Gastric varices
- Angiodysplasia
- Mallory-Weiss tear
- Boerhaave's syndrome
- Gastric carcinoma
- Esophagitis
- Esophageal carcinoma
- Dieulafoy's lesion

Epidemiology

- Found in up to 90% of cirrhotic patients
- Most commonly seen in alcoholics with cirrhosis
- Hepatic schistosomiasis (although rare in the US) is the second most common cause of esophageal varices worldwide
- Accounts for 10% of upper GI bleeds—most common causes of upper GI bleeding are peptic ulcers, gastritis, and mucosal tears

Signs/Symptoms

- Rupture of varices results in painless but massive hematemesis of dark brown blood
- "Coffee-ground" emesis or melena are less likely
- Signs of volume depletion, such as pallor, tachycardia, and orthostasis
- Physical signs associated with liver cirrhosis, including hepatomegaly, splenomegaly, ascites, jaundice, palmar erythema, clubbing of fingers, spider angiomata, parotid enlargement, Terry's nails, and bitemporal wasting

Diagnosis

- Endoscopy is diagnostic—should be performed immediately after patient is stabilized
- Even in patients with known varices (i.e., those with cirrhosis), endoscopy will show a nonvariceal source of bleeding in half of all cases

Treatment

- Initial management is aimed at stabilizing the patient
  - Fluid resuscitation and hemodynamic monitoring
  - Intubation of obtunded or inebriated patients
- Once stabilized, endoscopy to identify source
- IV octreotide is the first-line treatment
- Sclerotherapy and esophageal banding may be needed to control acute bleeds
- Vasopressin injection is effective (contraindicated in patients with angina) if octreotide is not available
- Somatostatin injection
- Balloon tamponade carries a risk of pulmonary aspiration—not used unless the patient continues to bleed after endoscopic treatment
- If bleeding continues, consider emergency procedures: transjugular intrahepatic portosystemic shunt (TIPS), porto-caval shunts, and/or hepatic transplantation

Prognosis/Clinical Course

- Variceal bleeding rarely subsides spontaneously; it nearly always requires intervention
- 40% mortality with the first episode of variceal bleeding if not adequately treated
- Recurrence occurs within one year in >50% of survivors; similar mortality rate for each episode
- Emergency surgery carries a 50% mortality rate
- Prophylactic sclerotherapy has been tried in patients with alcoholic cirrhosis but appears to offer no benefit
- In children, varices are usually due to extrahepatic obstruction

59. Esophageal Carcinoma

Etiology

- Squamous cell cancer results from dietary and environmental factors: Tobacco, alcohol, vitamins A and C deficiency, achalasia, sprue, tylosis, and diets high in pickled foods, nitrosamines, and mold
- Risk of adenocarcinoma increases 30- to 40-fold in cases of Barrett's esophagus (found in 10% of patients with chronic reflux disease)
- Barrett's esophagus: Columnar epithelium replaces the normal squamous epithelium of the distal esophagus following chronic inflammation from GERD; results in ulceration, bleeding, strictures, and esophageal carcinoma

Epidemiology

- Equal incidence of squamous and adenocarcinoma in US; worldwide, 90% of cases of esophageal carcinoma are squamous cell cancers
- Squamous cell carcinoma: Highest incidence in Iran and China
  – Adults over age 50; males > females; and blacks > whites
- Adenocarcinoma develops in Barrett's patients at a rate of 1% per year
  – Males > females; whites > blacks

Differential Dx

- Esophageal web or ring
- Benign stricture
- Dysphagia lusoria (obstruction from right subclavian artery passing behind esophagus)
- Achalasia
- Diffuse esophageal spasm
- Scleroderma
- GERD

Signs/Symptoms

- Insidious onset—most patients present at late stages of disease
- Progressive dysphagia for solids indicates the gradual development of an obstructive lesion
- Patients tend to alter their diets from solids to liquid foods
- Extreme weight loss
- Cough and hoarseness
- Choking and aspiration pneumonia after development of a tracheoesophageal fistula
- May also present with bleeding, chest pain, or vomiting

Diagnosis

- Barium study should be done if obstructive dysphagia is suspected
- Endoscopy with biopsy is diagnostic
- CT, bronchoscopy, and endoscopic ultrasound (most accurate) are used for staging and to evaluate for metastases and local invasion
- Squamous cell carcinoma tends to occur in the middle 1/3 of the esophagus; adenocarcinoma generally occurs in the lower 1/3

Treatment

- Surgical resection for lesions in the lower third of the esophagus restores patency but recurrence is common
- Radiation +/− chemotherapy is the most common treatment for squamous cell cancer; adenocarcinoma does not respond well to radiation
- Esophageal bougienage (dilation) or stenting can be used for palliative restoration of an adequate lumen (especially if extraesophageal metastases are present and cure is not possible)
- Laser therapy has been used to destroy intraluminal tumors

Prognosis/Clinical Course

- Although resectability has improved with advanced screening techniques, prognosis remains poor if the tumor is found in the late stages of disease
- Overall 5-year survival is just 5%
- About 1/4 of patients have resectable tumors; 10–20% do not survive surgery; 5-year survival rate with surgery is 5–20%
- Radiation therapy alone yields a 1-year survival rate of 20–40% and a 5-year survival rate of 5–15%
- Prognosis of adenocarcinoma has a 5-year survival rate of less than 30% but with early detection and resection of superficial lesions, survival increases to greater than 80%
- Squamous cell carcinoma has a much better prognosis than adenocarcinoma

60. Gastroesophageal Reflux Disease

Etiology

- Usually due to inappropriate LES relaxation: Recently ingested fat in duodenum, full stomach, smoking, chocolate, progesterone (pregnancy), supine position, caffeine, alcohol
- Often associated with hiatal hernia

Differential Dx

- Esophageal cancer
- Gastritis
- Gastric cancer
- Peptic ulcer disease
- Angina
- Costochondritis
- Pancreatitis
- Achalasia
- Diffuse esophageal spasm

Epidemiology

- Nearly half of patients have heartburn once per month
- Nearly 15% of patients take antacids twice per week

Signs/Symptoms

- Heartburn—GERD accounts for 3/4 of cases of noncardiac chest pain
- Persistent, nonproductive cough (second most common cause of chronic cough)
- Hoarseness due to reflux laryngitis, repetitive throat clearing, hiccups
- Full feeling in throat
- Exacerbation of asthma symptoms
- Dysphasia and odynophagia with advanced esophagitis and stricture
- Ear pain may be present
- Loss of dental enamel
- Night sweats

Diagnosis

- First test is a therapeutic trial unless "danger signs" are present
  - Lifestyle changes (see below)
  - Antacids
  - H_2 blockers or proton pump inhibitors
- Endoscopy (EGD) if above fails or "danger signs" are present
- Danger signs: Symptoms of nausea/vomiting, weight loss, blood in stool, true chest pain, dysphagia, anemia, long duration of symptoms, age >50
- Barium esophagram should be done before endoscopy if obstructive symptoms or dysphagia are present
- 24-hour intraesophageal pH monitor if normal EGD, but refractory symptoms that fail to respond to PPIs
- Bernstein test: Reproduction of symptoms with 0.1 M HCl infusion into esophagus—rarely used

Treatment

- Lifestyle changes
  - Sleep with head up
  - Lose weight
  - No food within 3 hours of bedtime
  - Dietary changes: Decrease or eliminate alcohol, caffeine, chocolate, fat, mint—especially in pm
  - No smoking
  - Eliminate medications that may decrease LES tone (i.e., Ca^{++}-channel blockers)
- Pharmacologic interventions
  - Antacids PRN
  - H_2 blockers or proton pump inhibitors
  - Prokinetics (metoclopramide)
- Severe GERD
  - PPIs indefinitely
  - Surgery: Laparoscopic or open fundoplication

Prognosis/Clinical Course

- Complications
  - Esophageal ulcers
  - Stricture: Treat with endoscopic dilation or bougienage
  - Bleeding (rarely serious)
  - Barrett's esophagus: Screen with endoscopy every other year

61. Gastritis

Etiology

- Acute erosive gastritis: Self-limited irritation of mucosa due to NSAIDs, alcohol, or severe physiologic stress (major surgery, burns, ventilator)
- Chronic gastritis
  - Type A: Less common; proximal stomach only; due to pernicious anemia, atrophic gastritis, achlorhydria, autoimmune disease, or radiation
  - Type B: Most common; distal stomach/antrum; due to *Helicobacter pylori* infection

Epidemiology

- Occurs in 50% of older patients
- Occurs in 30% of people infected with *H. pylori*

Differential Dx

- Peptic ulcer disease
- Gastric cancer
- Pancreatitis
- Cholecystitis
- GERD
- Gastroenteritis
- Esophageal cancer

Signs/Symptoms

- Burning epigastric pain
- Dyspepsia
- Nausea/vomiting
- Bleeding—hematemesis, shock
- Microcytic anemia in chronic gastritis

Diagnosis

- Endoscopy is diagnostic
- *H. pylori* testing
  - Gold standard is antral mucosa biopsy (rarely done)
  - Serologic test: ELISA-IgG
  - Urease breath test with radiolabeled urea
  - Cultures (specific but not sensitive)
- CBC: Anemia in chronic gastritis
- Secondary hypergastrinemia (gastrin >1000 pg/mL) due to decreased acid production in Type A chronic gastritis
- Schilling test if pernicious anemia is suspected

Treatment

- Manage hemodynamic instability in hemorrhaging patient
- Avoid offending agent
- H_2 blockers, antacids
- Sucralfate (binds to ulcer and forms protective barrier against acid)
- Many people are infected with *H. pylori* although few have symptoms—treat only if symptomatic
- Triple therapy
  - Omeprazole 20 mg, clarithromycin 500 mg, amoxicillin 1 g *or*
  - Bismuth, metronidazole, ampicillin/tetracycline
  - Never treat *H. pylori* infection with monotherapy
  - Treat for 10–14 days

Prognosis/Clinical Course

- Increased incidence of gastric ulcers and gastric cancer with chronic gastritis
- Acute gastritis generally heals within a few days

62. Peptic Ulcer Disease

Etiology

- Most common cause is *Helicobacter pylori* infection—causes 75% of duodenal ulcers
- Steroids and NSAIDs—1/4 of NSAID users develop ulcers (primarily gastric)
- Zollinger-Ellison syndrome—3–5% of duodenal ulcers
- Gastrinoma—causes increased acid production in stomach
- Crohn's disease of stomach/duodenum
- Smoking is not a cause but exacerbates ulcers and decreases healing
- Personality type and stress are questionable etiologic factors

Epidemiology

- Males = females

Differential Dx

- Gastritis
- Gastric cancer
- Angiodysplasia
- Esophageal or gastric varices
- Esophageal cancer
- GERD
- Pancreatitis
- Pancreatic cancer
- Cholecystitis
- Gastroenteritis
- Meckel's diverticulum

Signs/Symptoms

- Gnawing/burning epigastric or RUQ pain
- Gastric ulcers are exacerbated by eating
- Duodenal ulcers: Pain is decreased with meals but increased 2–3 hours after meal
- Signs and symptoms of anemia
- Bleeding will result in hematemesis and/or melena
- Perforated ulcer will result in onset of severe pain with rebound tenderness and guarding
- Many patients have no pain—they present only with bleeding

Diagnosis

- Make sure the patient is hemodynamically stable
  - If unstable—stabilize, then operate
  - If stable—give IV fluids, monitor urine output, and do EGD and *H. pylori* culture (NG tube is controversial)
- EGD is diagnostic; often therapeutic in many cases
- Upper GI series is cheaper than EGD but less sensitive and specific; also misses angiodysplasias
- EGD and UGI are contraindicated in suspected perforation—upright abdominal X-ray will show free air under diaphragm
- *H. pylori* testing:
  - Gold standard is antral mucosa biopsy (rarely done)
  - Serologic test: ELISA-IgG
  - Urease breath test with radiolabeled urea
  - Cultures: Specific but not sensitive
- Fasting serum gastrin test if Zollinger-Ellison is suspected

Treatment

- Eradicate *H. pylori* if present using triple therapy
  - Omeprazole 20 mg, clarithromycin 500 mg, amoxicillin 1 g *or*
  - Bismuth, metronidazole, ampicillin/tetracycline
  - Never treat *H. pylori* infection with monotherapy
  - Treat for 10–14 days
- Antacids, H$_2$ blockers, proton pump inhibitors
- Sucralfate: Mucosal protective agent; binds to ulcer and forms a protective barrier against acid
- Decrease or eliminate exacerbating factors: Smoking, NSAIDs (COX-2 inhibitors may be less ulcerogenic)
- Indications for surgery: Intractable bleeding, gastric outlet obstruction, perforation, Zollinger-Ellison syndrome
- Surgical interventions: Oversewing of ulcer, creation of an omental patch, vagotomy, or antrectomy

Prognosis/Clinical Course

- Bleeding ulcers may be treated with endoscopic electrocoagulation, angiography, or surgery
- Risk of malignant transformation with gastric ulcers

63. Gastric Cancer

Etiology

- 95% are adenocarcinoma
- Two primary tumor types
  - Intestinal: The more common type; grows as a cohesive tumor and eventually erodes through the stomach wall to nearby organs
  - Diffuse: A poorly differentiated cancer that has little cell cohesion; it grows outward along the submucosa of the stomach and widely envelopes the stomach without producing a discrete mass; also known as "linitis plastica"

Epidemiology

- Decreasing in frequency over the past century; previously the #1 cancer in US and worldwide—now #2 worldwide and #11 in US
- Males > females
- Median age of diagnosis: mid-60s
- Highest incidence in Japan, China, Chile, Ireland, and Russia
- Risk factors: *H. pylori,* PA, atrophic gastritis, postgastrectomy, tobacco, alcohol, low fruits/vegetables; salted, smoked, poorly preserved foods

Differential Dx

- Peptic ulcer disease
- Amyloidosis
- Gastritis
- Sarcoidosis
- Pancreatic cancer
- Menetrier's disease
- Gastric lymphoma
- Zollinger-Ellison syndrome
- Hyperplastic polyp
- Adenomatous polyp
- Inflammatory polyp
- Infections
- Metastasis
- Carcinoid
- Peutz-Jeghers syndrome

Signs/Symptoms

- Early tumors tend to be asymptomatic
- As tumor progresses:
  - Epigastric pain
  - Postprandial fullness
  - Anorexia
  - Nausea
  - Weight loss
  - Vomiting if pyloric tumor—due to gastric outlet obstruction
  - Dysphagia if tumor of cardia
  - Occult hemorrhage
  - Palpable abdominal mass with advanced tumors

Diagnosis

- Screening: No clear recommendation exists at this time
  - Double-contrast barium enema (barium + air) is least expensive option
  - Endoscopy (EGD) is most sensitive and specific; allows for biopsy and cytology
- Biopsy is diagnostic
- Abdominal CT: For staging and to look for metastases
- Endoscopic ultrasound: For staging and lymph node inspection
- Diagnostic laparoscopy and laparotomy: For precise staging to determine treatment and prognosis
- CBC may show iron-deficiency anemia
- Chest X-ray/CT: To look for lung metastases
- LFTs: To look for liver metastases

Treatment

- Surgery is the only potential cure
- Total gastrectomy for proximal lesions (body, cardia, fundus)
- Subtotal gastrectomy for distal lesions (pylorus, antrum)
- Lymphadenectomy is important; the extent of nodes resected depends on the type of cancer, its location, staging, and the preference of the surgeon
- Adjacent organs may be resected depending on the level of involvement and the preference of the surgeon (spleen, tail of pancreas, omentum, distal esophagus, duodenum)
- Palliative surgery is possible to relieve symptoms in incurable disease (such as gastric outlet obstruction, dysphagia, pain)
- Adjuvant chemotherapy and radiation are controversial; useful for palliation of symptoms rather than cure

Prognosis/Clinical Course

- Spread to nearby organs and metastases are rampant and often fatal
  - Direct spread to esophagus, duodenum, pancreas, spleen, peritoneum, colon, and liver
  - Mets to liver (most common), lung, brain, bone
  - Virchow node: Supraclavicular node mets
  - Krukenberg tumor: Ovarian node mets
  - Sister Mary Joseph node: Periumbilical metastases
  - Blumer's shelf: Mets to cul-de-sac
  - Malignant ascites
- Average 5-year survival in US <20%
- Average 5-year survival in Japan nearly 50% due to aggressive screening and surgical resection

64. Acute Pancreatitis

Etiology

- Due to inappropriate activation of pancreatic enzyme precursors within the pancreas, leading to autodigestion, necrosis, edema, and hemorrhage
- Most commonly caused by excessive alcohol intake or gallstones/biliary tract disease
- Other causes: Trauma, viral (mumps, Coxsackie, hepatitis), hypercalcemia, hypertriglyceridemia, drugs (sulfonamides, furosemide, thiazides, estrogens, tetracycline, valproate, chemotherapeutic agents, prednisone), ERCP

Differential Dx

- Biliary colic
- Acute cholecystitis
- Peptic ulcer disease
- Perforated viscus
- Small bowel obstruction
- Abdominal cancer
- Dissecting aneurysm
- Renal colic
- Diabetic ketoacidosis
- Ruptured ectopic pregnancy
- Mesenteric ischemia/thrombosis

Epidemiology

Signs/Symptoms

- Steady, severe epigastric pain beginning 1–4 hours after consumption of a large meal or alcohol
- Decreased pain when slumped forward
- Radiation to back
- Nausea and vomiting
- In severe disease: Epigastric guarding, rebound tenderness, fever, hypovolemia, tachycardia, shock, hypoxemia, ascites, abdominal distension from ileus, left-sided pleural effusion
- Grey-Turner's sign: Flank bruising
- Cullen's sign: Periumbilical bruising

Diagnosis

- Positive CT/MRI with increased serum amylase is diagnostic
  - Amylase >1000 suggests biliary disease (ultrasound may show gall bladder pathology)
  - Amylase of 200–500 suggests alcoholic pancreatitis
  - Patients with acute pancreatitis superimposed on chronic pancreatitis may not have increased amylase
  - Amylase-to-creatinine ratio may increase sensitivity
  - Other diseases may elevate amylase—obtain lipase also
- CT/MRI will also show possible biliary tract pathology
- Ultrasound is useful but may fail to visualize pancreatitis
- X–ray: Rule out perforation/obstruction; calcifications in the pancreas suggest chronic pancreatitis
- CBC: ↑ HCT due to hemoconcentration; leukocytosis
- Elevated LFTs, hyperbilirubinemia if biliary etiology
- ERCP if evidence of biliary obstruction

Treatment

- NPO for bowel rest until pain resides and abnormal tests are back to normal for 48 hours
- IV fluids: Replace fluids lost in vomiting, 3rd-spacing
- Antibiotics may reduce risk of abscess formation; also provide prophylaxis against cholangitis (may be caused by swollen pancreas head)
- Nasogastric suction to rest pancreas and control N/V
- Meperidine for pain (morphine is contraindicated—may cause spasm of sphincter of Oddi and worsen pancreatitis)
- ABG, CXR: Monitor for resp distress, pleural effusion
- Treat associated hypocalcemia and hyperglycemia
- Indications for surgery:
  - To confirm disease in severe pancreatitis that doesn't respond to treatment
  - To relieve biliary or pancreatic duct obstruction
  - Necrosis and sepsis

Prognosis/Clinical Course

- Mild cases resolve within a week
- Severe cases may result in shock, sepsis, DIC, ARDS, or ATN—mortality 20%–40%
- Ranson's criteria to assess severe cases: mortality <1% if fewer than 3 criteria; mortality nearly 100% if >6 criteria

On admission	Within 48 hours
– Age > 55	– HCT ↓ > 10%
– WBC > 16,000	– BUN increase > 5 mg/dL
– LDH > 350	– PaO_2 < 60
– SGOT > 250	– Calcium < 8
– Glucose > 200	– Base deficit > 4
	– Fluid deficit > 6

- Pancreatic abscess/pseudocyst may develop after 3–6 weeks
- Chronic pancreatitis may result

65. Chronic Pancreatitis

Etiology

- Alcohol abuse is the most common cause
- Other causes include cystic fibrosis, severe protein calorie malnutrition, hyperparathyroidism, obstruction of the pancreatic duct, idiopathic

Differential Dx

- Pancreatic cancer
- Other GI malignancy
- Biliary colic
- Cholecystitis
- Gastritis
- Peptic ulcer disease
- Abnormal aortic aneurysm
- Mesenteric ischemia

Epidemiology

Signs/Symptoms

- Similar signs and symptoms as acute pancreatitis
- Chronic epigastric pain—radiates to back
- Steatorrhea
- Signs of malnutrition
- Jaundice
- Glucose intolerance

Diagnosis

- Triad of pancreatic calcification, steatorrhea, and diabetes
- In contrast to acute pancreatitis, amylase and lipase are usually not elevated; leukocytosis is often absent
- ERCP and MRCP are the gold standards for diagnosis
- Ultrasound and CT are also effective for diagnosis
- Secretin stimulation test is very sensitive but not often available
- Abdominal X-ray: Calcifications of pancreas in 1/3 of cases
- Vitamin B_{12} deficiency
- Rule out pancreatic cancer: CEA, CA 19-9, biopsy if necessary

Treatment

- Avoid alcohol and fatty foods
- Replace enzymes and vitamins B_{12}, A, D, E, and K
- Antacids or H_2 blockers to decrease secretin release
- Narcotics are often used for pain
- Local resection or ductal dilation
- Insulin or hypoglycemic agent if diabetes is present

Prognosis/Clinical Course

- Poor prognosis if alcohol is the cause and patient continues to drink—50% mortality at 10 years
- Prognosis is good if the patient remains abstinent and replacement therapy is adequate
- Patients have an increased risk of pancreatic cancer

66. Pancreatic Cancer

Etiology

- Little is known about the causative agents—smoking is probably the greatest risk factor
- Mutations in *K-ras* are commonly found
- More than 90% of cases are ductal adenocarcinomas
- 70% occur in the head of the pancreas, 20% in the body, and 10% in the tail

Differential Dx

- Pancreatitis
- Other GI malignancies
- Lymphoma
- Cholecystitis
- Cholangitis
- Perforated ulcer
- Gastritis

Epidemiology

- 5th most common cancer-related mortality
- Males > females
- Blacks > whites
- Usually age >50

Signs/Symptoms

- Insidious onset of weight loss, fatigue, anorexia, gnawing abdominal/back pain
- Epigastric pain with radiation to back is probably the most common symptom but *painless jaundice* is a common presentation
- Pain may improve with bending forward
- Jaundice, dark urine, pale stools
- Courvoisier's sign: Palpable, enlarged gallbladder
- Diabetes mellitus
- Migratory thrombophlebitis

Diagnosis

- Elevation of tumor-associated antigens—CEA and CA 19-9
- Elevated alkaline phosphatase and bilirubin levels if bile duct is obstructed or if liver metastases are present
- CT should be first test
- Ultrasound, endoscopic ultrasound (most accurate for staging), and ERCP may enhance sensitivity of CT and are useful for staging
- Percutaneous or open biopsy

Treatment

- Resection is the only truly effective treatment
  - Total pancreatectomy
  - Distal pancreatectomy
  - Pancreaticoduodenectomy (Whipple's procedure)
- Chemotherapy may improve survival
- Radiation is only palliative
- Biliary division and stenting if biliary obstruction
- Pain medications as necessary
- Pancreatic enzyme replacement

Prognosis/Clinical Course

- Nearly all patients have advanced tumors and local or widespread metastases at the time of diagnosis
- Curative operations are only possible in 10–15% of patients—usually in tumors in the head of the pancreas that cause early jaundice but have not yet spread to lymph nodes
- Five-year survival is less than 2%
- Median survival in patients with unresectable cancer is less than 6 months
- Patients experience severe pain—medication should be used liberally for comfort

67. Hepatitis

Etiology

- Inflammation of the liver that may result in areas of necrosis
- Major causes: Hepatitis viruses, alcohol, drug-induced (isoniazid, methyldopa, ketoconazole, halothane, acetaminophen)
- Other causes: Autoimmune disease, EBV, CMV, yellow fever, herpes, rubella, adenovirus, TB, sarcoidosis, IBD, hemochromatosis, Wilson's disease
- May be acute or chronic (lasting >6 months)

Epidemiology

Differential Dx

- Cholecystitis
- Cholelithiasis
- Cholangitis
- Biliary cirrhosis
- Steatohepatitis
- Reye's disease
- Tetracycline toxicity
- Hemolytic anemia
- Dubin-Johnson syndrome
- Carcinoma (biliary, head of pancreas)
- Biliary atresia and strictures

Signs/Symptoms

- Disease varies from asx to debilitating
- Acute hepatitis
  - Jaundice, dark urine/light stools
  - Hepatomegaly
  - Fatigue, malaise, lethargy
  - RUQ pain
  - Nausea/vomiting
  - Fever, headache
- Liver failure
  - Edema due to hypoalbuminemia
  - Hepatic encephalopathy (confusion, stupor, coma, rigidity, asterixis)
  - Hyperestrogenemia—gynecomastia, palmar erythema, spider angiomata
  - GI bleeding (esophageal varices)

Diagnosis

- Elevated AST/ALT and bilirubin levels
- Normal or slightly elevated alkaline phosphatase level
- Viral markers (see specific hepatitis entries)
- Autoantibody measurements (see Autoimmune Hepatitis)
- Increased prothrombin time and coagulation disorders due to decreased production of Factors II, VII, IX, and X
- Hypoalbuminemia
- Hyperammonemia
- Biopsy may be diagnostic (although different causes of hepatitis often result in the same histologic appearance)
- Ultrasound: To look for dilated biliary ducts and gallstones
- Abdominal X-ray, CT/MRI, and ERCP may help rule out other diseases

Treatment

- See specific disease entries
- Removal of offending substances (e.g., alcohol, drug)
- End-stage liver failure is treated by liver transplant, if possible
- Vaccines and immune globulin are available for hepatitis A and B
- Treat acute complications as necessary
  - Lactulose (decreases protein absorption from gut) in encephalopathy due to hyperammonemia
  - Control GI bleeding
  - Correct coagulation and electrolyte disorders

Prognosis/Clinical Course

- Multi-organ failure, hepatorenal syndrome, hepatopulmonary syndrome, and hepatic encephalopathy are important complications
- Chronic hepatitis may result in cirrhosis and hepatocellular carcinoma
- Mortality is due to bleeding varices, sepsis, and hepatocellular carcinoma

68. Hepatitis A

Etiology

- Small, spherical RNA picornavirus with single-stranded RNA
- Only one serotype has been identified in humans
- Fecal-oral transmission
- Mean incubation period of 30 days
- Only acute disease—no carrier state; chronic manifestations of HAV infection are very rare

Differential Dx

- Other viral hepatitis
- Drug-induced hepatitis
- Shock liver
- Alcoholic hepatitis
- Autoimmune hepatitis
- Right-sided heart failure

Epidemiology

- About 30% of Americans have serologic evidence of past HAV infection (IgG)— more than 80% of elderly may be HAV IgG-positive
- Transmission is related to household size and sanitary conditions
- Mostly a disease of childhood
- Young children play a key role in community outbreaks

Signs/Symptoms

- Patients may be totally asymptomatic
- See Hepatitis for signs and symptoms
- Jaundice usually lasts to 2–4 months
- Nausea/vomiting may be present early in the course of the disease
- Anorexia, abdominal pain, diarrhea
- Arthralgias

Diagnosis

- Anti-HAV IgM indicates acute infection
- Anti-HAV IgG indicates past exposure—confers lifelong immunity
- Fecal HAV shedding occurs early in the course of the disease
- See the Hepatitis entry for tests used to rule out other causes of hepatitis

Treatment

- Self-limited
- Vaccine for prevention is important for high-risk groups
- Bed rest and symptomatic relief for nausea
- Liver transplantation for severe cases of fulminant hepatitis
- Members of the patient's household should be given immunoglobulin and HAV vaccine
- No role for steroids

Prognosis/Clinical Course

- Mortality <0.1% in young, healthy individuals
- Almost all cases resolve spontaneously
- Although acute HAV infection is associated with very little morbidity and mortality, it can be devastating in elderly patients with underlying chronic liver disease
- 1–5% of affected patients have fulminant hepatitis or aplastic anemia
- Vaccine has been approved for patients with other underlying chronic liver disease (i.e., hepatitis C)

69. Hepatitis B

Etiology

- Enveloped, spherical DNA virus—the only DNA virus that has been able to infect humans
- Multiplies using reverse transcriptase
- Transmission via blood and body fluids—sexual contact, IV drug use, hemodialysis and transfusions, tattoo and body piercing, unvaccinated health care workers
- Long incubation period—mean of 60–90 days

Differential Dx

- Other viral hepatitis
- Drug-induced hepatitis
- Shock liver
- Alcoholic hepatitis
- Autoimmune hepatitis
- Right-sided heart failure

Epidemiology

- 1.25 million carriers of HBV in US alone
- Development of persistent disease depends on age
  - <10% of adults with exposure to HBV will develop chronic disease
  - 50% of children will develop chronic disease
  - 90% of neonates will develop chronic disease

Signs/Symptoms

- May be asymptomatic in chronic carriers
- See Hepatitis for signs and symptoms of acute hepatitis and chronic liver failure
- Chronic viral hepatitis is defined as >6 months of histologic evidence of inflammation and necrosis—some chronic hepatitis patients are asymptomatic with only elevated liver enzymes; others exhibit the full spectrum of hepatitis symptoms

Diagnosis

- In acute infection:
  - HBsAg positive
  - HBV DNA positive
  - HBeAg indicates active replication and high infectivity—becomes elevated before onset of symptoms
  - Presence of Anti-HBe indicates decreased infectivity
  - Anti-HBc IgM—becomes elevated with onset of symptoms; absent in chronic disease
  - Anti-HBs IgG and anti-HBc IgG form when acute disease is over; they persist indefinitely
- In asymptomatic chronic carriers:
  - HBsAg positive
  - HBeAg negative; HBV DNA negative
- In chronic persistent disease:
  - HBsAg positive; HBeAg positive; HBV DNA positive
- See Hepatitis for further diagnostic tests

Treatment

- Interferon α-2b
  - Effective in 1/3 to 1/2 of patients
  - Daily treatment for 4 months
- Lamivudine
  - An orally administered, relatively cheap, and well-tolerated antiviral drug
  - Effective in 1/3 to 1/2 of patients
  - One year of treatment has been reported as optimal
- Liver transplantation

Prognosis/Clinical Course

- Test for the presence of coinfection or superinfection with hepatitis D
- Acute disease lasts weeks to months
- Most likely of the hepatitis viruses to produce an asymptomatic carrier state
- Hepatocellular carcinoma is linked to chronic HBV infection—200× higher risk of HCC
- About 10% of chronic HBV patients per year will develop cirrhosis
- Of patients who develop cirrhosis, 2–3% per year will develop hepatocellular carcinoma and 5–10% per year will decompensate and need liver transplantation

70. Hepatitis C

Etiology

- Single-stranded RNA flavivirus
- Multiple serotypes exist; thus a vaccine has not been effective
- Incubation period 15–120 days (mean 50 days)
- Transmitted via blood and body fluids—IV drug abuse has become the most common method of transmission followed by transfusions; sexual contact accounts for less than 5% of cases
- Acute disease is mild or asymptomatic but high rate of chronic disease
- Chronic disease with HCV results in cirrhosis and its sequelae

Differential Dx

- Other viral hepatitis
- Drug-induced hepatitis
- Shock liver
- Alcoholic hepatitis
- Autoimmune hepatitis
- Right-sided heart failure

Epidemiology

- The most common cause of chronic viral hepatitis in US
- 2% of U.S. population has been exposed to HCV
- As many as 85% of affected patients may develop chronic disease; the remaining patients will clear the virus from their bodies

Signs/Symptoms

- Most patients are asymptomatic for about 20 years from the time of exposure
- Patients may experience signs and symptoms of hepatitis or similar viral illness (see Hepatitis)
- Ultimately, signs and symptoms of cirrhosis develop in those patients with chronic disease (see Cirrhosis)

Diagnosis

- Anti-HCV antibody indicates past exposure; will remain positive even if the patient is cured of HCV infection and has no evidence of chronic disease
- HCV RNA level does not correlate with the patient's prognosis
- For patients who develop cirrhosis, regularly check RUQ ultrasound or abdominal CT and α-fetoprotein to monitor for hepatocellular carcinoma
- AST/ALT significantly elevated (usually 2–3× normal)
- See Hepatitis for further diagnostic tests

Treatment

- Ribavirin and interferon
- Maintain hydration and dietary intake
- Correct coagulation disorders
- Avoid alcohol
- Minimize use of acetaminophen (<3.5 g per day)

Prognosis/Clinical Course

- Most patients do well for 20–25 years before developing cirrhosis—only 25% become acutely symptomatic
- Patients with underlying liver disease—e.g., other hepatitis viruses, alcoholic liver disease, hemochromatosis—have a poorer prognosis and will become symptomatic more quickly
- 50% of chronic hepatitis patients will develop cirrhosis
- 2–3% of patients with cirrhosis will develop hepatocellular carcinoma each year

71. Hepatitis D

Etiology

- Spherical particle enveloped by hepatitis B surface antigen (HBsAg)—only infectious when encapsulated by this surface antigen
- HDV can only infect those who have HBV infection
  - Coinfection may occur when HBV is first acquired—usually results in complete recovery
  - Superinfection of HBV carrier—usually results in accelerated hepatitis and progression to chronic hepatitis within weeks
- Incubation period 30–50 days

Epidemiology

- Primarily drug addicts and hemophiliacs
- Transmission via blood and body fluids—sexual contact, IV drug use, hemodialysis and transfusions, tattoo and piercings, unvaccinated health care workers

Differential Dx

- Other viral hepatitis
- Drug-induced hepatitis
- Shock liver
- Alcoholic hepatitis
- Autoimmune hepatitis
- Right-sided heart failure

Signs/Symptoms

- May be asymptomatic in chronic carriers
- Signs and symptoms of hepatitis (see Hepatitis)

Diagnosis

- Anti-HDV IgM or IgG is consistent with infection
- Look for serum markers of hepatitis B

Treatment

- Interferon-α for at least one year

Prognosis/Clinical Course

- Rule out HDV superinfection in hepatitis B patients
- Similar prognosis as with HBV infection

72. Hepatitis E

Etiology

- Small, spherical RNA calcivirus
- Only one serotype has been identified in humans
- HEV causes only acute disease
- Disease is usually mild, except in pregnant women—acute liver failure has been reported in pregnancy
- Fecal-oral transmission; water-borne transmission
- Mean incubation period of 40 days

Differential Dx

- Other viral hepatitis
- Drug-induced hepatitis
- Shock liver
- Alcoholic hepatitis
- Autoimmune hepatitis
- Right-sided heart failure

Epidemiology

- No endemic foci of HEV has been identified in the US—HEV is considered an "imported" infection
- Affects primarily young and middle-aged adults
- Severe disease may occur in pregnant women

Signs/Symptoms

- Similar signs and symptoms as in other viral hepatitis syndromes (see Hepatitis)

Diagnosis

- Detection of anti-HEV antibodies or HEV RNA in clinical specimen is diagnostic
- During acute infection, both IgM and IgG antibody response occurs

Treatment

- Prevention is key—ensure clean water sources
- Usually self-limiting

Prognosis/Clinical Course

- No chronic disease state
- Mortality rate has been reported at 0.5–4%
- Pregnant women, particularly in the second and third trimesters, have poorer outcomes—mortality has been reported as high as 25%
- Frequency of abortion, stillbirth, and neonatal death is increased

73. Autoimmune Hepatitis

Etiology

- A chronic hepatitis resulting in cirrhosis and liver failure
- The pathogenesis of AIH is a loss of tolerance against one's own liver—likely a loss of cell-mediated immunity
- Viruses, drugs, and other chemicals may trigger AIH in genetically predisposed individuals

Differential Dx

- Viral hepatitis
- Drug-induced hepatitis
- Alcoholic hepatitis
- Wilson's disease
- α_1-AT deficiency
- Hemochromatosis
- Other autoimmune diseases—RA, SLE, and so on

Epidemiology

- Females >> males
- May present at any age but most commonly arises between ages 10–30
- Associated with other autoimmune diseases, such as RA, UC, Sjögren's syndrome, and thyroiditis

Signs/Symptoms

- About half of patients present with an abrupt onset of acute hepatitis—may mimic viral hepatitis
- Remainder of patients have insidious onset of jaundice, anorexia, fatigue, and amenorrhea
- Extrahepatic features may include arthritis, vasculitis, glomerulonephritis, colitis, and pericarditis

Diagnosis

- History and physical examination
- Elevated transaminases (AST/ALT usually <1000)
- Hypergammaglobulinemia (>2.5 g/dL)
- Autoantibodies are often present: ANA, anti-smooth muscle antibody, anti-liver kidney microsome, P-ANCA, SLA
- Cytopenia
- PT, bilirubin, and alkaline phosphatase may be normal (tend to be elevated later in the progression of the disease)

Treatment

- Glucocorticoids are the mainstay of therapy to diminish immune system attack on the liver
  - Prednisone 50 mg daily starting dose, then taper down to 10–20 mg daily
  - May add azathioprine to decrease the needed dose of prednisone

Prognosis/Clinical Course

- In patients with insidious onset of symptoms, advanced liver damage may occur by the time they seek medical intervention
- Severe cases may result in death within months; milder cases have limited morbidity and mortality
- Without treatment, 50% will die within 5 years
- With treatment, 20-year survival exceeds 80% and life expectancy is nearly normal
- 2/3 of patients will exhibit clinical, biochemical, and histologic remission after initial tx; 80% will relapse, requiring lifelong tx
- Some patients with complete remission may still progress to cirrhosis
- Death results from hepatic failure, encephalopathy and coma, infection, complications of cirrhosis, or HCC

74. Alcoholic Liver Disease

Etiology

- Acute: Fatty liver and alcoholic hepatitis—both reversible with abstinence
- Chronic: Cirrhosis—irreversible
- Due to excess alcohol intake over many years
  - Each drink contains 14 g of alcohol
  - Men: >40–60 g per day
  - Women: >30–40 g per day

Differential Dx

- Viral hepatitis
- Drug-induced hepatitis
- Shock liver
- Alcoholic hepatitis
- Autoimmune hepatitis
- Right-sided heart failure
- Hemochromatosis
- Wilson's disease
- α_1-AT deficiency

Epidemiology

- About 10% of the U.S. population abuses alcohol
- Very few of these people actually develop disease—genetic factors and diet play protective roles
- Alcoholic fatty liver in nearly 100% of heavy drinkers
- Alcoholic hepatitis in 10–35% of heavy drinkers

Signs/Symptoms

- Fatty liver: Asymptomatic hepatomegaly
- Signs and symptoms of hepatitis
- Signs and symptoms of cirrhosis
- Signs and symptoms of acute and/or chronic pancreatitis

Diagnosis

- History of alcohol abuse and physical signs of chronic hepatitis and/or cirrhosis—spider angiomata, ascites, encephalopathy, contracture of thenar muscles of hand, and so on
- CAGE questions
- Labs
  - Elevated liver enzymes with AST:ALT ratio of 2:1
  - AST not exceeding 400
  - Elevated alkaline phosphatase
  - Elevated bilirubin
  - Hypoalbuminemia
- Biopsy is diagnostic: may show Mallory bodies, fatty droplets, fibrosis, necrosis, PMNs

Treatment

- Early recognition and treatment of alcoholism
- Patient may need to be enrolled in a detox program
- Four-week course of prednisone for patients with alcoholic hepatitis or hepatic encephalopathy
- Thiamin, folate, and vitamin B_{12} supplementation

Prognosis/Clinical Course

- Liver disease will regress with abstinence unless irreversible cirrhosis has occurred
- Mortality of acute bout of alcoholic hepatitis may be as high as 50% in some populations
- 1/3 to 1/2 of patients with alcoholic hepatitis will develop cirrhosis with continued drinking
- Hepatic causes of death include hepatic failure, GI hemorrhage, infection, hepatorenal syndrome, and hepatocellular carcinoma

75. α_1-Antitrypsin Deficiency

Etiology

- An inherited deficiency of α_1-antitrypsin, the major serum protease inhibitor
- Results in unchecked action of elastase and other proteases at sites of inflammation; primarily manifested in the lungs and liver
  - Lung: Accelerated emphysema
  - Liver: Hepatitis, cholestasis, and cirrhosis

Differential Dx

- Viral hepatitis
- Drug-induced hepatitis
- Shock liver
- Alcoholic hepatitis
- Autoimmune hepatitis
- Wilson's disease
- Hemochromatosis

Epidemiology

- Autosomal recessive inheritance

Signs/Symptoms

- Prolonged jaundice in affected infants
- Neonatal hepatitis syndrome
- Mild transaminase elevation in toddlers
- Portal hypertension develops in mid-childhood/adolescence
- Cirrhosis ensues as patient becomes a young/middle-aged adult
- Hepatocellular carcinoma
- Emphysema

Diagnosis

- Phenotyping is essential
- Liver biopsy is diagnostic
- Serum α_1-antitrypsin is usually (but not always) decreased

Treatment

- No specific treatment available
- Avoidance of cigarette smoking is essential to decrease the progression of lung disease
- Screen for hepatocellular carcinoma
- Liver transplant when decompensation occurs—however, these patients are usually not good surgical candidates due to lung disease

Prognosis/Clinical Course

- Progressive liver dysfunction and failure in children has been treated with liver transplant, with survival approaching 90% at 1 year and 80% at 5 years
- Some patients will have a relatively slow rate of disease progression and can lead a normal life for an extended period of time (not smoking is imperative!)—such individuals may not develop lung injury until their seventh decade of life

76. Hemochromatosis

Etiology

- A disease of chronic iron overload
- The pathogenesis lies in a defective gene(s) that allow unregulated absorption of iron from the gut
- Excess iron is continually deposited in various organs, especially the liver, pancreas, heart, skin, and pituitary; free radicals are produced that interact with DNA
- Patients slowly accumulate iron from infancy but do not exhibit signs or symptoms of iron overload for several decades—thus patients are often diagnosed after significant tissue injury has already occurred

Differential Dx

- 2° hemochromatosis
  - Transfusions
  - Hemolytic anemias (thalassemia, sickle cell anemia)
  - Hemoglobinopathies
- Atransferrinemia
- Aceruloplasminemia
- Wilson's disease
- Chronic liver diseases

Epidemiology

- Autosomal recessive inheritance
- Primarily a disease of whites and those of northern European ancestry
- Symptoms begin in middle age—many patients are never diagnosed due to varying levels of penetrance
- Males accumulate iron more quickly because females regularly lose iron during menstrual periods

Signs/Symptoms

- Hepatic iron overload leads to chronic hepatitis, hepatomegaly, and possibly cirrhosis
- Pancreatic iron overload leads to diabetes mellitus
- Iron overload in the heart leads to CHF, arrythmias, and cardiomyopathy
- Iron deposition in the skin leads to a bronzed appearance
- Iron deposition in the pituitary leads to decreased trophic hormones—adrenal insufficiency, hypogonadism
- Iron deposition in the joints leads to arthritis

Diagnosis

- Elevated serum iron (>300 mg/dL)
- Elevated transferrin saturation (>50%)
- Elevated serum ferritin and RBC ferritin
- Elevated urinary iron excretion
- Diagnostic deferoxamine administration: Upon intramuscular administration of 500–1000 mg, urinary iron will be significantly elevated (>2 mg/24 hours)
- Liver biopsy is diagnostic
- MRI will show increased iron content in liver

Treatment

- Weekly phlebotomy until serum iron is normal; thereafter, less frequent phlebotomies must be continued for life
- Deferoxamine, an iron chelator, can be used if the patient does not tolerate phlebotomy
- Treat associated disease (e.g., diabetes, cardiac disturbance)
- Liver transplantation if cirrhosis occurs

Prognosis/Clinical Course

- Iron studies and genetic screening should be done in all 1° relatives of affected patients
- Severe sequelae (e.g., cirrhosis, CHF) appear in middle age in untreated patients
- Underlying liver disease, such as viral or alcoholic hepatitis, will speed progression of cirrhosis
- Cirrhosis will eventually occur in 100% of untreated patients; once cirrhosis ensues, 10-year survival is just 60% (even with liver transplant)
- Increased risk of hepatocellular carcinoma
- Many patients die of heart-related disease (arrhythmias, sudden cardiac death); phlebotomy does little to reverse iron overload of heart muscle

77. Wilson's Disease

Etiology

- Inherited disorder of copper metabolism—more than 60 different mutations have been identified
- Decreased biliary copper excretion, resulting in copper accumulation in the liver, brain, cornea, kidney, bones, joints, and other tissues

Differential Dx

- Viral hepatitis
- Hemochromatosis
- α_1-Antitrypsin deficiency
- Alcoholic liver disease
- Autoimmune hepatitis
- Primary biliary cirrhosis
- Isolated ceruloplasmin deficiency

Epidemiology

- Autosomal recessive transmission

Signs/Symptoms

- Patients may be totally asymptomatic
- Hepatic manifestations include chronic hepatitis and fulminant hepatitis; will proceed to cirrhosis if not diagnosed and treated early
- Extrahepatic manifestations
  - Basal ganglia: Parkinsonism, psychosis
  - Cornea: Keiser-Fleischer rings
  - Skeletal copper deposition

Diagnosis

- Diagnosis made by a combination of clinical and biochemical findings
  - Low serum ceruloplasmin
  - Slit-lamp examination for presence of Kayser-Fleischer rings in cornea
  - Elevated hepatic copper level on liver biopsy
- Liver biopsy is diagnostic but is not necessary if Kayser-Fleischer rings are present
- Elevated serum copper
- Elevated urinary copper excretion
- Elevated transaminases
- Hemolytic anemia

Treatment

- D-penicillamine: Chelates copper and increases urinary copper excretion
  - May cause vitamin B_6 deficiency—B_6 replacement is necessary
- Dimercaprol if patient cannot tolerate D-penicillamine or if neurologic symptoms predominate
- Zinc supplementation can decrease copper absorption from gut
- Decrease intake of high-copper foods—chocolate, shellfish, liver
- Liver transplantation for patients with fulminant hepatitis or cirrhosis

Prognosis/Clinical Course

- Without treatment, this disease is fatal by early adulthood
- Lifelong therapy is necessary to avoid rapid hepatic failure and neuropathology
- Strict compliance with pharmacotherapy is essential—monitor pill counts and urinary copper excretion

78. Portal Hypertension

Etiology

- Increased resistance to blood flow through the portal vein
- Prehepatic causes: Narrowed portal vein, occlusive thrombosis
- Intrahepatic causes: Cirrhosis (most common cause overall), biliary cirrhosis, schistosomiasis, sarcoidosis, tuberculosis, hepatic fibrosis
- Posthepatic causes: Hepatic vein obstruction (Budd-Chiari syndrome), IVC obstruction, right heart failure, constrictive pericarditis, restrictive cardiomyopathy

Differential Dx

Epidemiology

Signs/Symptoms

- Ascites
- Splenomegaly
- Hepatic encephalopathy
  - Mental status changes (confusion, stupor, coma)
  - Rigidity, hyperreflexia, seizures
  - Asterixis
- Portosystemic shunting
  - Hemorrhoids
  - Esophageal varices
  - Caput medusae
- Jaundice
- Edema
- Gynecomastia, palmar erythema, spider angiomata (due to decreased estrogen metabolism in liver)

Diagnosis

- Clinical evidence is usually diagnostic
- Measurement of portal vein pressure may be useful
- Ultrasound or CT
- Endoscopy to show esophageal varices
- Examination of ascites fluid may show PMNs if infection
  - Serum albumin – Ascites gradient (SAG) >1.1
  - Ascitic albumin <1.0 g/dL
  - Absolute neutrophil count >250 in spontaneous bacterial peritonitis

Treatment

- Determine and treat underlying cause
- Manage acute problems, such as bleeding varices

Prognosis/Clinical Course

- Esophageal varices can result in massive hematemesis and high mortality (>50%)
- Hepatorenal syndrome may result
- Hepatopulmonary syndrome may result
- Spontaneous bacterial peritonitis may result from infection of ascitic fluid

79. Cirrhosis

Etiology

- Irreversible destruction of liver architecture by nodules of fibrosis
- Results from the liver's attempt to repair its chronically damaged state
- Most cases due to chronic alcohol abuse or viral hepatitis; any chronic liver disease may result in cirrhosis (Wilson's disease, hemochromatosis, drugs—chronic usage or acute overdose, PSC, PBC, and so on); massive acute injury may result in cirrhosis as well

Differential Dx

- 1° or 2° biliary cirrhosis
- Noncirrhotic hepatic fibrosis

Epidemiology

- Most common causes in US are alcohol abuse and hepatitis C

Signs/Symptoms

- Firm, nodular liver
- S/S of portal hypertension—see Portal Hypertension
  - Ascites
  - Hepatosplenomegaly
  - Caput medusa
  - Esophageal varices
- S/S of liver failure
  - Jaundice
  - Spider angiomata
  - Palmar erythema
  - Gynecomastia
  - Testicular atrophy
  - Bruising and hypocoagulation
  - Dupuytren's contracture
- Hepatic encephalopathy

Diagnosis

- History and physical examination
- Ultrasound or abdominal CT
- Biopsy is diagnostic
- Liver enzymes are elevated early due to chronic liver disease but decreased when significant cirrhosis ensues
- Hypoalbuminemia and hypocholesterolemia
- Azotemia and electrolyte disturbances
- Increased prothrombin time
- Endoscopy to diagnose esophageal varices
- Elevated BUN/creatinine in hepatorenal disease
- Regularly check RUQ ultrasound or CT and α-fetoprotein to monitor for hepatocellular carcinoma

Treatment

- Treat the underlying liver disease
- Avoid alcohol regardless of the etiology of cirrhosis
- Hospitalize in acute deterioration to manage complications (e.g., encephalopathy, bleeding)
- Stabilize electrolytes
- Low-protein diet
- Lactulose—decreases protein absorption from gut, thereby decreasing the production of ammonia and the risk of azotemia and encephalopathy
- Slowly remove excessive ascites fluid—rapid removal may result in hepatorenal syndrome
- Liver transplantation

Prognosis/Clinical Course

- Most common cause of portal hypertension
- 50–75% of patients will have esophageal varices
  - 25% will develop bleeding varices
  - Nearly 50% of patients with bleeding varices will die in the hospital—only 1/3 will be alive one year after the initial bleeding episode
- Major complications—encephalopathy, ascites, bleeding varices—indicate poor prognosis

80. Hepatocellular Carcinoma

Etiology

- Many diseases that result in chronic liver disease and cirrhosis predispose to HCC:
  - Hepatitis B, C, and D (chronic HCV is the most common cause of HCC in the US)
  - Alcoholic liver disease
  - Hemochromatosis or Wilson's disease
  - *Aspergillus* toxin
- It is rare but possible for HCC to occur without existing cirrhosis

Differential Dx

- Hepatocellular adenoma
- Nodular hyperplasia
- Cyst
- Hemangioma
- Metastatic cancer
- Cholangiocarcinoma
- Gallbladder tumors
- Hepatic leukemia
- Hepatic lymphoma
- Liver abscess

Epidemiology

- Major cause of worldwide mortality
- Males >> females
- Tends to occur in fifth and sixth decades of life
- May grow and metastasize quickly

Signs/Symptoms

- Classic presentation is RUQ/epigastric pain (due to distention of the liver capsule by tumor and/or hemorrhage), abdominal swelling/ascites, and weight loss in a patient with existing cirrhosis
- Fever, malaise
- Enlarged, hard liver with irregular surface
- Vascular bruit may be heard

Diagnosis

- Onset of hepatic decompensation in a patient with known cirrhosis may signal the development of HCC
- Sudden hypoglycemia in cirrhotic patient
- Elevated alkaline phosphatase
- Elevated α-fetoprotein
- Liver biopsy is diagnostic
- Ultrasound, CT, or MRI
- Angiography

Treatment

- Prevent of chronic liver disease (i.e., universal vaccination for hepatitis B virus)
- Surgical resection of a lobe
- Removal of liver and transplantation

Prognosis/Clinical Course

- Survival is generally very poor—death may occur in as little as 6–8 weeks from diagnosis
- Spreads initially to remainder of the liver and to the inferior vena cava
- Surgical resection can increase survival time 10-fold or more
- Liver transplant has resulted in 70–80% five-year survival rates

81. Budd-Chiari Syndrome

Etiology

- Thrombosis of the hepatic vein, resulting in hepatic venous outflow
- Hypercoagulable states (such as protein C deficiency, protein S deficiency, antithrombin III deficiency) and malignancies account for most cases
- Also myeloproliferative disorders, polycythemia vera, OCP use, pregnancy, paroxysmal nocturnal hemoglobinuria

Epidemiology

- Rare

Differential Dx

- Impaired hepatic inflow
    - Hepatic artery thrombosis
    - Portal vein obstruction
- Impaired intrahepatic flow
    - Cirrhosis
    - Sinusoid occlusion
    - Schistosomiasis
    - Sickle cell disease
    - Circulatory collapse
- Impaired outflow
    - IVC obstruction
    - Right heart failure
    - Pericarditis
    - Cardiomyopathy
- Hepatitis
- Biliary cirrhosis

Signs/Symptoms

- Presentation depends on extent and rate of outflow obstruction
- Hepatomegaly and ascites are present in nearly 100% of patients
- Esophageal varices and splenomegaly are present in about 50% of patients
- Jaundice
- RUQ pain
- Patients may be relatively asymptomatic or have signs and symptoms of fulminant hepatic failure and/or cirrhosis

Diagnosis

- Angiography is the gold standard for diagnosis, although rarely done
- CT is most commonly used for diagnosis
- Ultrasound may have sensitivity >90% in the hands of experienced operators
- MRI is rarely needed; it can visualize absent hepatic veins or attenuated vessels with intraluminal thrombus formation
- Elevated transaminases
- Rule out underlying diseases such as myeloproliferative disorders and malignancies

Treatment

- Goal of treatment is to relieve venous obstruction and preserve hepatic function
- Medical therapy is generally ineffective
- Hepatic shunts, such as TIPS, have been used successfully
- Liver transplant for patients with cirrhosis
- Patients require lifelong anticoagulation

Prognosis/Clinical Course

- Without treatment, most patients will die within 3 years

82. Liver Abscess

Etiology

- Most often caused by *Entamoeba histolytica* or bacteria (*Streptococcus, Staphylococcus, Klebsiella, E. coli*)
- Liver infection is generally secondary to bacteremia, ascending cholangitis, or penetrating trauma

Differential Dx

- Amebic abscess
- Pyogenic abscess
- Hepatocellular carcinoma
- Liver metastasis
- Liver adenoma
- Cyst
- Hemangioma

Epidemiology

- Rare in US
- Most liver abscesses in US are bacterial
- Highest incidence in poor countries with poor sanitary conditions

Signs/Symptoms

- Intense, constant RUQ pain—may radiate to right shoulder
- Increased pain with cough, deep breathing, or when lie on right side
- May appear pale
- Fever/chills/night sweats

Diagnosis

- Leukocytosis >15,000
- Elevated alkaline phosphatase and transaminases
- Anti-amebic serum antibody is present in >90% of patients
- RUQ ultrasound is the preferred noninvasive imaging study
- CT
- Needle aspiration and culture
- Mild anemia
- Elevated bilirubin in some patients

Treatment

- Metronidazole × 2 weeks for *E. histolytica*
- Broad-spectrum antibiotics for bacterial infections
- Percutaneous drainage of abscess if great risk of rupture exists, if response to antibiotics is slow, or if pyogenic infection is suspected
- Surgical drainage for ruptured abscess

Prognosis/Clinical Course

- Clinical improvement is seen within 72 hours of initiation of antibiotics in >95% of patients
- Excellent prognosis with treatment
- Complications include rupture and subphrenic abscess formation

83. Primary Sclerosing Cholangitis

Etiology

- Inflammation, fibrosis, and stenosis of the bile ducts (especially extrahepatic ducts)
- The cause of PSC remains unknown despite extensive investigation; hypotheses focus on infectious, genetic, or immunologic mechanisms
- Secondary sclerosing cholangitis occurs with bile duct injury (stones, gallbladder surgery) or bile duct ischemia
- PSC is a premalignant condition of the biliary tree—nearly 50% of patients will develop cholangiocarcinoma

Differential Dx

- Biliary cirrhosis
- Biliary strictures
- Biliary trauma (surgery)
- Biliary ischemia
- Acute cholangitis
- Autoimmune cholangitis
- Choledocholithiasis
- Hepatitis
- Pancreatic head cancer

Epidemiology

- 70% of patients have ulcerative colitis (about 5% have Crohn's disease)
- Overall, about 5% of all UC patients develop PSC
- Males >> females
- Mean age of diagnosis 40 years

Signs/Symptoms

- Spectrum of disease varies from asymptomatic alkaline phosphatase elevation to full cirrhosis
- RUQ pain
- Jaundice and pruritis
- Fatigue
- Nausea
- Signs and symptoms of ulcerative colitis or Crohn's disease may be present

Diagnosis

- ERCP is the gold standard
- Jaundice and elevated alkaline phosphatase in a young male must raise suspicion of PSC
- Elevated alkaline phosphatase for longer than 6 months is the hallmark of disease
- Elevated bilirubin
- ANA, AMA, and ASMA may be elevated in some patients
- Hypergammaglobulinemia

Treatment

- No medical treatment is effective
- Stent placement and biliary drainage may help alleviate symptoms but do not decrease mortality
- Antibiotics to treat superimposed bacterial cholangitis
- Liver transplant is effective—recurrence in about 20% of cases

Prognosis/Clinical Course

- Progression to liver failure within 10–15 years
- Acute cholangitis may occur
  - Charcot's triad: Fever, jaundice, and RUQ pain

84. Primary Biliary Cirrhosis

Etiology

- A chronic disease of cholestasis secondary to granulomatous destruction of intrahepatic bile ducts
- Etiology of PBC is unknown but most likely of immunologic cause (associated with many other immunologic diseases, such as Hashimoto's thyroiditis, scleroderma, and inflammatory arthritis)
- 2° biliary cirrhosis occurs due to prolonged extrahepatic obstruction

Differential Dx

- 2° biliary cirrhosis
- Sclerosing cholangitis
- Ascending cholangitis
- Drug-induced cholestasis
- Hepatitis
- Autoimmune cholangitis
- Sarcoidosis
- Choledocholithiasis
- Biliary atresia

Epidemiology

- Primarily a disease of middle-aged women (>90% of patients are women)

Signs/Symptoms

- Pruritis and persistent fatigue are usually the presenting symptoms
- Evidence of advanced liver disease, such as jaundice and ascites, presents later in the course of PBC
- Hepatosplenomegaly
- Steatorrhea
- May be associated with:
  – Osteoporosis
  – Fat-soluble vitamin deficiency (A, D, E, K)
  – Hypercholesterolemia
  – Malabsorption
  – Renal tubular acidosis

Diagnosis

- Elevated alkaline phosphatase and bilirubin
- Positive AMA antibodies in >90% of patients
- Positive ANA in some patients
- Transaminases are usually normal or mildly elevated— if >200–300, look for other causes
- Biopsy is diagnostic
- Ultrasound or ERCP

Treatment

- Ursodeoxycholic acid may be effective
- Liver transplantation

Prognosis/Clinical Course

- Generally takes 15–20 years before the development of cirrhosis, although some patients deteriorate in a matter of years
- Liver transplantation yields excellent results

85. Cholecystitis

Etiology

- Inflammation of the gallbladder due to infection or obstruction
- About 95% of all cases are caused by gallstones

Differential Dx

- Peptic ulcer disease
- Hepatitis
- Liver abscess
- Pancreatitis
- Carcinoma of the liver or bile ducts
- Carcinoma of the gallbladder
- Cholangitis

Epidemiology

- Due to the high correlation of cholelithiasis with cholecystitis, the epidemiology is similar: Female, fertile, fat, forty
- Other risk factors include use of oral contraceptives, bile stasis, cirrhosis, hyperlipidemia, and chronic hemolysis

Signs/Symptoms

- Right upper quadrant pain/tenderness
- Fever
- Nausea/vomiting
- Right subscapular pain (referred from diaphragm)
- Gallbladder is palpable and painful in one-third of cases
- Murphy's sign: Pain upon palpation of the gallbladder while taking a deep breath

Diagnosis

- Appropriate history and physical is highly suggestive of gallbladder disease
- Ultrasound is the gold standard
    - Thickened gallbladder wall (greater than 3 mm)
    - Distended gallbladder
    - Pericholecystic fluid
    - Gallstones/ductal stones
- CT is somewhat less accurate and much more expensive
- Leukocytosis
- Elevation of LFTs, amylase, bilirubin, and alkaline phosphatase may be present

Treatment

- IV fluids
- Nasogastric decompression, if necessary
- Antibiotics
- Surgery: Laproscopic or open cholecystectomy

Prognosis/Clinical Course

- Very good prognosis if treated early
- Complications include abscess formation, perforation, gallstone ileus, and formation of a cholecystenteric fistula
- Although many people have asymptomatic cholelithiasis, few cases will result in cholecystitis; however, once infection occurs, surgery to remove the gallbladder is indicated as cholecystitis will nearly inevitably recur

86. Malabsorption Syndromes

Etiology

- Abnormal digestion resulting in malabsorption of one or many nutrients:
  - Insufficient gastric mixing: Gastrectomy
  - ↓ Enzymes: CF, pancreatitis, liver failure, lactase or IF deficiency
  - Decreased acidity: Zollinger-Ellison syndrome, subtotal gastrectomy
- Impaired absorption:
  - Damaged absorptive surface: Infection, sprue, Whipple's disease, drugs/alcohol, amyloidosis, Crohn's disease, ischemic colitis
  - Decreased absorptive surface: resection, infarcted bowel, volvulus

Differential Dx

- Eating disorders
- Irritable bowel syndrome
- Infectious diarrhea
- Drug-induced diarrhea (quinidine, colchicine, vitamins, amiodarone, clindamycin)

Epidemiology

Signs/Symptoms

- Osmotic diarrhea and steatorrhea
- Bulky, greasy stools
- Bloating, distention, flatus
- Weight loss and anorexia
- Glossitis, carpopedal spasm
- Vitamin/mineral deficiencies
- Amenorrhea in fat malabsorption
- Osteopenia in calcium or vitamin D malabsorption
- Tetany in calcium deficiency
- Coagulation disorders in vitamin K deficiency
- Neuropathy in vitamin B_{12} deficiency
- Edema and ascites in protein deficiency

Diagnosis

- Diarrhea, weight loss, and anemia suggest malabsorption
- 72-hour fecal fat analysis
- Xylose absorption test: Measures intestinal absorptive capacity
- Intestinal biopsy and culture: To diagnose infection, carcinoma, patency of absorptive surface
- Small bowel follow-through: To diagnose sprue, Whipple's disease, fistulas, stasis, blind loop, diverticulosis, Crohn's disease
- Pancreatic function tests
- H_2 breath test: To diagnose lactose intolerance
- Schilling test for vitamin B_{12} absorption
- Measure levels of iron, folate, gastrin (Zollinger-Ellison syndrome), cortisol (Addison's disease), sweat chloride (cystic fibrosis)

Treatment

- Treat underlying cause
  - Enzyme replacement
  - Supplementation
  - Antibiotics for infections and bacterial overgrowth syndromes
  - Disease-specific diet (eliminate gluten, lactose, alcohol, etc.)

Prognosis/Clinical Course

87. Bowel Obstruction

Etiology

- Small bowel obstruction: Most commonly due to adhesion, hernia, tumors
- Large bowel obstruction: Most commonly due to colon cancer, volvulus, or diverticulitis
- Obstruction may be partial or complete; acute or chronic
- Obstruction may be mechanical (e.g., adhesion, hernia) or paralytic/impaired motility (e.g., trauma, surgery, hypokalemia, peritonitis)
- Obstruction may be simple or strangulating (cuts off arterial/venous flow)

Epidemiology

Differential Dx

- Colon cancer
- Intraperitoneal cancer
- Crohn's disease
- Hernia
- Adhesions
- Foreign bodies
- Bezoars
- Hirschsprung's disease
- Volvulus
- Fecal impaction
- Diverticular disease
- *Ascaris* infestation
- Intussusception
- Large polyp
- Lipoma
- Gallstone ileus

Signs/Symptoms

- Crampy, intermittent abdominal pain
- Distention
- Vomiting
- Constipation
- Mechanical obstruction: High-pitched bowel sounds with peristaltic rushes and tinkles
- Ileus: Decreased or absent bowel sounds

Diagnosis

- History and physical
- Flat and upright abdominal X-rays are often diagnostic
  - Excess air in small bowel; no air in colon
  - Air–fluid levels in distended loops of bowel
  - Normal bowel distal to obstruction
  - If ileus, diffuse gas
- If strangulated bowel, leukocytosis will be present
- Gastrograffin enema to diagnose colonic obstruction

Treatment

- IV fluids
- NG suction
- Correct electrolyte abnormalities
- Serial physical examinations and radiographs with further workup if symptoms do not resolve in 2 days
- Monitor urine output
- Treat underlying causes: Lysis of adhesions, reduction and repair of hernia, resection of tumor, and so on
- Indications for surgery to repair obstruction: Strangulated bowel, complete obstruction, partial obstruction with worsening course

Prognosis/Clinical Course

- Strangulated bowel can become necrotic and gangrenous in as little as 6 hours—accurate and quick diagnosis is essential

88. Ischemic Bowel Disease

Etiology

- Ischemic colitis: Non-occlusive (never embolic); usually affects IMA
  – May be due to CHF, hypercoagulable states, decreased intestinal flow
- Chronic mesenteric ischemia (intestinal angina)
  – Due to atherosclerotic narrowing of mesenteric arteries
- Acute mesenteric ischemia: Due to acute loss of blood flow through small intestine; usually embolic (history of valve disease, arrythmias)
- Mesenteric venous thrombosis: Associated with hypercoagulable states

Differential Dx

- Gastroenteritis
- Ulcerative colitis
- Crohn's disease
- Bowel obstruction
- Carcinoma

Epidemiology

- Elderly patients
- History of atherosclerotic disease, embolic sources

Signs/Symptoms

- Ischemic colitis
  – Sudden LLQ pain
  – Reddish, loose stool
  – Urge to defecate
- Intestinal angina
  – Abdominal pain following meals
  – Abdominal bruit
  – Wt loss—cannot tolerate full meals
- Acute mesenteric ischemia
  – Sudden onset of severe pain, vomiting, diarrhea, occult blood
  – Physical exam may be benign
- Mesenteric venous thrombosis
  – Pain out of proportion with exam
- Peritonitis may be present: Fever, tachycardia, rebound tenderness, guarding

Diagnosis

- Ischemic colitis
  – Barium enema: "Thumbprinting" is diagnostic
  – Colonoscopy—do not attempt if signs of peritonitis
- Intestinal angina
  – Classic triad of abdominal pain with meals, abdominal bruit, and weight loss
  – Angiography
  – Doppler ultrasound
- Acute mesenteric ischemia
  – Angiography—do not attempt if suspect perforation or if patient is rapidly declining
  – Exploratory laparotomy in critically ill patients
  – X-ray: Dilated loops of bowel
  – Leukocytosis, acidosis, hypotension, shock may result
- Mesenteric venous thrombosis
  – CT is diagnostic

Treatment

- Ischemic colitis
  – Bowel rest (no intake, NG tube)
  – IV fluids
  – Antibiotics if leukocytosis
  – Resection of involved segment if necessary
- Intestinal angina
  – Nitroglycerin may provide relief
  – Surgical revascularization (bypass) or angioplasty
- Acute mesenteric ischemia
  – Laparotomy to reestablish perfusion
  – Thrombolytics if not a surgical candidate
- Mesenteric venous thrombosis
  – Thrombolytics
  – Long-term anticoagulation

Prognosis/Clinical Course

- Ischemic colitis: Fibrosis and stricture formation are common complications; 50% have complete resolution
- Signs of perforation include acidosis, elevated ALT, and elevated amylase

89. Appendicitis

Etiology

- Obstruction of lumen of appendix by fecalith → distention of appendix and ↑ intraluminal pressure → venous engorgement and arterial ischemia → bacterial invasion of wall → inflammation → appendicitis → necrosis → rupture → peritonitis

Epidemiology

- 10% of people in US develop appendicitis at some time
- 2nd most common cause in US of severe, acute abdominal pain that requires surgery (#1 is hernia)
- Peak in 2nd and 3rd decades of life but can occur at any age
- Male > female

Differential Dx

- Gastroenteritis
- Perforated peptic ulcer
- Meckel's diverticulitis
- Acute cholecystitis
- Mesenteric lymphadenitis
- Intestinal obstruction
- Crohn's disease
- Ileitis
- Diverticulitis
- Renal colic
- Ectopic pregnancy
- Ruptured ovarian follicle
- PID/TOA
- Mittelschmertz

Signs/Symptoms

- Periumbilical and/or epigastric pain that soon localizes to RLQ
- Anorexia
- Nausea/vomiting
- Low-grade fever (>38.3° C [101°F] suggests perforation)
- RLQ tenderness at McBurney's point
- If rebound or generalized tenderness, appendix may have ruptured with ensuing peritonitis
- Rovsing's sign: Pain in RLQ caused by palpation of LLQ
- Psoas sign: Pain upon passive extension of right leg
- Obturator sign: Pain upon passive internal rotation of flexed leg

Diagnosis

- Leukocytosis
- Abdominal X-ray: May be able to see fecalith in RLQ
- Ultrasound: Diagnostic if positive but cannot rule out appendicitis if negative
- CT: To locate abscess formation
- Must rule out pelvic syndromes in females

Treatment

- IV fluids
- Appendectomy is treatment of choice
  - Surgery is emergent, as perforation can occur within 24 hours of onset of symptoms
  - Antibiotics against enteric organisms (gram-negative organisms and anaerobes) should be given preoperatively, intraoperatively, and postoperatively: Ampicillin plus sulbactam or 3rd generation cephalosporin

Prognosis/Clinical Course

- Rapid recovery and low mortality with early diagnosis and treatment
- Rupture, abscess formation, and/or peritonitis complicate treatment; repeat operations and long recovery may follow

90. Ulcerative Colitis

Etiology

- Chronic, relapsing inflammatory disorder of rectum and colon; idiopathic origin
- In contrast to Crohn's disease:
  - Diffuse, continuous mucosal inflammation (versus skip lesions in Crohn's disease)
  - Inflamed areas *do not* alternate with uninvolved areas
  - No small bowel involvement
  - No granuloma formation; microabscesses are produced
  - Limited to mucosa/submucosa

Epidemiology

- Male > female
- Family history is important: 10× greater risk in 1st degree relatives
- Bimodal peak: Ages 20–35 and 50–65
- Higher incidence than Crohn's disease
- Higher incidence in Jews; lower incidence in African Americans
- Genetic? Infectious? Immune-related?

Differential Dx

- Infectious colitis (*E. coli, Campylobacter, Shigella, Salmonella,* or other organism)
- Crohn's disease
- Colorectal cancer
- Malabsorption syndromes
- Diverticulitis
- Ischemic colitis

Signs/Symptoms

- Intermittent bouts of bloody, mucous diarrhea with periods of constipation
- Lower abdominal pain and cramps—relieved by defecation
- Fever and weight loss may occur
- Tenesmus and constipation with proctitis
- Extraintestinal manifestations: Sclerosing cholangitis, arthritis, erythema nodosum, ankylosing spondylitis, uveitis, venous thrombosis, pyoderma gangrenosum
- Failure to thrive in affected children
- Rectum is always involved (if colon is spared, then called "ulcerative proctitis")

Diagnosis

- Colonoscopy with biopsy is diagnostic; also used to rule out cancer
- Pathology: Friable mucosa, pseudopolyps, microabscesses, normal serosa
- Barium enema will show ulceration, pseudopolyps, and "lead pipe" appearance of colon in end-stage cases
  - Barium enema is contraindicated in toxic megacolon
- Upper GI series with small bowel follow-through
- Proctoscopy
- Stool cultures: Blood, mucus, leukocytes; rule out infection
- P-ANCA: Positive in 75%
- LFTs: Elevated (especially alkaline phosphatase) if cholangitis
- Although small bowel is not affected in UC, "backwash ileitis" may occur

Treatment

- Daily medication
  - Sulfasalazine: Induces remission in >50%
  - Mesalamine
  - Hydrocortisone enema
  - Antidiarrheals and bulking agents
- Flare-ups
  - Bowel rest (no oral intake, NG tube)
  - IV fluids
  - Steroids
  - Metronidazole
- Colectomy is curative for UC (not so for Crohn's disease)
  - Indications for surgery: Dysplasia or carcinoma, perforation, toxic colitis, hemorrhage, intractable disease, inability to wean off steroids
  - About one-third of patients undergo colectomy

Prognosis/Clinical Course

- Area of involvement increases in only 10% of cases (versus contiguous spread in Crohn's disease)
- Chronic, relapsing course (in some patients, first attack is last)
- Complications
  - Toxic megacolon in 10% of cases
  - Strictures, obstruction, perforation
  - Hypokalemia
  - Hemorrhage and shock
- Colon cancer: Higher risk than in Crohn's
  - ↑ risk with degree of involvement
  - 2% risk at 10 years, 2% risk/year thereafter
  - Annual screening colonoscopy
  - Proctitis alone carries no cancer risk
- Nicotine may be effective to decrease relapses

91. Crohn's Disease

Etiology

- Chronic granulomatous disease (although only 1/3 of cases actually present with granulomas)
- May affect any part of GI tract, from mouth to anus—primarily the ileum
  – 30% colon only; 40% small intestine only; 30% both
- Alternating areas of disease with normal mucosa (skip lesions)
- Full thickness of colonic wall involved (versus only mucosa in UC)
- Ulcerating lesions that may progress to fistula, structures, or obstruction

Differential Dx

- Infectious colitis (*E. coli, Campylobacter, Shigella, Salmonella,* or other organism)
- Ulcerative colitis
- Colorectal cancer
- Malabsorption syndromes
- Diverticulitis
- Ischemic colitis
- Appendicitis

Epidemiology

- Bimodal incidence: Age 20–30 most common, also >50 years
- Female > male

Signs/Symptoms

- Initial symptoms: Abdominal pain, fever, weight loss, anal disease
- Colicky pain
- Steatorrhea if ileum significantly affected or resected
- Occult blood
- Melena
- Diarrhea
- RLQ mass if extensive ileum involvement— may mimic appendicitis
- Arthritis in 10% of cases (enteropathic arthropathy)

Diagnosis

- Abdominal X-ray
- Endoscopy: Inflammatory changes, rectal sparing, skip lesions
- Biopsy: Inflammation; granulomas are characteristic but rare
- Anemia, leukocytosis
- Small bowel follow-through: "String sign" indicates lumen of ileum compressed from edematous bowel wall (looks like thin string of contrast)

Treatment

- Daily treatment
  – Sulfasalazine, 5-acetylsalicylic acid, mesalamine
- Flare-ups
  – Bowel rest (no oral intake, NG tube)
  – IV fluids/total parental nutrition
  – Steroids
  – Antibiotics
- Surgery is used only for severe disease or for complications (perforation, fistula to other organs, abscess, obstruction, intractable disease)
  – Disease recurs around areas of surgery; adhesions and obstructions also result
  – Most patients need repeat surgery within 8 years
- Best surgery is full colectomy and ileostomy
- Vitamin B_{12} if extensive ileum involvement
- Immunomodulants (i.e., 6-MP) and infliximab

Prognosis/Clinical Course

- Less responsive to treatment than UC—difficult to get patients off steroids
- High recurrence rate: once in remissions, most cases will recur within 3 years
- Complications
  – Nephrolithiasis
  – Hypocalcemia (due to vitamin D malabsorption)
  – Vitamin B_{12} deficiency
  – Adhesions, strictures, fistulas, obstruction
- Increased risk of cancer but not as high as in UC—screening colonoscopy should be done every other year

92. Diverticular Disease

Etiology

- Diverticulosis: Asymptomatic outpouchings of the colon
- Diverticulitis: Infection and inflammation of a diverticulum; microperforations usually present; *no bleeding*
- Diverticular bleeding: Most common cause of lower GI bleeding in the elderly (#2 is angiodysplasia)
- Associated with low-fiber diet → ↓ bulk of stool → ↑ force generated by colonic peristalsis → outpouching of focal weaknesses in colon wall
- Sigmoid is most common area of colon affected

Differential Dx

- Colon cancer
- Volvulus
- Angiodysplasia
- Ulcerative colitis
- Crohn's disease
- Appendicitis
- Pelvic cancer
- PID

Epidemiology

- Presence of diverticuli increases with age; majority of people over age 50 have diverticuli
- Often more severe in younger persons

Signs/Symptoms

- Diverticulosis: Usually asymptomatic
  - Alternating diarrhea and constipation
  - Lower abdominal pain, relieved by bowel movement
- Diverticular bleeding
  - Generally painless
  - Signs of lower GI bleeding
- Diverticulitis
  - LLQ pain: ↑ with bowel movement
  - May have inflammatory mass in LLQ
  - Tenderness; rebound tenderness indicates perforation
  - Fever
  - No occult bleeding
- Periumbilical symptoms are possible as sigmoid colon curves toward the midline

Diagnosis

- Triad of LLQ pain, fever, and leukocytosis in acute diverticulitis
- CT is diagnositic
- Flexible sigmoidoscopy/colonoscopy is also diagnostic
- Abdominal X-ray: Diverticula appear as "thumbprints" along colon
- Upright abdominal X-ray: Free air under diaphragm if perforation has occurred
- Ultrasound will also show diverticula

Treatment

- Diverticulosis: High-fiber diet
- Diverticular bleeding
  - Stabilize the patient
  - Rule out upper GI bleeding: NG tube, EGD, BUN/creatinine >30 (digested blood raises BUN)
  - Identify bleeding source: Colonoscopy, angiography, or Tc-tagged RBC scan
  - Sigmoidectomy if intractable bleeding
- Diverticulitis
  - Bowel rest
  - Broad-spectrum antibiotics to cover gram-negative organisms and anaerobes (metronidazol plus ciprofloxacin is a good choice)
  - Percutaneous abscesses drainage if necessary
  - Colonic resection is indicated after the second bout of diverticulitis or after the first bout in young patients

Prognosis/Clinical Course

- In patients >50 years, follow up with flexible sigmoidoscopy or colonoscopy (after the acute event resolves) to rule out cancer
- Although most patients are advised to have a sigmoidectomy or colectomy after two bouts of diverticulitis, young patients should have the affected colon removed after the initial bout as recurrences in young patients are nearly inevitable

93. Colon Cancer

Etiology

- 98% are adenocarcinomas
- Almost always arise from adenomatous polyps
  - High-risk polyps tend to be >2 cm, villous, sessile
- Polyps may be benign, premalignant, or malignant
- Lynch syndrome (hereditary nonpolyposis colon cancer)
  - Colon cancer in three 1st degree relatives over 2 or more generations with someone diagnosed before age 50
  - Also increased risk ovarian/uterine cancer

Differential Dx

- Diverticulitis
- Volvulus
- Ulcerative colitis
- Crohn's disease
- Infection
- Pelvic cancer
- PID
- Ischemic colitis

Epidemiology

- 2nd most common cancer in incidence and mortality
- Incidence increases with age (peak = 60–70 years)
- Rectal cancer is more common in males; right-sided cancer is more common in females
- Risk factors: Family history, Crohn's, UC, adenomatous polyps, low-fiber diet, familial polyposis syndromes (FAP, Gardner, Peutz-Jeghers)

Signs/Symptoms

- Change in bowel habits, ↓ stool size
- Fatigue, weakness, weight loss
- Abdominal discomfort
- Inguinal lymphadenopathy
- If obstruction: N/V, fever, tachycardia, no bowel movements or flatus
- Right-sided cancers
  - Postprandial discomfort
  - Possible right-sided mass
  - S/S of iron-deficiency anemia
- Left-sided cancers
  - Alternating diarrhea and constipation
  - ↑ Risk of obstruction due to ↓ lumen size
  - Hematochezia
  - Possible left-sided mass
- Rectal cancer: Tenesmus; mass on DRE

Diagnosis

- Iron-deficiency anemia in older males is considered colon cancer until proven otherwise
- Screening: Annual PE with digital rectal exam
  - Stool guiac for occult blood
  - After age 50: Sigmoidoscopy every 3–5 years or colonoscopy every 10 years
  - High-risk patients: Yearly colonoscopy
- Barium enema to look for polyps
- Colonoscopy is diagnostic: Allows for biopsy and removal of early lesions
- CT: Not necessary but may help evaluate lesions
- CEA levels: Not for screening; useful as follow-up to evaluate for recurrences or metastases
- Look for distant metastases: CXR, LFTs, alkaline phosphatase, renal function
- U/A: Enterovesical fistula may occur

Treatment

- Best treatment is prevention: Identify early polyps with sigmoidoscopy or colonoscopy and remove them
- Surgery is curative for early cancers (Duke's A and B)
- Surgery plus chemotherapy (5-fluorouracil + levamisole) for Duke's C
- Surgery for palliation only in Duke's D
- Radiation before surgery for rectal lesions
- Treat metastases as necessary

Prognosis/Clinical Course

- Duke's staging
  - A: Confined to mucosa/submucosa; 95% 5-year survival
  - B: Extends to muscularis (B1) or through serosa (B2); 70–80% 5-year survival
  - C: Extends to regional lymph nodes (C_1: 1–4 nodes; C_2: 5+ nodes); 30–60% 5-year survival
  - D: Metastases (liver especially; also lung, brain, bone); 5% 5-year survival
- Follow-up after resection
  - CEA every 2 months; stool guiac every 6 months; colonoscopy at 1 year

Renal
Disease

JOSEPH H. BREZIN, MD, FACP

94. Acute Renal Failure

Etiology

- Prerenal failure is caused by renal hypoperfusion, most often due to dehydration, excessive diuresis, CHF, or any type of shock
- Intrarenal (parenchymal disease): Acute tubular necrosis; acute glomerulonephritis; atherosclerosis/thromboembolism; interstitial nephritis (β-lactams, H_2 blockers, NSAIDs), acyclovir, methotrexate, etc
- Postrenal obstruction: Prostate enlargement, bladder or ureteral obstruction (tumors, stones, lymph nodes, clot, fibrosis)
- Vascular: renal artery stenosis, aortic dissection, renal v. thrombosis

Differential Dx

- Differentiate between possible causes of acute renal failure—see the Etiology section
- Chronic renal failure

Epidemiology

- Prerenal causes account for about 1/3 of cases; intrarenal causes account for about 1/2 of cases (ATN is most common cause overall); postrenal causes account for 10%; major vascular causes account for <5%
- ATN often develops in hospital settings and is multifactorial (hypoperfusion, myoglobin, nephrotoxins, and prerenal causes)

Signs/Symptoms

- Patient may be anuric, oliguric (<30 mL/hour of urine output), or nonoliguric
- Signs and symptoms of uremia:
    - Lethargy
    - Encephalopathy, HA, confusion
    - Anorexia
    - Nausea/vomiting
    - Fluid overload, edema, heart failure
    - Hypertension
    - Metabolic acidosis
    - Hyperkalemia and arrhythmias
    - Pericarditis/friction rub
    - Asterixis
    - Fever may indicate a secondary infection

Diagnosis

- Defined as a rise in BUN and creatinine, measured over hours to days (creatinine rising >0.5 when baseline is ≤3 mg/dL and rising >1.0 when baseline is >3.0)
- Clinical history: Look for presence of possible etiologies and evaluate time course of renal failure (i.e., renal failure occurs immediately with exposure to cis-platinum; occurs 5–14 days after methicillin use; etc)
- Obtain urine sodium and creatinine to determine fractional excretion of sodium (FENa): used to distinguish prerenal causes from intrarenal parenchymal causes
- Urine sediment: Presence of RBC casts, ATN casts, pyuria, crystalluria, and bacteria indicates an intrarenal parenchymal etiology; unremarkable sediment indicates vascular disease, prerenal azotemia, or postrenal obstruction
- Ultrasound/CT: Look for obstruction/hydronephrosis
- Angiography (for vascular occlusion) and MRA
- Biopsy if prolonged episode of ARF or nephritic syndrome

Treatment

- Correct hydration, lytes, and optimize hemodynamics
    - Always save 10–20 mL urine for urinalysis and FENa before giving fluids and diuretics
- Discontinue offending agents if possible
- Attempt diuresis with high-dose loop diuretics
- Dialysis or continuous hemodiafiltration (alternative to dialysis) for symptoms of uremia, fluid overload, or hyperkalemia
- Specific treatments as indicated (i.e., nephrostomy for ureteral obstruction, plasma exchange in TTP-HUS, steroids in rapidly progressive glomerulonephritis)

Prognosis/Clinical Course

- Sudden, often reversible, interruption of renal function; prognosis depends on etiology
    - Prerenal azotemia is reversible by definition
    - Patients with oliguric ATN usually recover in 1–3 weeks
    - Patients with contrast nephropathy recover in 3–7 days
- Mortality in hospital-acquired ATN is still over 50% in surgical patients, due to multi-organ failure
- Early response to a rise in creatinine may lead to prevention of ATN in the prerenal patient
- Note: FENa = $(U_{Na} \times S_{Cr}/S_{Na} \times U_{Cr}) \times 100$

95. Acute Tubular Necrosis

Etiology

- Injury or obstruction of the tubule of the nephron; most common cause of acute renal failure; often due to ischemic injury or nephrotoxins:
  - Ischemia: Due to hemorrhage, sepsis (even without hypotension), hypotension/shock from any cause, prolonged dehydration, obstetric complications, or cardiopulmonary bypass
  - Pigmenturia (myoglobin in rhabdomyolysis, hemoglobin in hemolysis)
  - Drugs/toxins: Aminoglycosides, contrast agents with iodine, amphotericin B, cis-platinum, cyclosporine, NSAIDs, herbal remedies

Epidemiology

- Predisposing conditions include chronic renal insufficiency (especially due to diabetes mellitus and multiple myeloma), recovery from a prior episode of ATN, use of ACE inhibitors or NSAIDs prior to the renal insult (impair autoregulation of renal blood flow and GFR), underlying CHF, hypoxia, and a severe state of sepsis or injury with cytokine formation and cellular oxidative stress

Differential Dx

- Other causes of intrinsic renal failure
- Prerenal failure
- Postrenal failure

Signs/Symptoms

- Often presents in critically ill patients with significant comorbidities
- Decreased urine output
- Signs and symptoms of uremia
- Fever may signal secondary infection

Diagnosis

- Oliguria (<30 mL/hour) in 30–40% of cases
- Rising BUN and creatinine levels
- FENa >1% [FENa = $(U_{Na} \times S_{Cr}/S_{Na} \times U_{Cr}) \times 100$]
- Urinalysis: Coarse granular casts in 75–80% of cases and renal epithelial cells
- Specific etiologic presentations
  - Focal muscle weakness/swelling in rhabdomyolysis
  - Hypokalemia and renal tubular acidosis with amphotericin
  - Hypokalemia and hypomagnesemia with cis-platinum
- Biopsy is rarely needed; may show minimal tubular necrosis

Treatment

- Prevention is always the best strategy: Hydration and N-acetylcysteine can prevent or mitigate contrast nephropathy in high-risk patients; avoid prolonged exposure to potentially nephrotoxic drugs; avoid NSAIDs in patients with underlying renal disease
- Respond quickly to a decrease in urine output
- Prerenal azotemia promptly responds to hydration and hemodynamic support with pressors
- May respond to loop diuretics, with an increase in urine output but not GFR
- IABP, dialysis/CVVH
- No proven benefit from low-dose dopamine
- Atrial natriuretic peptide may be helpful in oliguric patients
- Nesiritide has not been well studied as yet

Prognosis/Clinical Course

- Recovery in 3–7 days from contrast nephropathy
- Recovery in 1–3 weeks from ischemic, toxic, or pigment-induced ATN
- More profound ischemia and the presence of comorbidities are associated with delayed recovery of up to 6 weeks
- Mortality may be as high as 50–70%
- Death is often due to secondary infection, heart failure, or multiple-organ failure
- A progenitor cell in the proximal tubule is capable of regeneration in the presence of growth factors and the absence of inflammatory cytokines

96. Nephritic Syndrome (Glomerulonephritis)

Etiology

- Injury, inflammation, and necrosis of glomeruli, resulting in abrupt onset of renal failure with rising serum creatinine, HTN, hematuria, proteinuria
- Most common etiologies include IgA nephropathy, post-streptococcal glomerulonephritis (PSGN), glomerulonephritis associated with bacterial endocarditis, Goodpasture's syndrome, SLE, hepatitis C, vasculitis (Wegener's, PAN, Churg-Strauss, HSP), thrombotic microangiopathy (TTP-HUS), idiopathic rapidly progressive glomerulonephritis, glomerulonephritis of HIV, and acute "allergic" interstitial nephritis

Differential Dx

- Acute tubular necrosis
- Various causes of acute renal failure
- Atheroembolic renal disease

Epidemiology

- PSGN occurs 1–3 weeks after streptococcal pharyngitis or impetigo; peak age 2–6 years; sporadic or epidemic
- GN can occur any time in the course of hepatitis C or bacterial endocarditis
- SLE is 8 × more common in women but the incidence of nephritis is the same in men; 20% risk of flare-up in pregnancy

Signs/Symptoms

- Hematuria (microscopic or macroscopic); dark urine
- Proteinuria
- Mild to severe hypertension
- Peripheral edema
- Oliguria or anuria in severe cases
- Signs and symptoms of uremia
- Associated pulmonary hemorrhage in Goodpasture's, SLE, or vasculitis

Diagnosis

- Active urine sediment with RBCs, WBCs, casts, protein
- Hypertension
- Subacute or rapidly progressive renal failure
- Renal biopsy is diagnostic
- Serologic studies
  - Antistreptolysin (post-streptococcal GN)
  - ANA, cANCA, pANCA
  - Serum complement for low C_3 (post-streptococcal, SLE, mixed cryoglobulinemia, MPGN)
  - Hepatitis B and C serologies
  - HIV
  - Anti-GBM antibody
- Associated clinical features (nasal septum, eye, and pulmonary involvement in Wegener's disease; rash and arthritis in SLE)
- Microangiopathic hemolytic anemia with schistocytes, increased LDH, and thrombocytopenia in TTP-HUS

Treatment

- Appropriate clinical picture should dictate prompt drawing of serologies, pulse methylprednisolone, plasmapheresis, dialysis, and renal biopsy
- Diuretics, antihypertensive treatment, and dialysis for uremia and fluid/electrolyte imbalances
- Pulse methylprednisolone (1 g) in all forms of crescenteric glomerulonephritis (Goodpasture's syndrome, SLE, Wegener's/vasculitis, idiopathic)
- Plasmapheresis in Goodpasture's syndrome, TTP-HUS, and mixed cryoglobulinemia
- IV cyclophosphamide in SLE and Wegener's disease/vasculitis
- Antibiotic/antiviral treatment in bacterial endocarditis, HIV, and other infectious causes
- Interferon-α in hepatitis C

Prognosis/Clinical Course

- Prognosis depends on biopsy results; chronic pathology (glomerular sclerosis, interstitial fibrosis, fibrotic crescents) indicates poorer prognosis
- Rapidly progressive forms of glomerulonephritis have poorer prognosis
- Excellent prognosis for post-streptococcal GN
- Good prognosis with long-term treatment of SLE and Wegener's disease/vasculitis

97. Nephrotic Syndrome

Etiology

- Increased permeability of glomerulus → significant protein excretion
- Often due to primary renal disease, secondary to infection, renal manifestations of systemic disease, or idiopathic
  - Primary renal disease: Minimal change nephropathy, idiopathic membranous nephropathy, IgA nephropathy, membranoproliferative nephritis, and focal sclerosing glomerulosclerosis (FSGS)
  - Renal manifestation of systemic disease: Amyloidosis, diabetes, SLE
  - Secondary to infection (HIV, hepatitis B and C), lymphoma, NSAIDs

Differential Dx

- CHF of various etiologies
- Cirrhosis
- In the edematous patient, always check the urine for proteinuria—many cases undergo a full workup for CHF and cirrhosis before referral to a nephrologist!

Epidemiology

- Minimal change disease accounts for >75% of cases in children <10, 50% in children >10, and 15–20% of adult cases without systemic etiologies
- Membranous in 25% of adults (most frequent in white males)
- FSGS in 30% of cases (more aggressive in blacks)

Signs/Symptoms

- Peripheral and/or periorbital edema (due to decreased oncotic pressure from protein loss)
- Other manifestations/complications
  - Hyperlipidemia with lipiduria (oval fat bodies and fatty casts)
  - Hypercoagulable state leading to DVT, thromboembolism, or renal vein thrombosis
  - Infections, due to loss of IgG in urine

Diagnosis

- Proteinuria (>3.5 g/day)
- Hypoalbuminemia
- Hyperlipidemia
- Urine sediment to detect nephrotic elements (finely granular casts, oval fat bodies, fatty casts) and associated nephritic elements (dysmorphic RBCs, RBC/WBC casts)
- Serologic studies for viral and systemic diseases
- Renal biopsy is diagnostic and should be done in most adult cases
- Clinical response to steroids in young children is suggestive of minimal change disease

Treatment

- Fluid/electrolyte management
- Careful diuretic prescription
- Statins are useful to control symptoms and prevent complications of hyperlipidemia
- ACE inhibitors or angiotensin receptor blockers may reduce proteinuria and slow progression
- Minimal change disease: Prednisone × 14–16 wks
- Membranous nephropathy
  - 1/3 of cases remit spontaneously
  - Treatment depends on stage, complications, and duration of disease
  - Treat with cytotoxic drugs (cyclophosphamide or chlorambucil) and steroids
- FSGS: High-dose steroids or cyclosporin
- Treatment of primary infection or malignancy and stopping suspect drugs is crucial

Prognosis/Clinical Course

- Prognosis depends on the specific underlying disease; it may resolve with few complications, as in minimal change disease, or progress to renal failure, as is common in membranous nephropathy
- This disease is the most symptomatic renal syndrome; patients complain of edema and can often identify its onset precisely

98. Acute Interstitial Kidney Disease

Etiology

• Acute interstitial nephritis (AIN) is a cell-mediated inflammation, most commonly due to drugs (e.g., β-lactam antibiotics, sulfonamides including diuretics, NSAIDs, cimetidine, ciprofloxacin, allopurinol, rifampin); myeloma kidney with tubular casts; heavy metal exposure (lead, mercury, cadmium); ischemic papillary necrosis and inflammation in sickle cell disease; or nephrocalcinosis in hypercalcemic disorders and Type 1 RTA

Differential Dx

• Chronic interstitial nephritis
• Glomerulonephritis
• Acute renal failure of various etiologies
• Hypertensive nephrosclerosis

Epidemiology

• Analgesic nephropathy requires years of heavy use with a mixture of aspirin and acetaminophen/phenacetin
• Check for occupational exposure to lead, mercury, or cadmium (e.g., alkaline battery workers)

Signs/Symptoms

• Signs and symptoms of renal failure
• Fever
• Rash
• Flank pain in some cases
• Skeletal pain and severe anemia in myeloma

Diagnosis

• Clinical history is important
• Pyuria, hematuria, and eosinophiluria; WBC casts
• Ultrasound: Results depend on the underlying etiology (small irregular kidneys in analgesic nephropathy, normal to large echodense kidneys in myeloma, renal calcification in nephrocalcinosis, and so on)
• Renal biopsy
• Anemia, hypercalcemia, elevated total protein, and back pain suggest multiple myeloma; confirm with protein electropheresis and bone marrow biopsy
• Nephrotic syndrome may occur with NSAID use
• Prominent hyperuricemia and tophaceous gout in lead nephropathy

Treatment

• Stop incriminating drugs
• Two-week trial of prednisone 1 mg/kg/day
• Management of acute or chronic renal failure, including dialysis, if necessary

Prognosis/Clinical Course

• Full recovery if diagnosis is made promptly before severe interstitial fibrosis develops
• Stabilization or partial recovery sometimes occurs with successful treatment of myeloma
• Interstitial disease should be considered in unexplained renal failure in ambulatory or hospitalized patients receiving multiple drugs
• Responsible for 10% of cases of acute renal failure

99. Chronic Kidney Disease*

Etiology

Formerly called chronic renal failure or chronic renal insufficiency
- End-stage renal disease (ESRD) due to gradual loss of renal function or sudden onset of rapidly progressive renal disease
- May develop on top of acute renal failure
- Diabetic nephropathy accounts for nearly 50% of cases; hypertension (25%); glomerulonephritis (10%); renal cystic disease; other urologic pathology (congenital disease, obstruction); myeloma; amyloid; atheroemboli; Fabry's disease; HUS; analgesic abuse; idiopathic

Epidemiology

- Current dialysis population of 250,000
- >50,000 people have functional renal transplants
- NHANES III estimated that 10.9 million Americans had CKD with serum creatinine >1.5 and 800,000 had creatinine >2.0
- The incidence of diabetes as an etiology exceeds 60% in hispanics
- Blacks and Native Americans have 3 × higher risk

Differential Dx

- Acute renal failure

Signs/Symptoms

- GFR of 25–50: Few symptoms
- GFR of 10–25
  - Hypertension
  - Anemia (↓ erythropoeitin production)
  - Fluid retention
  - Hyperkalemia
  - Metabolic acidosis (anion gap)
  - Hyperphosphatemia and hypocalcemia, resulting in secondary hyperparathyroidism with bone pain
- GFR <10: ESRD; signs of uremia
  - Anorexia, nausea, vomiting, wt loss
  - Metabolic encephalopathy (poor attention, slowing on EEG, asterixis)
  - Pruritis   – Peripheral
  - Pericarditis   neuropathy
                             – Bleeding

Diagnosis

- Serum creatinine is used as a rough indicator
- There are several estimates of GFR, such as $[(140 - \text{age}) \times (\text{weight in kg})]/72 \times P_{Cr}$
- Normal GFR is > 90 at age 40 (serum creatinine 0.8–1.2)
- Mild CKD: GFR 50–90 (creatinine 1.0–2.5)
- Moderate CKD: GFR 25–50 (creatinine 1.2–4)
- Severe CKD: GFR 10–25 (creatinine (2–8)
- ESRD: GFR < 10 (creatinine 4–15)
- Differentiate from acute, reversible renal failure by persistence over time (>3 months) and failure to respond to hydration, discontinuation of medications, and specific treatments
- Renal imaging (ultrasound is the best initial screen), urinalysis, and renal biopsy to determine etiology
- Follow CBC, electrolytes, calcium, parathyroid hormone level and correct abnormalities as necessary

Treatment

- Protect kidneys: Control BP to ≤ 130/75 and use ACE inhibitors or angiotensin receptor blockers in maximum tolerated doses in diabetic patients or patients with excessive proteinuria (≥1 g/day)
- Treat specific disease entities (i.e., SLE, myeloma)
- Assess and treat for reversible factors: Adverse drug effects, obstruction, infection, fluid imbalance
- Dietary restrictions: Fluid and sodium restriction to prevent secondary HTN; protein restriction (extreme protein restriction is not proven to be helpful); phosphate/potassium restriction
- Treat anemia with iron replacement and recombinant erythropoietin (Hb target of 11–12 g/dL)
- Phosphate binders (Ca^{++}-containing or non-Ca^{++}) and calcitrol when phosphate <5.5 mg/dL
- Use diuretics judiciously
- Dialysis and renal transplant

Prognosis/Clinical Course

- Renal disease is inexorably progressive
- The rate of GFR decline can be reduced or even halted with aggressive blood pressure control using ACE inhibitors or angiotensin receptor blockers in diabetic and nondiabetic renal disease with proteinuria
- Early treatment in diabetics with preserved GFR is the key to success
- CKD is a major independent risk factor for cardiovascular mortality
- Plan for creation of AV fistulas (for dialysis) 6–12 months before the projected date of ESRD and educate the patient about transplant and all dialysis options (hemodialysis, peritoneal)

100. Adult Polycystic Kidney Disease

Etiology

- Adult PKD is caused by autosomal dominant mutations at *PKD1* (chromosome 16) and *PKD2* (chromosome 4); these genes encode polycystins, which interact to alter cellular differentiation, proliferation and transport, and apoptosis
- Focal clusters of cysts do not develop until adulthood; it is thought that random mutations in the normal allele of tubular cells initiate the process
- An autosomal recessive form is caused by mutations on chromosome 6, involves more tubular segments, and frequently causes renal failure in childhood

Differential Dx

- Multiple simple cysts
- Tuberous sclerosis
- Von Hippel-Lindau disease
- Renal cell carcinoma
- Chronic renal failure of other etiologies

Epidemiology

- Adult PKD does not usually present clinically until the fourth or fifth decade but can be detected earlier by ultrasound or CT scan; although the gene is expressed 100% of patients, they may present earlier or be asymptomatic even at age 80
- Affects only 0.1% of the population but is responsible for 8% of ESRD
- Family history in 60% of cases

Signs/Symptoms

- Flank pain due to cyst enlargement or infection, symptoms of a UTI, and/or associated kidney stones
- Gross hematuria
- Increased abdominal girth with palpable abdominal mass
- Frequently associated with hypertension and progressive kidney failure
- Also associated with hepatic cysts, intracerebral aneurysms, aortic aneurysms, diverticulosis, and abdominal/inguinal hernias

Diagnosis

- Positive family history in 60% of cases
- Clinical signs and symptoms
- Renal imaging (ultrasound or CT) reveals enlarged kidneys with multiple cysts (criteria vary with age) in each kidney
- DNA linkage analysis in at least 2 family members is more than 99% accurate
- MRA to detect intracerebral aneurysms is reserved for patients with a notable family history of this complication, persistent/severe headaches, and/or associated neurological symptoms

Treatment

- Analgesia
- Bed rest for hematuria
- Aggressive treatment of infection and stones
- Treatment of hypertension is important but does not affect progressive kidney failure
- Kidney replacement
- Genetic counseling is available for patients and families; screening can be considered after age 18

Prognosis/Clinical Course

- End-stage renal disease develops in 45% of cases by age 60
- Persistent urinary tract/cyst infections accelerate the progression of ESRD
- *PKD1* mutation is associated with a greater incidence of gross hematuria and earlier development of renal failure

101. Nephrolithiasis

Etiology

- Calcium oxalate stones are most common (65%); others include calcium phosphate, uric acid, and struvite (magnesium ammonium phosphate)
- Most often due to increased concentration of stone-forming material in urine either due to increased excretion or decreased urinary volume
- Calcium-containing stones are due to ↑ urinary calcium/oxalate excretion (i.e., excess calcium absorption from bone in primary hyperparathyroidism)
- Uric acid stones are common in patients with gout
- Struvite stones are usually due to urea-splitting organisms such as *Proteus*

Epidemiology

- Incidence in US is less than 0.5%; lifetime incidence is 10%
- Males > females
- Whites > blacks
- Young to middle-aged adults
- Paradoxically, high dietary calcium intake may decrease the risk of stones as it forms ligands with dietary oxalate and phosphate

Differential Dx

- Pyelonephritis
- Papillary necrosis
- Renal cell carcinoma
- Transitional cell carcinoma
- Back injury/spasm
- Broken ribs
- Herpes zoster
- Dissecting aortic aneurysm
- Biliary colic
- Pancreatitis

Signs/Symptoms

- Severe, acute, colicky flank pain
- Hematuria (stone in kidney) often with radiation to testicle or labia
- Severe, acute urethral pain (stone passing through urethra)
- Nausea/vomiting are common
- Dysuria, urgency, and frequency are less common
- Obstruction of ureter may result in anuria or acute renal failure in patients with a single functioning kidney; rarely, bilateral ureteral obstruction may occur
- Fever/chills and other constitutional symptoms if infection complicates the picture
- CVA tenderness

Diagnosis

- A history of flank pain and the presence of microscopic or gross hematuria mandates imaging studies
- Urinalysis, urine pH, and urine culture
- Spiral CT and abdominal films may be diagnostic if the stone is radio-opaque (Ca^{++}-containing stones, struvite, cysteine)
- Ultrasound and intravenous pyelogram for radiolucent stones, to better localize stones, and to detect obstruction
- Search for etiology of stone, especially if recurrent
  - Strain urine and send stone to the lab if possible
  - 24-hour urine collection for volume, pH, calcium, citrate, oxalate, phosphorus, uric acid, ammonium, magnesium
  - Serum chemistries and parathyroid hormone evaluation
  - Consider many systemic diseases that can contribute to development of urolithiasis (e.g., gout, enzyme deficiencies, malignancy, sarcoidosis)

Treatment

- Surgically active stone disease (passing a stone) is treated with hydration and analgesics (NSAIDs, narcotics)
- Stones too large to pass require external shock wave lithotripsy, cystoscopic or ureteroscopic laser lithotripsy, stenting, basket retrieval, or urolithotomy
- Admit to hospital if patient is unable to keep fluids down or pain is not adequately managed
- Treat infection if present (see UTI entry for choices)
- Prevention via increased water intake (>3 L/day)
- Directed treatment depending on type of stone
  - Limit sodium intake and thiazide diuretics for Ca^{++}-containing stones with hypercalciuria
  - Dietary oxalate reduction if hyperoxaluria
  - Alkalinize urine and allopurinol if hyperuricosuria
  - Penicillamine for cystinuria

Prognosis/Clinical Course

- 90% of stones <4 mm pass spontaneously
- <10% of stones >6 mm pass spontaneously
- Prognosis depends on the type of stone and the primary cause for stone formation
- Recurrence is very common—14% at one year after first stone and 75% at 20 years
- All patients should be counseled to increase water intake after passing their first stone

102. Renal Cell Carcinoma

Etiology

- Simple cysts account for 70% of renal masses
- Solid renal masses include benign tumors, such as angiomyolipoma and oncocytoma, and malignant tumors, such as renal cell carcinoma, transitional cell carcinoma, and metastatic cancers (breast, lung, ovarian)
- Renal cell carcinoma accounts for >90% of renal malignancies in adults (Wilm's tumor is the most common etiology of intra-abdominal mass in neonates and infants)
- Most renal masses arise from the proximal tubule epithelium

Differential Dx

- Renal cyst
- Angiomyolipoma
- Oncocytoma
- Metastatic cancer
- Transitional cell carcinoma
- Sarcoma
- Lymphoma
- Pyelonephritis
- Renal abscess

Epidemiology

- Renal cell carcinoma accounts for 2% of all cancers
- Males > females
- Ages 50–70
- About 25% of cases are metastatic at diagnosis (to lung, brain, or bone)
- Risk factors include von Hippel Lindau disease, acquired renal cystic disease associated with end-stage renal failure, smoking, obesity

Signs/Symptoms

- Classic triad
  - Hematuria
  - Abdominal pain
  - Abdominal or flank mass
- Other symptoms include fever, night sweats, and weight loss
- Symptoms of anemia and hypercalcemia may be present
- Signs and symptoms of metastases to lung, brain, and/or bone may infrequently be the presenting finding

Diagnosis

- CT of abdomen and pelvis is often diagnostic—any solid renal mass should be assumed malignant until proven otherwise
- MRI is useful to evaluate the renal vein and inferior vena cava for metastases
- Urinalysis and urine cytology
- Chest X-ray and/or chest CT to evaluate for pulmonary metastases
- Bone scan to evaluate bone metastases

Treatment

- Nephrectomy (partial or complete) is the definitive cure
  - Partial nephrectomy may be sufficient for peripheral tumors <4 cm
  - Partial nephrectomy for patients with only one kidney
- Radiation and chemotherapy are *not* useful
- Interferon-α, interleukin-2, and allogenic stem cell transplants are used in refractory cases

Prognosis/Clinical Course

- Staging
  - Stage 1: Confined within renal capsule; >60% 5-year survival
  - Stage 2: Extending through capsule but only to Gerota's fascia; >60% 5-year survival
  - Stage 3: Renal vein, inferior vena cava, and/or local lymph node spread
  - Stage 4: Distant metastases; mean survival of 1 year; <10% 5-year survival
- Spontaneous remissions have been reported

Infectious Disease

JOSE DELGADO, MD

103. Sepsis

Etiology

- A systemic response to infection that compromises organ perfusion and may lead to multiorgan failure
- Release of endotoxin (generally by gram-negative bacteria) → induces production of tumor necrosis factor and interleukins → triggers systemic inflammatory response and hypotension
- Most commonly due to gram-negative rods (*Pseudomonas, Serratia, Klebsiella, E. coli*); also gram-positive organisms, fungi (*Candida*), and viruses

Differential Dx

- Cardiogenic shock
- Neurogenic shock
- Hypovolemic shock

Epidemiology

- Leading cause of death in hospitalized patients
- Increased incidence in immunosuppressed, neutropenic patients, IV line carriers, elderly, diabetics, asplenic patients, and alcoholics
- Mortality rises with the number of organs involved
- Incidence: 400,000 cases per year

Signs/Symptoms

- Fevers/chills
- Hypotension
- Hyperventilation
- Hypothermia
- Mental status changes
- Tachycardia, cardiovascular collapse, decreased SVR, normal pulmonary wedge pressure
- Local signs of infection (i.e., cough, SOB, dysuria, diarrhea, heart murmur, signs of cellulitis, and abdominal pain, depending on initial cause of infection)
- End organ failure may ensue (lung, kidney, heart)

Diagnosis

- Clinical diagnosis is based on the finding of hypotension that is unresponsive to fluid resuscitation
- Workup is directed to find infectious focus
  – CXR
  – Blood cultures × 2
  – Urinalysis and culture
  – CT scan of potentially affected areas
  – Culture of infected lines or devices
  – Lumbar puncture if meningitis or CNS involvement is suspected
  – Pulmonary artery catheterization if hemodynamic questions arise
- Leukopenia, thrombocytopenia, DIC may be present

Treatment

- Direct antibiotic treatment against primary infection
- Remove any indwelling catheters or other medical devices if possible
- Drain associated abscess
- Hemodynamic support is essential—vasopressors include norepinephrine and dopamine
- Supportive therapies as needed: Dialysis, continuous hemofiltration, mechanical ventilation, plasmapheresis

Prognosis/Clinical Course

- Mortality increases as organ failure increases

104. Cellulitis

Etiology

- Infection of skin and soft tissues
- Generally caused by gram-positive bacteria, especially *Streptococcus* group A or *Staphylococcus aureus* (*Haemophilus influenzae* is more common in children)
- Infection causes local cytokine release, which mediates local and systemic signs and symptoms

Epidemiology

- Very common complication in diabetes patients and patients with poor vascular circulation
- Immunosuppression, trauma, and poor hygiene are risk factors
- Animal bite may cause infection by direct inoculation
- Erysipelas and impetigo are more common superficial skin infections in children

Differential Dx

- Sunburn
- Contact dermatitis
- Skin cancer
- Acne
- Folliculitis
- Necrotizing fasciitis
- Lymphangitis
- DVT
- Arterial or venous insufficiency
- STDs
- HSV or shingles
- Post-radiation changes

Signs/Symptoms

- Redness and warmth of affected skin and soft tissues due to local inflammatory changes
- Tender lymphadenopathy, lymphangitis, and abscess may be present
- Systemic symptoms include fever, rigors, and possible change in mental status in elderly

Diagnosis

- Clinical diagnosis
- Blood cultures required in patients with systemic symptoms
- CBC: Leukocytosis with left shift
- Local X-ray if osteomyelitis is suspected
- Check renal function in diabetics and elderly before the administration of antibiotics
- Head CT required in periorbital or orbital cellulitis to evaluate extension of infection to venous sinuses
- Direct cultures are generally not helpful; if desired, do a punch biopsy with the specimen placed in non-bacteriostatic saline and send for culture
- Diagnosis of streptococcal cellulitis can be supported by ASO, anti-hyaluronidase, or anti-deoxyribonuclease tests, although they are not routinely used

Treatment

- Antibiotic coverage of *Streptococcus* group A and *S. aureus*
- IV or oral antibiotics (depending on severity) for 7–14 days
    - Cephalexin 500 mg po QID
    - Amoxicillin/clavulanate 250–500 mg po TID
    - Nafcillin 1–2 g IV q 4 hours
    - Cefazolin 1 g IV TID
    - Clindamycin 600 mg IV TID
- May involve unusual or resistant organisms; adjust therapy as needed
- Recommendations for diabetics
    - Ampicillin/sulbactam 3 g IV QID
    - Strict glucose control

Prognosis/Clinical Course

- Generally excellent prognosis
- Spontaneous resolution over a few weeks
- Complications
    - Local abscess formation
    - Osteomyelitis
    - Lymphatic obstruction
    - Periorbital or orbital infection
    - Cavernous sinus thrombosis
    - Brain abscess

105. Infectious Diarrhea

Etiology

- Diarrhea is an increased number or amount of bowel movements
- May be acute (<5 days) or chronic
- Caused by (there are additional causes in AIDS patients):
  - *Salmonella*
  - *Staphylococcus aureus* toxin
  - *Shigella*
  - *Giardia*
  - *E. coli*
  - *Clostridium botulinum*
  - *C. perfringens*
  - *C. difficile*
  - *Campylobacter jejuni*
  - *Vibrio cholerae* toxin
  - *Viral (Norwalk, rotavirus)*
  - *Yersinia*
  - *Entamocha histolytica*
  - *Bacillus cereus*

Differential Dx

- Ischemic bowel
- Colon cancer
- Irritable bowel
- Inflammatory bowel disease
- Appendicitis
- Diverticulitis
- Malabsorption syndrome (bacterial overgrowth, short gut, sprue)
- Laxative abuse
- Whipple's disease
- Drug-induced diarrhea (quinidine, colchicine, amiodarone, clindamycin)
- Endocrine (hyperthyroidism, VIPoma, gastrinoma)

Epidemiology

- Isolation of pathogens is possible in about half of cases
- Most common transmission is food-borne or fecal-oral
- Associated with recent travel, eating out, uncooked food, seafood, poorly refrigerated food

Signs/Symptoms

- Increased frequency or quantity of bowel movements
- Dysentery (bloody, mucous stools associated with rectal tenesmus) may be present (especially seen in *E. histolytica* infection)
- Dehydration (hypotension, orthostasis, tachycardia)
- Low-grade fever
- Flatulence with foul-smelling stool (especially in *Giardia* infection)
- Weight loss
- Anal excoriations
- Abdominal cramps

Diagnosis

- Diagnosis is often based on clinical presentation and epidemiology
- WBCs in stool indicates invasive/bacterial diarrhea or inflammation of mucosa (inflammatory bowel disease)
- Stool cultures and ova/parasite screens
- Test for *C. difficile* toxin in stool
- Stool osmolar gap
  - Gap > 50 indicates osmotic diarrhea due to laxatives, malabsorption, or other sources
  - Gap < 50 indicates secretory diarrhea, which may be bacterial/viral toxin mediated

Treatment

- Treatment is primarily supportive
- Avoid Imodium; kaopectate is acceptable
- If proof of bacterial cause, treat specific to pathogen
  - *Shigella:* Quinolone or TMP/SMX × 5 days
  - *C. difficile:* Metronidazole is first-line therapy; if ineffective, oral vancomycin for 10 days
  - *C. jejuni:* Erythromycin/tetracycline × 5 days
  - Treat *Salmonella only* if systemic symptoms, bacteremia, or HIV-positive
  - Only enterotoxigenic *E. coli* (traveler's diarrhea) is treatable with antibiotics—antibiotics for enteroinvasive *E. coli* may result in HUS
  - *Vibrio cholera:* Tetracycline × 10 days
  - *Giardia:* Metronidazole × 3–5 days
  - *E. histolytica:* Metronidazole × 14 days

Prognosis/Clinical Course

- Good prognosis with supportive measures
- Patients may develop acute renal failure secondary to hemolytic-uremic syndrome
- Carrier status develops with *Salmonella* and *C. difficile*

106. Influenza

Etiology

- Acute respiratory illness caused by influenza viruses
- High morbidity and mortality in high-risk populations
- Influenza A is responsible for most cases; influenza B is often the cause of epidemics
- Human-to-human transmission via respiratory particles

Differential Dx

- Atypical pneumonia (especially *Mycoplasma*)
- Severe streptococcal pharyngitis
- Other viral illnesses

Epidemiology

- Multiple epidemics and pandemics have been reported
- Most common in urban areas
- Winter is "flu season"
- Higher risk in elderly, patients with cardiac or pulmonary disease, diabetes, IgA deficiency, HIV, immunodeficiencies of any type, and health care workers

Signs/Symptoms

- High fever
- General malaise with myalgias
- Severe frontal headache
- Cough
- Chest congestion
- Sore throat
- Photophobia and pain with eye motion
- Cervical lymphadenopathy
- Patient may have cardiac (myocarditis) or CNS involvement (encephalitis, meningitis)
- In bacterial superinfection: SOB, chest tightness, prostration

Diagnosis

- Clinical exam and epidemiologic history are most important
- Rapid influenza test (immunofluorescence) is very good for initial guidance; 50–80% sensitivity; take swabs from nose and throat
- Chest X-ray to rule out bacterial superinfection (most commonly *Streptococcus pneumoniae* and *Staphylococcus aureus*); may see micronodular calcifications and diffuse atypical infiltrates
- Monitor ABG carefully for hypoxemia
- CBC may show leukopenia or lymphocytosis

Treatment

- In general, symptomatic treatment is best
- Amantadine (effective only for influenza A) and rimantadine decrease the severity and length of infection in <50% of patients if started in the first 48 hours of symptoms
- Inhaled antivirals (zanamivir) also decrease the length of infection if used early
- Benefits of antivirals may appear only in younger populations
- Major goal of treatment for high-risk populations is to keep ideal oxygenation and prevent bacterial superinfection
- Do not use aspirin—may result in Reye's syndrome

Prognosis/Clinical Course

- Prognosis is excellent in younger populations
- Poorer prognosis in the elderly and in patients with comorbidities
- Vaccination should be administered in any high-risk population during the fall of every year

107. Lyme Disease

Etiology

- An infection by a spirochete, *Borrelia burgdorferi*
- Transmitted by a vector (ticks)
- *Ixodes scapularis* (deer tick) is the principal vector in the US

Differential Dx

- Cellulitis
- Fibromyalgia
- Rheumatoid arthritis
- CVD
- Meningitis
- HIV
- Multiple myeloma

Epidemiology

- Most common vector-borne infection in the US
- Most common in the Northeast and Midwest

Signs/Symptoms

- Stage I: Erythema migrans
  - Cutaneous annular lesion with clear center and reddish periphery
  - Begins at area of bite, then migrates
- Stage II: 2–4 weeks after stage I
  - Hematogenous spread occurs
  - HA, fatigue, sore throat, fever/chills, muscle aches, joint aches, hepatitis
  - Neurologic: Meningitis, Bell's palsy, polyneuropathy (toe drop)
  - Cardiovascular: Carditis, AV block
- Stage III: Months to years later
  - Frank arthritis (knees especially), encephalopathy (loss of memory, mood changes, sleep changes)
  - Acrodermatitis chronica atrophicans

Diagnosis

- Diagnosis is made by stage
- Stage I
  - Presence of erythema migrans plus history is enough for diagnosis
- Stage II
  - History suspicious of disease
  - Lumbar puncture may show lymphocytic pleocytosis
  - Examine CSF for IgM and IgG
  - EKG for suspected heart block
- Stage III
  - Serologies in suspicious patients (ELISA and Western blot)

Treatment

- Stage I
  - Oral antibiotics for 21 days: Doxycycline is the antibiotic of choice; others include amoxicillin and cefuroxime
- Stages II and III
  - IV antibiotics give faster resolution, but oral doxycycline can be used
  - IV ceftriaxone or penicillin G for 30 days if arthritis, AV block, or progressive neurologic involvement
  - Pacemaker may be necessary

Prognosis/Clinical Course

- Excellent prognosis after treatment
- Most patients eventually recover without sequelae
- Patients may continue to suffer arthritis even after treatment
- Vaccination now available
  - Decreases infection by 50% after 2 doses and 75% after 3 doses
  - Should be used only in high-risk patients who have repetitive exposure to ticks

108. Neutropenic Fever

Etiology

- Fever with a total neutrophil count (neutrophils plus bands) <500/mm^3
- Most common organisms
  - Gram-negative organisms (especially from GI source): *E. coli, Pseudomonas, Serratia, Enterobacter*
  - Gram-positive organisms: *Staphylococcus, Streptococcus*
  - Fungi: *Candida, Aspergillus, Mucor,* and others

Differential Dx

Epidemiology

- Most common in hematopoietic and lymphoid malignancies and following chemotherapy

Signs/Symptoms

- Fever and associated symptoms
- An infectious focus may be found, including sinusitis, skin lesions, mucositis, pneumonia, UTI, line infection, endocarditis, vaginal lesions, or perirectal abscess

Diagnosis

- Fever >38.2°C (101°F) and neutrophil count <500/mm^3
- Attempt to find focus of infection
  - Blood cultures × 2; culture lines if present
  - Chest X-ray: Note that it may be difficult for patients with neutropenia to produce infiltrates
- Urinalysis and cultures
- Sputum cultures
- Sinus X-ray if signs of sinusitis
- Lumbar puncture if signs of meningeal irritation or altered mental status
- Consider viral cultures for CMV and/or herpes

Treatment

- Neutropenic diet and isolation are recommended
- Treat the primary cause of neutropenia
- Guide choice of antibiotic by culture results
  - Initial treatment against gram-negatives: IV ceftazidime, cefepime, piperacillin plus aminoglycoside, or imipenem plus aminoglycoside
  - Cover gram-positive organisms (with vancomycin) if signs of line infection or shock
  - If fever continues for 4–7 days after antibiotics have begun, treat with amphotericin to cover fungi
  - Acyclovir if herpes simplex infection is suspected (gancyclovir for CMV)
  - Patients with hematologic malignancies have a higher incidence of encapsulated organisms (pneumococci, meningococci, *Haemophilus*)
- Colony-stimulating factor if neutrophil count <100, pneumonia, hypotension, sepsis, or fungal infection

Prognosis/Clinical Course

- Good prognosis if treated early and sepsis is prevented
- Patient usually recovers in 7–10 days after neutropenia is resolved

109. Osteomyelitis

Etiology

- Infxn of bone and marrow due to direct inoculation or hematogenous spread
- Majority of cases are due to hematogenous spread—in theory, may result from any bacteremic episode; other causes include spread from contiguous tissues in patients with poor circulation (i.e., diabetics due to foot ulcers, patients with PVD), after orthopedic surgery and prostheses
- *Staphylococcus aureus* causes 50% of cases; also *E. coli*; Group B strep; *Serratia* and *Pseudomonas* in IV drug use; *Salmonella* if hemoglobinopathies; TB (usually in spine—Pott's disease); *Pasteurella* in cat/dog bite

Epidemiology

- Common infection with high morbidity
- Risk factors include immunodeficiency, asplenia, diabetes mellitus, and IV drug use
- Important cause of fever of unknown origin

Differential Dx

- Cellulitis
- Fracture
- Stress fracture
- Bone metastasis
- Primary bone tumor
- Postoperative hematoma
- Soft tissue abscess
- Paget's disease
- Avascular necrosis
- Suppurative arthritis

Signs/Symptoms

- Most commonly affected areas include the back/spine, foot, and toe
- Fever/chills
- Pain and point tenderness in the involved area
- Redness, warmth, crepitus, and pus drainage may be present
- Loss of function
- Soft tissue abscess may be present
- Hypotension if septic shock develops

Diagnosis

- CBC may show leukocytosis with left shift
- X-ray is the first tool for diagnosis
- Bone scan if X-ray is not conclusive: 95% sensitive but does not differentiate infection from fractures or tumors
- CT is useful to determine the extent of disease
- MRI to evaluate osteomyelitis of the spine; will also evaluate for possible epidural abscess
- Needle aspiration and blood cultures to isolate pathogen
- Surgical debridement may be diagnostic and therapeutic
- Wound cultures have a low yield because they are often contaminated with multiple pathogens
- Presence of gas or crepitus in wound may indicate anaerobic infection, which is common in contiguous spread from diabetic foot ulcers
- Any ulcer more than 2 weeks old should raise a suspicion of osteomyelitis

Treatment

- Treat empirically—be sure to cover *S. aureus*
  - IV nafcillin or 1st generation cephalosporin is a good choice for uncomplicated infections
  - Obtain cultures before beginning treatment
  - Narrow antibiotic choice once definitive cultures are completed
- If anaerobes are suspected→ Unasyn or clindamycin
- If gram-negative organisms are suspected→ 3rd generation cephalosporin plus aminoglycoside; other options are a quinolone, Unasyn, or Zosyn
- If patient looks septic, treat with broad-spectrum antibiotics until cultures return
- Treat all cases for 4–6 weeks with IV or oral quinolone
  - PICC lines may not be advisable in some patients (i.e., drug abusers)
- Operative treatment may be necessary to debride necrotic tissue and drain associated abscess

Prognosis/Clinical Course

- Prognosis is good if detected early
- If antibiotics are not effective, check for sensitivity or uncommon pathogens
- If patient does not respond to therapy, amputation may be necessary
- Educate patient to prevent further episodes, especially in the case of diabetics with recurrent foot lesions

110. Septic Arthritis

Etiology

- Acute infection of the synovial space
- Hematogenous spread is most common
- Usually bacterial; fungi and viruses may produce a more chronic picture
  - *Staphylococcus aureus* is the most common cause
  - Group B *Streptococcus* is most common in infants
  - *N. gonorrhoeae* is most common in sexually active young adults
  - Also *Streptococcus pneumoniae, S. pyogenes,* TB, *Pasteurella* (dog/cat bites), and gram-negative rods (esp *Pseudomonas* and *E. coli*)

Epidemiology

- Women are at higher risk during menses

Differential Dx

- Fracture
- Hemarthrosis
- Foreign body
- Rheumatoid arthritis
- Osteoarthritis
- Avascular necrosis
- Meniscal rupture
- Disseminated TB
- Reactive arthritis
- Reiter's syndrome
- Gout
- Lyme disease
- Pseudogout

Signs/Symptoms

- Fever/chills
- Mono- or oligoarticular arthritis
- Warmth, redness, and tenderness around the affected joint
- Decreased range of motion
- Signs of synovitis
- Knee is most commonly involved joint

Diagnosis

- Arthrocentesis
  - More than 75,000 white blood cells with a predominance of PMNs
  - Generally positive Gram stain
  - Absence of crystals
  - Purulent fluid
  - Low pH
- Synovial fluid cultures (for gonorrhea; also culture urethra/cervix, rectum, and pharynx)
- CBC: Leukocytosis with left shift

Treatment

- Initial empiric coverage with IV 3rd generation cephalosporin (cefotaxime, ceftriaxone) to cover *S. aureus* and *N. gonorrhoeae*
- Definitive antibiotics once pathogen is isolated and cultured
- Treatment usually lasts for 14 days (3–4 weeks for pyogenic organisms)

Prognosis/Clinical Course

- Excellent prognosis when antibiotics are started early; more damage to synovium with delayed treatment
- Orthopedics should be involved as surgical intervention may be indicated
- If *N. gonorrhoeae* is the causative organism, treat for *Chlamydia* infection as well and screen for other STDs

111. HIV

Etiology

- HIV-1 is a retrovirus that infects CD4 T-helper cells resulting in humoral and cellular immune deficiency and the development of multiple opportunistic and nonopportunistic infections
- AIDS is defined as a CD4 T-helper cell count <200 or the presence of any AIDS-defining infection
- HIV-2 infection occurs in West Africa; it has a longer latent period
- Transmitted by blood products, sex, IV drug use, perinatal infection, breast feeding, and open wound–fluid interchange

Epidemiology

- More than 50 million people are infected worldwide
- 90% are heterosexual
- Nearly 1 million people are infected in the US yearly
- Transfusion risk = 1:1,000,000
- Occupational risk after needle stick << 1%

Differential Dx

- CD4 > 500: *Candida* vaginitis, meningitis
- CD4 200–500: Bacterial pneumonia, thrush, anemia, cervical cancer, ITP, lymphoma
- CD4 < 200: PCP, miliary TB, histoplasmosis, coccidiomycosis, NHL, PML, HIV dementia
- CD4 < 100: Disseminated herpes, pharyngeal *Candida,* toxoplasmosis, cryptoccocosis
- CD4 < 50: CNS lymphoma, disseminated CMV/MAI
- Herpes simplex, Zoster, TB may occur any time

Signs/Symptoms

- Initial presentation during serum conversion is a flu-like syndrome that occurs within 12 weeks of infxn: Fever, chills, cough, myalgias, adenopathy
- Asymptomatic period of 2–10 or more years after initial immune response as CD4 T-helper cell counts decline
- Once CD4 cells are sufficiently depleted, patients experience multiple opportunistic infections
  – Presents as URIs, UTIs, diarrhea, TB, meningitis, skin infections, abscesses, lymphoma, squamous cell cancer, Kaposi's sarcoma
  – New onset of thrombocytopenia and Bell's palsy are characteristic of HIV infection

Diagnosis

- Positive ELISA test and Western blot are diagnostic
- Viral load test and CD4 counts every 3–6 months to follow the course of the disease
- Routine CBC, creatinine, and LFTs to follow possible side effects of medications
- Other diagnostic tests depend on the presenting opportunistic infection
- All HIV-positive patients should be screened for STDs
- Obtain baseline PPD, RPR, hepatitis B serologies, toxoplasma serology, CMV, VZV, CXR, Pap smear
- See also the HIV-Related Lung Disease entry

Treatment

- Strict adherence to antiretrovirals is essential
- Antiretrovirals include nucleoside reverse transcriptase inhibitors (AZT, ddI, d4T, 3TC), non-nucleoside reverse transcriptase inhibitors (e.g., efavirenz), and protease inhibitors (e.g., indinivir)
- Begin asymptomatic treatment when CD4 <350 or viral load >30,000
- "Triple therapy" is the rule (to avoid/prolong resistance): Initial combinations include indinivir + ZDV + lamivudine, nelfinavir + d4T + ddI, indinivir + ZDV + ddI, efavirenz + ddI + ZDV
- Once PCP, *Cryptococcus* infection, or CMV retinitis develops, long-term antimicrobial suppression is recommended
- Treat positive PPDs (>5mm) with isoniazid for 9 months or rifampin plus pyrazinamide 2 months

Prognosis/Clinical Course

- Once the patient begins antiviral therapy, follow CD4 count and viral load every 3 mo and follow resistance studies of medications
- Good prognosis as long as CD4 count remains elevated and viral resistance does not develop
- Regular full physical exam, Pap smear, and ophthalmic and dental examinations
- Since introduction of triple antiviral therapy, life expectancy has increased considerably
- Poor prognostic factors are the development of progressive multifocal leukoencephalopathy (PML) and malignancies
- Complications include psychosis, HIV dementia, wasting syndrome, depression, severe anemia, and ITP
- Psychiatric and family support is strongly encouraged

112. Anthrax

Etiology

- Caused by *Bacillus anthracis,* a gram-positive rod
- Three types of anthrax:
  - Cutaneous anthrax (>95% of cases): Introduction of spores into subepidermal tissue through a skin lesion (e.g., cut, scrape, insect bite)
  - Pulmonary anthrax: Inhalation of airborne spores
  - GI anthrax: Ingestion of spores, most commonly in contaminated food

Epidemiology

- Primarily a disease of animals
- Nearly all cases occur by contact with infected animals or animal products; human-to-human transmission is rare
- Highest rates occur in Africa, the Middle East, and Asia

Differential Dx

- Cutaneous anthrax
  - Erysipelas
  - Boil
  - Syphilis
  - Cellulitis
- GI anthrax
  - Gastroenteritis/food poisoning
  - Acute abdomen of various etiologies
  - Streptococcal pharyngitis
  - Neck abscess/infection

Signs/Symptoms

- Cutaneous anthrax
  - 3–4 days after infection, a painless, reddish papule forms that becomes surrounded by erythema and vesicles
  - Systemic symptoms may develop
- Pulmonary anthrax
  - Influenza-like initial symptoms (fever, chills, fatigue, HA, cough, myalgias)
  - Sudden development of dyspnea, cyanosis, mental status changes, coma, and possible death occur over 24 hours
- GI anthrax
  - Oropharyngeal infection: Sore throat, dysphagia, fever, lymphadenopathy
  - Intestinal infection: Nausea, vomiting, fever, abdominal pain, hematemesis, bloody diarrhea, ascites

Diagnosis

- History of exposure and clinical presentation
- Definitive diagnosis by isolation of bacteria from cutaneous vesicles, sputum, vomitus, feces, and/or ascites fluid
- Blood cultures may be positive in any form of anthrax
- Chest X-ray in pulmonary anthrax shows a widened mediastinum due to enlarged mediastinal lymph nodes, diffuse patchy infiltrates

Treatment

- Begin antibiotics promptly—penicillin is the treatment-of-choice
  - Oral penicillin for 5–7 days in mild cutaneous infections
  - IV penicillin in severe cutaneous infections, pulmonary anthrax, and GI anthrax
  - Alternative drugs include ciprofloxacin, tetracycline, erythromycin, chloramphenicol, and many others
- Intubation and ventilatory support may be necessary in pulmonary anthrax
- ICU admission may be necessary in pulmonary and GI infections
- Plasmapheresis may be effective to clear the toxin from blood
- Vaccine is available for individuals at high risk

Prognosis/Clinical Course

- All forms of anthrax may be fatal
  - Cutaneous anthrax is usually self-limiting
  - Pulmonary anthrax is often fatal
  - GI anthrax, especially oropharyngeal infection, may result in sepsis, shock, and death (with or without treatment)
- Meningitis and sepsis are dangerous complications of all three forms of anthrax
  - Nearly 100% of cases of meningitis are fatal

113. Smallpox

Etiology

- Caused by a variola virus
- Incubation of about 2 weeks following exposure; during this time, there are no symptoms and the virus is not contagious
- Most infectious early in the course of disease, but transmission may occur at any time during illness; spread is by respiratory droplets, especially during face-to-face contact, coughing, and so on
- Virus spreads from the respiratory tract to blood and internal organs and skin

Differential Dx

- Chickenpox
- Influenza

Epidemiology

- Epidemics throughout history have been extremely devastating
- Routine vaccination ended in 1972
- Eliminated from the world in 1977

Signs/Symptoms

- Initial symptoms include high fever, fatigue, headache, and backache; nausea and vomiting may be present
- A characteristic rash follows 2–3 days later
    - Especially prominent on face, extremities, and mucous membranes of the mouth and nose
    - Progresses from reddish macules to papules to pus-filled vesicles to crusting scabs
    - All lesions appear in the same stage of development (as opposed to chickenpox)
    - Scabs fall off in 3–4 weeks
- Blindness may occur

Diagnosis

- Primarily diagnosed by examination of characteristic rash by trained personnel
- Must distinguish rash from chickenpox
    - Lesions of chickenpox tend to be more superficial
    - Chickenpox are more prominent on the trunk than on the face or extremities
    - In chickenpox, lesions of various stages exist together; in smallpox, lesions are at the same stage of development

Treatment

- Patients should be isolated until rash/scabs disappear
- No proven treatment; antivirals are in development
- Supportive care: IV fluids, analgesics, and antipyretics
- Antibiotics for secondary bacterial infections
- Vaccine
    - The available vaccine is made of live vaccinia virus, which is closely related to the variola virus
    - The vaccine may prevent or diminish the severity of illness in exposed individuals
    - Must be administered within 4 days of exposure, before rash develops
    - Contraindicated in pregnancy, history of eczema, and immunosuppression/immunocompromised

Prognosis/Clinical Course

- Most patients recover; death occurs in up to 30% of cases
- Some rare forms of smallpox are even more lethal
- Deep scars may remain ("pockmarks"), especially on the face
- Infection control procedures are essential, including decontamination of instruments, clothing, bedding, and so on; protective clothing and masks for medical personnel and caregivers; vaccines for those at risk

Endocrine Disorders

SCOTT KAHAN, MD

114. Syndrome of Inappropriate ADH

Etiology

- ADH is secreted in response to high plasma osmolality; ADH augments water reabsorption, effectively diluting the intravascular compartment
- However, low plasma osmolality should diminish ADH release—SIADH occurs when there is interference in this osmotic suppression of ADH, resulting in unchecked water reabsorption
- Because normal sodium excretion exists in this setting of impaired water excretion, a low-volume, highly concentrated urine is produced and serum hyponatremia results

Epidemiology

- Excess ADH production may be secondary to tumors (i.e., oat cell carcinoma of lung), infection (especially lung and brain infections), CNS disorders (head injury, masses, stroke), or drugs (i.e., chlorpropamide, carbamazepine, clofibrate, exogenous vasopressin, nicotine, oxytocin, SSRIs, MAO inhibitors)

Differential Dx

- Cerebral Na^+ wasting syndrome
- Dehydration
- Diarrhea/vomiting
- Diuretic use
- Adrenal deficiency
- Polydipsia
- Post-op hyponatremia
- Hypothyroidism
- Beer potomania
- Drugs (thiazides, ACE inhibitors)
- CHF
- Liver disease
- Nephrotic syndrome
- Advanced renal failure

Signs/Symptoms

- Signs and symptoms of hyponatremia:
  - Lethargy
  - Anorexia
  - Confusion
  - Headache
  - Nausea/vomiting
  - Focal neurologic deficits
  - Convulsions
  - Coma
  - Gradual development of hyponatremia may be asymptomatic

Diagnosis

- Hyponatremia (Na^+ <135 mmol/L)
- Clinical euvolemia: Absence of signs and symptoms of hypovolemia (tachycardia, orthostasis, dry mucus membranes) and hypervolemia (edema, ascites)
- Urinary sodium excretion >20 mmol/day despite serum hyponatremia
- Urine osmolality > serum osmolality
- Serum osmolality <275 mOsm/kg
- Low uric acid
- Water-load test: Determines if patient can excrete a water load by producing dilute urine—a patient with SIADH would not be able to excrete >90% of a 20 mL/kg water load in 4 hours and/or could not dilute urine output to <100 mOsm/kg

Treatment

- Treat underlying syndrome (i.e., thyroid replacement in hypothyroidism, steroids in mineralocorticoid deficiency)
- Fluid restriction (<1000 mL/day) to correct hyponatremia: Intake should be less than urinary plus insensible losses (~500 mL/day in adults)
- Hypertonic saline (3–5%) if severe hyponatremia (Na^+ <120 mmol/L)
- Demeclocycline: Inhibits ADH action on tubules (i.e., leads to an induced nephrogenic diabetes insipidus) and, therefore, decreases water reabsorption
- Loop diuretics if severely decreased urine output

Prognosis/Clinical Course

- Severe hyponatremia may be fatal
- Too rapid correction of hyponatremia may be fatal
- Established hyponatremia (>24–48 hours) should be carefully and slowly corrected; haphazard sodium infusion may lead to central pontine demyelinosis, a neurologic disorder resulting in spastic quadriparesis, ataxia, abnormal extraocular movements, swallowing dysfunction, mutism

115. Diabetes Insipidus

Etiology

- A syndrome of either decreased secretion or ineffective action of antidiuretic hormone, resulting in an inability to reabsorb water
- Nephrogenic DI: ↓ action of ADH due to insensitivity of renal tubules
- Central DI: Decreased secretion of ADH from pituitary gland
- Secondary DI: Due to inhibition of ADH secretion by excessive intake of fluids (primary polydipsia)—may be psychogenic (i.e., schizophrenia, OCD), dipsogenic (due to abnormal thirst—i.e., infections, head trauma, drugs), or iatrogenic (overzealous IV fluid administration)

Epidemiology

- 50% idiopathic
- 50% due to head trauma, brain tumors, or neurosurgery
- Central DI is more common than nephrogenic DI

Differential Dx

- Central: Head trauma, neoplasms (brain, heme), infections, granulomas (neurosarcoid), toxins, inflammatory diseases (SLE, scleroderma), vascular (internal carotid aneurysm), pregnancy, idiopathic
- Nephrogenic: Drugs (Li$^+$, tetracyclines, amphotericin, aminoglycosides), metabolic (hypercalcemia, hypokalemia), vascular (sickle cell, ATN), neoplasms, amyloidosis, pregnancy, gene defects, idiopathic

Signs/Symptoms

- Polyuria (up to 20 L/day in severe cases)
- Urinary frequency
- Enuresis
- Nocturia
- Excessive thirst
- Dehydration may occur but usually increased fluid intake compensates for large urinary water losses

Diagnosis

- Diagnosis is based on serum *hyper*tonicity with inappropriate urine *hypo*tonicity
- Urinalysis: Specific gravity <1.010; osmolality <300 mOsm/kg (serum osmolality > urine osmolality)
- 24-hour urine >50 mL/kg of body weight
- H$_2$O deprivation test: Overnight water restriction followed by injection of ADH
    - Normal response: Increase in urine concentration during the water restriction with no response to the ADH injection (because the body has already responded to water restriction by release of ADH)
    - Nephrogenic DI: No increase in urine concentration during water restriction; no response to ADH injection
    - Central DI: No increase in urine concentration during water restriction, but positive response to ADH injection

Treatment

- Nephrogenic DI
    - Thiazide diuretics and/or amiloride
    - Low-salt diet
    - Prostaglandin inhibitors (i.e., indomethicin)
- Central DI
    - DDAVP: A synthetic analog of ADH that has a three- to fourfold longer duration of action; it will increase urine concentration and decrease urine volume
    - Chlorpropamide: Potentiates effects of ADH on renal tubules
    - Diuretics may also be used
- Secondary DI: Treat underlying cause

Prognosis/Clinical Course

- Good prognosis if the underlying cause is treated (i.e., resection of pituitary tumor, eradication of infection, removal of drug)
- Lifelong treatment may be necessary
- Irreversible renal damage, adrenal insufficiency, or severe dehydration may result

116. Diabetes Mellitus

Etiology

- Type 1: Destruction (possibly autoimmune) of insulin-producing β cells of pancreas, resulting in significant insulin deficiency; patients require insulin
- Type 2: Due to impaired insulin secretion ("burnout" of β cells), insulin resistance (at level of peripheral insulin receptors), and increased hepatic glucose production; patients may or may not require insulin
- Glucose is toxic to nerve cells (resulting in neuropathy), blood vessels (resulting in heart disease, kidney disease, peripheral vascular disease, and hypertension), retinal cells (blindness) and many other cell types

Epidemiology

- Affects about 10% of the U.S. adult population
- Type 1 accounts for <10% of cases; HLA-associated
- Type 2 accounts for >90% of cases; genetic predisposition; risk increases with increased age and weight
- Affects males and females roughly equally
- Blacks, Native Americans, and Hispanics have much higher rates

Differential Dx

- Insulin resistance syndrome (syndrome X)
- Gestational diabetes
- Pancreatic disease (pancreatitis, pancreatic tumors, infection)
- Systemic disease resulting in pancreatic insufficiency (hemochromatosis, cystic fibrosis, hormonal changes)

Signs/Symptoms

- Polyuria, polydipsia, polyphagia
- Fatigue
- Frequent infections (UTI, osteomyelitis, cellulitis, otitis media)
- End-organ symptoms after long-term, poorly controlled disease
  - Retinopathy: Blindness, cataracts
  - Nephropathy: Glomerulosclerosis, nephrotic syndrome, renal failure, HTN
  - Atherosclerosis: CAD, PVD (foot ulcers, gangrene), CVA
  - Autonomic neuropathy: Orthostatic hypotension, gastroparesis, urinary retention, neurogenic bladder, impotence, arrythmias
  - Peripheral neuropathy: ↓ sensation, Charcot joints
  - Hypertension

Diagnosis

- ADA criteria for diagnosis: Symptoms of diabetes plus random blood glucose >200 mg/dL *or* fasting blood glucose >126 [best test] *or* blood glucose >200 during oral glucose tolerance test (2 hrs after glucose load)
- Fasting blood glucose (>8 hours fasting):
  - Blood glucose <110 is normal
  - 110–125 is considered impaired fasting glucose (IFG)
  - ≥126 is considered diabetes
- Screen all patients >45 every 3 years (earlier if have RFs)
- Hemoglobin A_{1c}: Reflects glucose control over past 3 mo
- Serum insulin: Greatly decreased in Type 1 DM; initially increased in Type 2, but falls as β cells "burn out"
- Signs and symptoms of end-organ damage
- Renal function: Microalbuminuria (30–300 mg/24 hrs) signifies early-stage nephropathy; BUN/creatinine increase as renal function decreases

Treatment

- Carefully integrate low-sugar diet, exercise, insulin
- Oral agents
  - Sulfonylureas: ↑ Insulin secretion from β cells
  - Biguanides (metformin): ↓ hepatic glucose production, weight loss
  - Thiazolidinediones: ↓ insulin resistance
  - α-Glucosidase inhibitors: ↓ carb absorption
  - Orlistat: ↓ fat absorption from gut
- Insulin preparations
  - Rapid-acting, short duration: Regular, Lispro
  - Intermediate-acting, medium duration: NPH, lente
  - Long-acting: Ultralente, Glargine
  - Combinations: 70/30 (70% NPH/30% regular)
- Aspirin, antihypertensives (especially ACE inhibitors because renal-protective), statins, heart meds

Prognosis/Clinical Course

- Acute complications
  - Diabetic ketoacidosis (Type 1)
  - Non-ketotic hyperosmolar coma (Type 2)
  - Hypoglycemia
- Chronic complications: end-organ disease
  - #1 U.S. cause of end-stage renal failure, nontraumatic leg amputation, and adult blindness
- Morbidity is especially due to MI, CVA, renal failure, and infections
- Regularly monitor glucose, lipids (LDL <100), HbA_{1c} (<7), renal function, BP (<130/85), and peripheral neuropathy
- Syndrome X: The gradual development (over 10–15 years) of hyperinsulinemia and insulin resistance before the onset of overt diabetes

117. Hyperthyroidism

Etiology

- Oversecretion of thyroid hormone due to:
  - Nodular hyperplasia of thyroid
  - Damage to thyroid—DeQuervain's thyroiditis, lymphocytic thyroiditis
  - Diffuse overproduction of thyroid hormone: Graves' disease (autoantibodies to TSH receptor stimulate thyroid hormone production)
- 1° hyperthyroidism is due to dysfunction (overfunction) of the thyroid gland itself
- 2° hyperthyroidism is due to overstimulation of the thyroid gland by excess TSH production (TSH-dependent hyperthyroidism)

Epidemiology

- Females > males
- Most common in ages 20–50
- >50% of cases due to Graves' disease

Differential Dx

- 1° hyperthyroidism
  - Graves' disease
  - Solitary adenoma
  - Iodine ingestion
  - Struma ovarii
  - Toxic multinodular goiter
  - TSH-secreting pituitary adenoma
  - Functioning thyroid cancer
- 2° hyperthyroidism
  - Pituitary adenoma
  - HCG-secreting tumor
  - Gestational thyrotoxicosis
  - Thyroid hormone resistance syndrome

Signs/Symptoms

- Heat intolerance and sweating
- Hyperactivity, irritability, nervousness
- Weight loss
- Diarrhea
- Weakness, fatigue
- Tremor
- Tachycardia, palpitations, Afib
- Enlarged thyroid/goiter
- Neck pain
- Lid lag/lid retraction
- Gynecomastia
- Loss of libido
- Menstrual irregularities
- Graves' disease: Proptosis, pretibial myxedema, exophthalmos

Diagnosis

- Thyroid function tests: Increased free T_4, total T_4, and T_3
  - 1° hyperthyroidism: Increased T_4 with *decreased* TSH
  - 2° hyperthyroidism: Normal/increased T_4 with *increased* TSH
- Radionucleotide thyroid scan: Low uptake (<5%) suggests hyperthyroidism is due to damage of thyroid or exogenous thyroid hormone ingestion; increased uptake suggests Graves' disease
- Antimicrosomal and thyroid peroxidase antibodies are present in Graves' disease and lymphocytic thyroiditis
- Antithyroglobulin antibodies are present in Graves' disease (present in any autoimmune thyroid disorder)
- EKG: Atrial fibrillation/sinus tachycardia
- Head CT/MRI may show pituitary tumor

Treatment

- Graves' disease or thyroid adenoma
  - Radioactive iodine (^{131}I) to ablate thyroid tissue is often the definitive treatment (do not use in pregnancy)
  - Antithyroid drugs to interfere with thyroid hormone production: Methimazole, propylthiouracil (PTU)
  - Thyroidectomy
- DeQuervain's thyroiditis: NSAIDs, β-blockers, prednisone if severe pain is present
- Thyroiditis generally improves on own in a few weeks—treat symptoms with β-blockers (propranolol)

Prognosis/Clinical Course

- Risk of subsequent hypothyroidism with resection and radioactive iodine treatments
- Nearly 30% of cases of Graves' disease go into remission within 2 years; therefore, medical management is preferred to surgery
- Thyroid storm: abrupt onset of severe hyperthyroidism
  - Especially occurs in Graves' disease patients
  - May die of arrhythmias

118. Hypothyroidism

Etiology

- Decreased production of thyroid hormone due to Hashimoto's disease, postpartum thyroiditis, drugs (e.g., lithium, interferon, sulfonamides, amiodarone), pituitary dysfunction, congenital dysplasia of the thyroid gland, or other causes

Epidemiology

- Females > males
- Iodine deficiency is most common worldwide cause
- Hashimoto's thyroiditis is most common U.S. cause

Differential Dx

- Primary hypothyroidism
    - Hashimoto's thyroiditis
    - Iodine deficiency
    - Congenital
    - Radiation to neck
    - Thyroidectomy
    - Radioactive thyroid ablation therapy
    - Drugs (e.g., Li^+, IFN-α)
    - Infiltrative diseases (amyloid, sarcoid, hemochromatosis)
- Secondary hypothyroidism
    - Hypopituitarism
    - Isolated TSH deficiency
    - Hypothalamic disease
    - Bexarotene treatment

Signs/Symptoms

- Weakness, lethargy, fatigue
- Poor concentration/memory
- Weight gain despite poor appetite
- Cold intolerance
- Dry skin, coarse hair, hair loss
- Constipation
- Dyspnea
- Hoarseness
- Hearing loss
- Parasthesias
- Bradycardia
- Menstrual irregularities
- Delayed deep tendon reflex relaxation
- Goiter
- Myxedema (puffy face and extremities)

Diagnosis

- Thyroid function tests
    - 1° hypothyroidism: Decreased T_4 with *elevated* TSH
    - 2° hypothyroidism: Decreased T_4 with *low/normal* TSH
- Thyroid peroxidase antibodies are present in autoimmune hypothyroidism
- Fine-needle aspirate may be used to confirm the diagnosis and/or rule out cancer
- Anemia may be present
- Elevated CPK, elevated cholesterol, and elevated triglycerides may be present

Treatment

- L-thyroxine (T_4): 1.0–1.6 μg/kg per day
    - Start slow and adjust dose based on TSH level

Prognosis/Clinical Course

- Follow TSH levels annually
- Myxedema coma (severe hypothyroidism)
    - Precipitated by hypoventilation, infection, CHF, MI, CVA, poor compliance with thyroid replacement
    - Results in respiratory insufficiency, hypothermia, hypoglycemia, seizures, coma
    - Treat rapidly with 0.5 mg bolus of T_4 followed by normal daily dose
- Cretinism: Untreated congenital hypothyroidism, resulting in physical and cognitive abnormalities

119. Thyroid Cancer

Etiology

- Especially associated with radiation to head/neck
- Four primary types
  - Papillary (75% of cases): Well differentiated; usually curable
  - Follicular (10%): Common in iodine-deficient areas; functions like normal thyroid tissue; often curable
  - Medullary (10%): Cancer of calcitonin-producing cells; associated with MEN II syndromes
  - Anaplastic (5%): Poorly differentiated; aggressive; poor prognosis

Epidemiology

- Females > males
- Risk increases with age
- Factors that suggest a thyroid nodule is malignant
  - Rapid growth
  - Family history
  - Male gender
  - Age <20 or >70
  - History of head/neck radiation
  - Not suppressed by L-thyroxine
  - "Cold" nodule: No uptake of ^{123}I
  - Fixed to underlying structures

Differential Dx

- Adenoma
- Sarcoma
- Toxic adenoma (functioning)
- Metastatic tumor
- Cyst
- Parathyroid growth
- Goiter
- Papillary carcinoma
- Follicular carcinoma
- Medullary carcinoma (may be a part of MEN)
- Anaplastic carcinoma
- Lymphoma (may be associated with Hashimoto's thyroiditis)

Signs/Symptoms

- Often presents as a solitary nodule, although benign lesions make up the majority (85%) of thyroid nodules
- Malignant thyroid tissue is generally nonfunctional; however, follicular cancer does function like normal thyroid tissue and may result in symptoms and signs of hyperthyroidism

Diagnosis

- Radioactive iodine (^{123}I) uptake scan: "Hot" nodule (those that readily take up iodine) are almost never malignant; 10–20% of "cold" nodules are malignant
- Fine-needle aspirate: Diagnostic for thyroid cancer (except follicular cancer because this diagnosis depends on evidence of invasion to adjacent structures)
- Ultrasound: Used to detect nodules, guide FNA, distinguish between solid and cystic lesions, and aspirate cystic lesions

Treatment

- Except for the anaplastic type, treatment is based on surgical excision (near-total thyroidectomy) followed by radioactive ^{131}I ablation of the remaining thyroid tissue and potential metastases
- TSH suppression therapy: Patients are then treated indefinitely with T_4 hormone to suppress TSH stimulation of the thyroid gland
  - TSH suppression may also be used to shrink benign tumors
- Radiation and chemotherapy may be used palliatively for patients with advanced medullary cancer, but neither offers a survival advantage
- Anaplastic: Radiation and radioactive ^{131}I may be used but neither is particularly effective

Prognosis/Clinical Course

- Follow-up after treatment
  - Total body thyrogen (recombinant TSH) scan
  - Neck ultrasound
  - Thyroglobulin to follow for recurrence of papillary and follicular carcinomas
  - Calcitonin to follow medullary carcinoma
- Papillary: Slow-growing; generally only regional metastases (bone, lung); few recurrences after removal; most caught early, when survival is high (>90%)
- Follicular: >50% 20 year survival
- Medullary: <50% 20 year survival
- Anaplastic: Early metastases; high mortality; death within 6 months

120. Addison's Disease

Etiology

- Primary adrenocortical insufficiency (cortisol and aldosterone deficiency) is most commonly due to autoimmune destruction of the adrenal cortex
- Secondary adrenal insufficiency (not considered Addison's disease) is due to inadequate ACTH stimulation of the adrenal cortex due to hypopituitarism or suppression of pituitary ACTH by excess steroid administration
    - Same symptoms as in Addison's disease except no pigmentation changes and no hyperkalemia

Epidemiology

- Males = females
- May occur at any age
- Rare, although secondary adrenal insufficiency due to steroid administration is common

Differential Dx

- 2° adrenal insufficiency
- Autoimmune destruction of adrenal cortex
- Infections, especially TB (also fungal infection, CMV, AIDS)
- Amyloidosis
- Sarcoidosis
- Hemorrhage
- Adrenoleukodystrophy
- Congenital adrenal hypoplasia
- ACTH receptor mutations
- Drugs (mitotane, metyrapone, ketoconazole, aminoglutethimide)

Signs/Symptoms

- Weakness and fatigue
- Weight loss
- Abdominal pain, anorexia, nausea, vomiting
- Hyperpigmentation of skin and mucous membranes (patient will complain of a recent, progressive increase in pigmentation)
- Hypotension and orthostatic hypotension

Diagnosis

- ACTH stimulation test is diagnostic
    - Measures cortisol release from adrenal cortex 1 hour after taking 250 μg of cosyntropin (synthetic ACTH)
    - Normal response: Increased cortisol levels and urinary corticoids
    - Response in Addison's disease: Cortisol levels (and aldosterone) do not increase sufficiently
    - 2° adrenocortical insufficiency: Cortisol levels remain low but aldosterone levels are normal
- Serum: Hyperkalemia, hyponatremia, hypoglycemia, eosinophilia
- EKG: Signs of hyperkalemia may ensue, including peaked T waves, prolonged PR interval, and heart block

Treatment

- Synthetic cortisol replacement
    - Hydrocortisone 15–30 mg/day (2/3 in the morning, 1/3 at night)
    - Avoid adrenal crisis: Increase dose of hydrocortisone supplementation during periods of stress, illness, surgery, and so on to mimic the normally increased release of cortisol during stressful times
- Aldosterone replacement
    - Fludrocortisone 0.05–0.1 mg/day
- Increased sodium intake

Prognosis/Clinical Course

- Adrenal crisis: Acute exacerbation of adrenal insufficiency due to stresses that necessitate increased levels of cortisol
    - Typical causes include infection, fever, shock, surgery, trauma, and gastrointestinal upsets
    - Symptoms: Nausea, vomiting, severe abdominal pain, lethargy, somnolence, dehydration, and hypotension
    - Treatment: Immediate cortisol infusion (100 mg bolus and 10 mg/hour) and correction of sodium and water deficits

121. Cushing's Syndrome

Etiology

- Hyperfunctioning of adrenal cortex, resulting in hypersecretion of cortisol
- Cortisol acts as an insulin antagonist, causing increased blood glucose, protein catabolism, and lipolysis; also has mild aldosterone-like effects, causing sodium retention and water diuresis
- Due to iatrogenic steroid administration or ACTH hypersecretion resulting in adrenal hyperplasia and hypercortisolism (most often due to pituitary ACTH-releasing tumors or ectopic ACTH)

Differential Dx

- Adrenal hyperplasia
- Adrenal neoplasm
- ↑ ACTH due to pituitary tumor (Cushing's disease)
- Ectopic ACTH (especially lung and thymus tumors)
- Iatrogenic steroid administration
- Prolonged steroid use
- Prolonged exogenous ACTH use
- Hypothalamic hyperfunctioning
- Pseudocushing's

Epidemiology

- Cushing's *disease* is hypercortisolism due to pituitary tumor

Signs/Symptoms

- Central obesity
- "Buffalo hump" and increased supraclavicular fat pads
- Moon facies
- Purple abdominal striae
- Acne, hirsutism
- Edema
- HTN due to cortisol effects on vasculature and Na^+ retention
- Impaired glucose tolerance: May have frank diabetes
- Osteoporosis
- Muscle weakness/fatigue
- Oligomenorrhea/amenorrhea
- Impotence/loss of libido
- Personality changes

Diagnosis

- Hyperglycemia
- Loss of diurnal cortisol levels
- Leukocytosis
- Elevated 24-hour urine cortisol
- Dexamethasone suppression tests: Dexamethasone will suppress adrenal release of cortisol in normal patients
  - Overnight dexamethasone suppression test should be initial test: 1 mg at midnight should decrease morning cortisol to <5 μg/dL
  - Low-dose suppression test should be done if overnight test yields cortisol >5: Administer 0.5 mg every 6 hours for 2 days → elevated blood or urine cortisol confirms the diagnosis of Cushing's syndrome
  - High-dose suppression test to establish etiology of Cushing's syndrome: 2 mg every 6 hours for 2–3 days → cortisol suppression occurs in Cushing's *disease* (pituitary tumor) but not in other forms of Cushing's syndrome
- Look for tumors: CT of adrenal glands, head, and chest

Treatment

- Adrenal adenoma: Resection with temporary postoperative cortisol replacement
- Adrenal carcinoma: Resection or symptomatic treatment with adrenal inhibitors (mitotane, ketaconazole, metyrapone, aminoglutethimide)
- Pituitary tumor
  - Transsphenoidal pituitary surgery is often successful (65–90% cure rate)
  - Pituitary irradiation in children
  - Bilateral adrenalectomy with permanent steroid replacement
- Ectopic ACTH tumors: Treat underlying cause

Prognosis/Clinical Course

- Pseudocushing's: Signs and symptoms of chronic alcoholism, obesity, and depression can mask as symptoms of Cushing's syndrome

122. Hyperaldosteronism

Etiology

- Aldosterone stimulates the Na/K pump in the kidney → elevated aldosterone results in increased sodium reabsorption and increased potassium and hydrogen excretion, which results in a state of hypokalemic alkalosis, often with HTN
- 1° hyperaldosteronism is due to adrenal causes that directly secrete aldosterone (i.e., increased aldosterone but normal renin)
- 2° hyperaldosteronism is due to extra-adrenal causes that activate the renin-angiotensin-aldosterone system (aldosterone *and* renin are increased)

Epidemiology

- Females > males
- Usually ages 30–50
- Accounts for 1% of cases of hypertension
- 2° hyperaldosteronism is normal in pregnancy (estrogen increases renin activity and release)

Differential Dx

- 1° hyperaldosteronism
  - Adrenal adenoma (Conn's syndrome)
  - Adrenal hyperplasia
  - Adrenal cancer
  - Liddle's syndrome
- 2° hyperaldosteronism
  - ↓ renal perfusion due to renal vasoconstriction, atherosclerosis, nephrosclerosis, etc
  - Renin-producing tumors
  - Edematous states (CHF, cirrhosis, nephrotic syndrome)
  - Bartter's syndrome
  - Gitelman's syndrome
  - Idiopathic

Signs/Symptoms

- Excess sodium reabsorption:
  - Volume expansion
  - HTN—usually diastolic
  - Edema is absent in 1° disease
- Potassium wasting:
  - Muscle weakness
  - Tetany
  - Fatigue
  - Paresthesias
  - Dilute urine
- Hydrogen wasting:
  - Metabolic alkalosis
- Headache
- Polyuria, polydipsia
- Possible signs of long-standing HTN (heart disease, kidney disease, retinal changes)

Diagnosis

- Hypokalemia (make sure patient is not on a K^+-wasting diuretic) and hypernatremia due to sodium retention and water loss
- Metabolic alkalosis and increased bicarb (b/c H^+ loss)
- Diastolic hypertension
- 1° hyperaldosteronism: Increased aldosterone with *decreased* renin
- 2° hyperaldosteronism: Increased aldosterone with *increased* renin
- Aldosterone will remain increased during sodium loading
- Abdominal CT/MRI: May visualize adrenal adenoma
- Adrenal vein catheterization: To determine differences in aldosterone concentration between the left and right adrenal glands (↑ aldosterone on side of adenoma)
- EKG: LVH due to HTN; signs of hypokalemia (prominent U waves, premature contractions, arrhythmias)
- U/A: Proteinuria may be present

Treatment

- Adrenal adenoma (Conn's syndrome): Resection (possibly laparoscopic)
- Other causes
  - Aldosterone antagonists (spironolactone, triamterene, or amiloride) to decrease potassium and hydrogen wasting and decrease hypertension
  - Sodium restriction and antihypertensives as necessary

Prognosis/Clinical Course

123. Hyperparathyroidism

Etiology

- 1° hyperparathyroidism: Excess parathyroid hormone (PTH) due to causes within the parathyroid gland (adenoma—90% of cases, hyperplasia, carcinoma)
- 2° hyperparathyroidism: Caused by overstimulation of the parathyroids due to decreased serum calcium; usually due to chronic renal failure → ↓ vitamin D activation → ↓ Ca^{++} absorption from gut and ↓ Ca^{++} release from bone → ↓ serum calcium → parathyroid stimulation and PTH release
- PTH increases blood calcium by stimulating breakdown of bone, increasing absorption from the gut, and decreasing renal excretion

Epidemiology

- Females > males
- Usually > age 50
- May occur several decades after ionizing radiation to neck
- May have family history

Differential Dx

- Causes of hypercalcemia
  - 1° hyperparathyroidism
  - Pseudohyperparathyroidism (ectopic PTH)
  - Hyperthyroidism
  - Malignancies
  - Immobilization (i.e., Paget's disease)
  - Sarcoidosis
  - Granulomatous disease (i.e., tuberculosis)
  - Excess vitamins A or D
  - Thiazide diuretics
  - Milk-alkali syndrome
  - Familial hypocalciuric hypercalcemia
  - Lithium

Signs/Symptoms

- Hypercalcemia—most cases of hypercalcemia are relatively asymptomatic (fatigue and other nonspecific symptoms may be present)
- "Stones, bones, abdominal groans, and psychic overtones" is the classic presentation, but these symptoms are not too common in clinical practice
  - *Stones:* Renal stones in 50%
  - *Bones:* Osteitis fibrosa cystica (bone pain, fractures, osteoporosis)
  - *Groans:* Abdominal pain, nausea/vomiting, constipation, anorexia, PUD, pancreatitis
  - *Psychic overtones:* Psychosis, depression, fatigue, anxiety

Diagnosis

- Correct calcium for albumin level: Ca + 4 − albumin
- 1° hyperparathyroidism
  - Diagnosis is based on serum calcium >10.5 mg/dL with elevated PTH
  - Serum phosphate is decreased
  - Urine levels of calcium and phosphate are increased
  - Ultrasound and CT of parathyroid may show adenoma
  - Radiographs often show bone fractures
- 2° hyperparathyroidism
  - Decreased serum calcium with elevated PTH
  - Renal function tests: BUN, creatinine, and GFR may indicate renal failure
- Pseudohyperparathyroidism
  - Elevated serum calcium and elevated PTHrP
  - Look for malignancy: X-ray/CT of lung, pancreas, breast

Treatment

- 1° hyperparathyroidism
  - Alendronate/pamidronate
  - Estrogen therapy
  - Oral phosphate to bind calcium ($CaPO_4$ deposits in tissues)
  - Increased fluid intake to ↑ excretion of Ca^{++}
  - Definitive treatment: Parathyroidectomy
- 2° hyperparathyroidism
  - Correct renal failure if possible
  - Phosphate-binding antacids
  - Calcium and vitamin D supplementation
  - Calcium-rich dialysis
  - Alendronate/pamidronate
  - Parathyroidectomy
- Pseudohyperparathyroidism: IV pamidronate; treat underlying cancer

Prognosis/Clinical Course

- Risks of parathyroid surgery include postoperative hypocalcemia and its associated signs and symptoms, loss of airway, hoarseness, and damage to nearby nerves

124. Hypocalcemia

Etiology

- Most common causes:
  - Hypoparathyroidism: Removal of or damage to parathyroid gland during surgery, inherited hypoparathyroidism, congenital absence of parathyroid gland (DiGeorge syndrome)
  - Pseudohypoparathyroidism: Resistance to PTH action
  - Vitamin D deficiency: 1,25 D_3 increases dietary Ca^{++} absorption
  - Renal disease: Decreased formation of 1,25 D_3
- Abnormal calcium levels disturb membrane potentials

Epidemiology

Differential Dx

- Hypoparathyroidism
- Pseudohypoparathyroidism
- Vitamin D deficiency
- Renal failure
- Renal tubular disease
- Hypoalbuminemia
- Hypomagnesemia
- Hyperphosphatemia
- Acute pancreatitis
- Septic shock
- Drugs (e.g., mithramycin, rifampin, phenytoin)
- Osteitis fibrosa cystica
- Bone metastases (from lung, breast, prostate, or other areas) may readily uptake Ca^{++}

Signs/Symptoms

- Latent tetany (mild hypocalcemia)
  - Muscle cramping and weakness
  - Circumoral paresthesias
  - Chvostek's sign: Twitch of facial muscle upon tapping on facial nerve (anterior to ear)
  - Trousseau's sign: Carpopedal spasm upon inflating BP cuff
- Overt tetany (severe hypocalcemia)
  - Paresthesias: Lips, tongue, hands, feet
  - Spontaneous facial spasm and carpopedal spasm
  - Stridor
  - Seizures
  - Arrhythmias
- Chronic hypocalcemia: Brittle nails, dry skin, coarse hair, enamel defects of teeth, cataracts (calcification of lens)

Diagnosis

- Serum: Ca^{++} <8.5 mg/dL, increased phosphate
  - Be sure to correct calcium for albumin level (calcium + 4 − albumin)
  - Mild hypocalcemia 7–8 mg/dL
  - Severe hypocalcemia <7 mg/dL
- Parathyroid hormone
  - Low if hypoparathyroidism is the cause of the hypocalcemia
  - High otherwise (because hypocalcemia is a stimulus for PTH secretion)
- Vitamin D_3 (25,OH D_3) level may be decreased
- X-ray: Look for bone metastases

Treatment

- Calcium repletion
  - 10 mL of 10% calcium gluconate
- Oral calcium supplementation (2 g per day)
- Treat the underlying cause
  - Replete magnesium in hypomagnesemia
  - 1,25 D_3 (calcitrol) in renal failure, hypoparathyroidism, pseudohypoparathyroidism

Prognosis/Clinical Course

125. Multiple Endocrine Neoplasia

Etiology

- Type 1 ("the three P's"): Parathyroid tumors in >90% of MEN I patients, pancreatic tumors in 50–75%, pituitary gland tumors in 50–60%
- Type 2a (Sipple's syndrome): Medullary carcinoma of thyroid in nearly 100%, pheochromocytoma in 50%, hyperparathyroidism in 25–50%
- Type 2b: Mucosal neuromas in nearly 100%, pheochromocytoma in 60%, medullary carcinoma of thyroid in 90%

Differential Dx

- Isolated thyroid, parathyroid, pancreatic, pituitary, or adrenal tumors
- Multiple myeloma
- Secretogogous malignancies (e.g., breast, lung)

Epidemiology

- Strong familial relationship; genes mapped to chromosomes 10, 11
- Type 1: Onset any time in life, usually 20s–40s
- Type 2: Signs often begin in childhood

Signs/Symptoms

- Type 1
  - Hyperparathyroidism: Hypercalcemia, nephrolithiasis, renal failure, osteoporosis (see hyperparathyroidism)
  - Hyperpituitarism: Cushing's disease, acromegaly, HA, visual disturbances (see Pituitary Disorders)
  - Hyperinsulinism: Hypoglycemia
  - Hypergastrinism: PUD, steatorrhea
- Type 2a
  - Calcitonin excess: $\downarrow Ca^{++}$, $\downarrow PO_4^-$
  - Pheo: HTN, hypertensive crises, HA, fever, palpitations (see Pheochromocytoma)
- Type 2b
  - Marfanoid appearance
  - Mucosal neuromas: Glistening bumps on lips, tongue, mouth, eyelids, cornea, conjunctivae; GI and skeletal abnormalities

Diagnosis

- Type 1
- Genetic testing of patients at risk is now available
- Annual screening of genetic carriers
  - PE: Signs and symptoms of PUD, chronic diarrhea, nephrolithiasis, hypoglycemia, visual field defects, and acromegaly
  - Labs: Ca^{++}, PTH, gastrin, prolactin, pituitary CT (if indicated)
- Types 2a and 2b
- Genetic testing is available (mutation in *RET* gene is diagnostic)—prophylactic thyroidectomy in affected patients due to fatal nature of medullary thyroid cancer
- Annual screening
  - Pheo: 24-hour urine catecholamines; CT/MRI of adrenal glands
  - Thyroid: Measure calcitonin levels after infusion of Ca^{++}
  - Parathyroid: Measure PTH, Ca^{++}, and PO_4^-

Treatment

- Type 1
  - Surgical removal of pituitary and parathyroid tumors
  - Surgical removal of pancreatic tumors if possible or total pancreatectomy
  - Diazoxide to treat hypoglycemia
  - Proton pump inhibitors or H_2 receptor blockers to treat hypergastrinemia and peptic ulcer disease
- Types 2a and 2b
  - Surgical removal of pheochromocytoma, thyroid carcinoma, and parathyroid carcinoma
  - Pheochromocytoma should be resected first

Prognosis/Clinical Course

126. Pheochromocytoma

Etiology

- An adrenal tumor that produces, stores, and secretes catecholamines (norepinephrine > epinephrine)
- May also secrete opioids, endothelin, erythropoeitin, neuropeptide Y, or adrenomedullin
- Usually <10 cm in diameter
- Usually benign but malignant in 10% of cases

Epidemiology

- Important, correctable cause of secondary HTN (0.1% of cases)
- 80% unilateral (R > L); 10% bilateral; 10% extra-adrenal (neck, mesenteric ganglia, thorax, bladder)
- May be familial—especially if bilateral
- Associated with MEN IIa and IIb, von Recklinghausen's neurofibromatosis, von Hippel-Lindau syndrome

Differential Dx

- Essential HTN
- Cocaine use
- Other secondary HTN
- MI/CAD (false elevation of catecholamines)
- Autonomic epilepsy
- Anxiety attack
- Clonidine withdrawal
- Chemodectoma (carotid body tumor)
- Ganglioneuroma (sympathetic neuronal tumor)
- Extra-adrenal pheo
- Intracranial lesion (posterior fossa tumor, SAH)
- MAO inhibitor use

Signs/Symptoms

- Hypertension is the most common sign
  - 1/2 of cases present with sustained HTN
  - 1/2 present with episodic HTN
  - HTN is poorly responsive to medications
- Headache, sweating, palpitations, nervousness, tachycardia, fever
- Weight loss
- Hyperglycemia
- Orthostatic hypotension due to blunted sympathetic responses
- *Hypo*tension/shock may occur with surgery or trauma
- Arrythmias
- Signs of heart failure/cardiomyopathy
- Angina or MI is possible (with or without underlying CAD)

Diagnosis

- 24-hour urine sample for catecholamines, metanephrines, and vanillylmandelic acid is generally diagnostic
- Plasma catecholamines are much less reliable
- Pharmacologic tests are also less reliable
  - Clonidine suppression test may be used as a confirmatory test: will ↓ catecholamines in normal subjects but not patients with pheochromocytoma
  - Glucagon stimulation test
- CT/MRI to locate tumor for resection
- EKG: Nonspecific ST-T wave changes, prominent U waves, bundle branch block, left ventricular strain patterns
- Increased amylase with normal lipase—may mimic appendicitis
- Increased hematocrit, calcium, or ESR is possible

Treatment

- Definitive cure is resection
  - Catecholomine-receptor blocking agent (phenoxybenzamine) must be used during surgery to prevent hypertensive crisis
  - Surgery results in 75% cure rate; 25% still have HTN but it is generally controllable with medical therapy; ~3% mortality
- Medical management: Nitroprusside, calcium-channel blockers, and ACE inhibitors to decrease blood pressure
- Unresectable or malignant tumors may be treated with tyrosine hydroxylase to decrease catecholamine production

Prognosis/Clinical Course

- Hypertensive crises occur in >50% of cases
  - Caused by anything that shifts abdominal contents; may be without an apparent precipitating factor
  - Sudden onset of high BP and tachycardia
  - HA, profuse sweating, palpitations
  - Sense of impending doom
  - May occur for minutes to hours
  - Also possible: Chest pain, abdominal pain, N/V, pallor or flushing
  - Attacks may be frequent or separated by several months
- Severe drug reactions with opiates, histamine, ACTH, glucagon, methyldopa, TCAs
- 15–20% develop cholelithiasis
- Five-year survival after surgery >95%; <10% recur

127. Pituitary Disorders

Etiology

- Hyperpituitarism: Most often due to pituitary adenoma
  - Excess GH = Acromegaly
  - Excess ACTH = Cushing's disease
  - Excess prolactin = Galactorrhea
- Hypopituitarism: Panhypopituitarism or selective hyposecretion of specific pituitary hormone(s)
- Central diabetes insipidus: Decreased ADH secretion (see Diabetes Insipidus)

Epidemiology

Differential Dx

- Hypopituitarism
  - Pituitary adenoma
  - Hypothalamic tumor
  - Sheehan's syndrome
  - Sarcoidosis, amyloidosis
  - Trauma/surgery
  - Tuberculosis
  - Hemochromatosis
  - Chronic alcoholism
- Hyperpituitarism
  - Cushing's syndrome
  - Acromegaly
  - Polycystic ovarian syndrome
  - Congenital adrenal hyperplasia

Signs/Symptoms

- Hyperpituitarism:
  - Growth hormone: HA, swelling of hands and feet, coarse facial features, moist skin, perspiration, macroglossia, HTN, prognathism, arthritis, enlarged organs, hyperglycemia, menstrual irregularities
  - Prolactin: Galactorrhea, amenorrhea, HA, ↓ libido, hot flashes
  - ACTH: Cushing's disease
- Hypopituitarism:
  - LH/FSH deficiency: Amenorrhea, infertility, impotence, testicular atrophy
  - TSH deficiency: Hypothyroidism
  - ACTH: Hypoadrenalism (see Addison's Disease)
  - GH: Somatostatin deficiency syndrome
  - Visual field defects may occur by compression of the optic chiasm by a tumor

Diagnosis

- Hyperpituitarism
  - Clinical findings
  - Visual field deficits
  - Plasma growth hormone level: Determine GH response to 75 g glucose load; >10 mg/dL suggests acromegaly (normal <5)
  - Plasma prolactin levels elevated
  - Skull CT/MRI with contrast to visualize tumor
- Hypopituitarism
  - Skull CT/MRI with contrast to visualize tumor
  - Measure free T_4 for hypothyroidism
  - Insulin tolerance test to evaluate ACTH, GH, prolactin function: Measure GH, cortisol, and glucose before and after administration of insulin bolus
  - Measure TRH, GnRH

Treatment

- Pituitary adenoma: Transsphenoidal resection; radiation is second-line therapy
- Prolactin adenoma
  - May not require surgery
  - Bromocriptine: Dopamine agonist; inhibits prolactin production
- Panhypopituitarism
  - Resection of adenoma
  - Hormone replacements: Cortisol, thyroid hormone, estrogen, testosterone
- Acromegaly: Inhibition of growth hormone via administration of somatostatin; dopamine agonists

Prognosis/Clinical Course

Neurologic Disease

J. BRAD BELLOTTE, MD

128. Alzheimer's Disease

Etiology

- A progressive dementia with insidious onset, characterized by atrophy of the cerebral cortex
- Primarily affects older individuals (there is a familial form that affects younger patients)
- Dementia is a state of global cognitive decline that impairs normal social and occupational functioning; normal consciousness is preserved
- Genetic mutations have been implicated, such as $\epsilon 4$ polymorphism of the apolipoprotein gene on chromosome 19

Epidemiology

- 70% of cases of dementia are due to Alzheimer's disease (vascular infarcts are traditionally considered the next greatest cause of dementia, although this is controversial)
- Prevalence <1% younger than age 65; 30–40% of population > age 85
- Incidence is slightly higher in women than in men

Differential Dx

- Pick's disease
- Parkinson's disease
- Multi-infarct dementia
- Infectious (i.e., Creutzfeldt-Jakob disease)
- Metabolic (i.e., Wilson's disease, hypercalcemia, hyper/hypothyroidism, vitamin B_{12} deficiency)
- Chronic alcohol abuse
- Tertiary syphilis
- Subdural hematoma
- Drugs (e.g., sedatives, neuroleptics, anticholinergics)
- Depression ("pseudo-dementia")

Signs/Symptoms

- Memory impairment
- Loss of reasoning abilities
- Difficulties with activities of daily living
- Decline in language function
- Decline in cognition
- Visuospatial disturbances
- Agitation

Diagnosis

- History and physical exam
- Definitive diagnosis can be proven only by autopsy: Neurofibrillary tangles and neuritic plaques are seen on microscopic examination
- Probable diagnosis can be inferred in patients who have a progressive deterioration in cognitive ability, without known neurologic or medical problems
- Possible diagnosis may be inferred in patients with progressive deterioration in cognitive ability, but who have other medical problems present
- Serum chemistries, calcium, vitamin B_{12}, TSH, and CSF studies to exclude other causes of dementia
- CT/MRI will show atrophy of the cerebral and identify possible vascular infarcts
- EEG
- Neuropsychological testing
- Urinalysis to rule out urosepsis

Treatment

- There is no cure—treatment is palliative
- Tacrine and donepezil are anticholinesterase drugs that improve cognitive function
- Selegiline and α-tocopherol may delay progression of the disease
- Treat depression as necessary

Prognosis/Clinical Course

- Follows a progressive course
- Mean of 10 years elapses from onset of symptoms to death

129. Stroke

Etiology

- Ischemic strokes constitute >80% of cases
  - Thrombosis of an atherosclerotic vessel
  - Embolism secondary to Afib or paradoxical emboli (DVT with patent foramen ovale results in the embolus bypassing the lungs to enter arterial circulation)
  - Small vessel lacunar infarction: Usually due to long-standing systemic disease such as HTN or DM
- Hemorrhagic strokes account for 15–20% of cases: Intracerebral hemorrhage or subarachnoid hemorrhage

Epidemiology

- Risk factors: Increasing age, atrial fibrillation, hypercoagulable states, HTN, diabetes, smoking, atherosclerosis and elevated serum lipids, arteritis, hyperuricemia, hypothyroidism, organ transplant, low cardiac output, recent MI (2.5% of MI patients will have a CVA within 1–2 weeks), carotid stenosis, TIA/prior stroke, inactivity
- Ranks in the top four causes of death in most countries

Differential Dx

- Seizure
- Cardiac causes
- Hypoglycemia
- Syncope
- Renal/hepatic failure
- Drugs
- Migraine
- Labyrinthan disorders
- Intracranial mass/tumor
- Psychogenic

Signs/Symptoms

- Acute onset of focal neurologic deficits (of patients presenting to ER with a new focal deficit, 95% are of vascular origin)
- Symptoms are usually preceded by transient ischemic attack (neurologic changes lasting less than 24 hours)
- Symptoms vary by the area of circulation affected
  - Carotid circulation: Visual, language, motor or sensory disturbances
  - Vertebro-basilar: Visual, CN deficits, eye movement disturbances, motor, coordination, sensory, drop attacks, altered consciousness
- Signs of embolus source: Carotid bruit, heart murmur, irregular heart beat

Diagnosis

- History and physical examination
- Emergent CT scan to rule out hemorrhage: Infarcts appear as low-density areas (dark); blood appears more dense (white)
- MRI is more sensitive than CT, especially early in the course and in posterior fossa events
- CT/MRI only shows the stroke, but may not delineate the etiology; full workup may include:
  - Cardiac workup (e.g., EKG, echocardiogram)
  - Carotid ultrasound
  - MRA to evaluate the intra- and extracranial vasculature
  - Additional tests include CBC (r/o polycythemia or anemia), glucose (r/o hypoglycemia), chemistries (r/o hyponatremia and metabolic disturbances), ESR, serum lipids, uric acid, thyroid function tests, hypercoagulable workup; EEG may be done if a seizure disorder is suspected
- Angiography if diagnosis is in doubt

Treatment

- Thrombolytic therapy: Recombinant tissue plasminogen activator (rTPA) must be given within 3 hours of onset of symptoms—only in ischemic stroke
- In those not receiving thrombolytic therapy
  - Avoid excess glucose: Hyperglycemia may extend the ischemic zone
  - BP management: Elevated BP helps to maintain cerebral perfusion; do not lower below 180 mm Hg
  - Heparin is commonly used, but has not been shown to improve outcome
- Emergency surgery may be indicated for release of mass effect associated with swelling
- Modify risk factors: Carotid endarterectomy for carotid stenosis, aspirin or anticoagulation in Afib or hypercoagulable states, manage HTN, and so on
- Hemorrhagic stroke: Mannitol, hyperventilation, head elevation may decrease elevated intracranial pressure

Prognosis/Clinical Course

- Leading cause of severe neurologic disability
- Stroke is usually not fatal, but leaves victims with lasting neurologic disability
  - About 1/4 of affected patients die before leaving the hospital
  - About 1/4 are transferred to nursing homes or rehabilitation units
  - About 1/2 are discharged home
- Addressing modifiable risk factors is important as patients are at risk for future cerebrovascular and coronary events
- The systemic nature of atherosclerotic disease is emphasized by the fact that nearly 50% of stroke victims will succumb to a subsequent MI

130. Subarachnoid Hemorrhage

Etiology

- The most common cause of subarachnoid hemorrhage is trauma
- Of nontraumatic SAH, 80% of cases are due to ruptured intracerebral aneurysms; other causes include arterovenous malformation (AVM), tumor, perimesencephalic hemorrhage, and pituitary apoplexy

Differential Dx

- Migraine
- Meningitis
- Intracerebral hemorrhage

Epidemiology

- Aneurismal SAH
  - 6–28 cases per 100,000 population per year in US
  - Peak age 55–60
- Conditions associated with aneurysms: Connective tissue diseases, AVM, family history, bacterial endocarditis
- Risk factors for aneurismal rupture include HTN and tobacco use

Signs/Symptoms

- The classic presentation is a patient complaining of a sudden onset of the worst headache of his or her life
- Nausea
- Photophobia
- Neck pain
- Altered mental status
- Syncope
- Coma
- Hypertension
- Ocular hemorrhage (Terson syndrome)

Diagnosis

- History and physical examination
- Noncontrast CT of the brain should be the first test done: Acute blood will appear bright white in the subarachnoid spaces of the brain (95% sensitive for detecting subarachnoid blood)
- If CT is negative, proceed with lumbar puncture:
  - Xanthochromia: Yellowish tint of CSF due to blood breakdown products
  - Elevated red cell count, usually >100,000 RBC/mm^3
  - Increased opening pressure
  - Leukocytosis with elevated protein
- Cerebral angiogram is the gold standard: Will demonstrate the source of the bleeding in 85% of cases
- Initial lab studies should include coagulation studies, EKG, chest X-ray, chemistries, and blood type/screen
  - Further cardiac studies may be warranted—as many as 20% of patients may suffer concurrent MI

Treatment

- Airway, Breathing, Circulation
- Minimize external stimulation
- Control blood pressure with medications as needed
- Treat hydrocephalous with ventriculostomy, if necessary
- Surgically secure the aneurysm
- Transcranial Doppler exams and frequent neurological exams to watch for the development of vasospasm
  - Hypertension, hypervolemia, hemodilution (HHH therapy) to combat vasospasm
  - Nimodepine (a calcium-channel blocker) may be administered to prevent vasospasm

Prognosis/Clinical Course

- Overall 45% mortality—10% will die before reaching the hospital
- If the aneurysm is not secured, >20% will rebleed during the first 2 weeks
- Only 30% of those who have had their aneurysm repaired after a rupture will return to the same quality of life as they had before
- Older patients fare worse than younger patients
- Secondary vasospasm (severe narrowing of intracranial vessels) is a feared complication
  - Occurs in 30% of cases
  - Presents 4–14 days after SAH
  - Results in increased intracranial pressure, headache, ischemia
  - Up to 10% mortality

131. Normal-Pressure Hydrocephalus

Etiology

- Dilatation of the cerebral ventricles
- Due to prior CNS insults, such as subarachnoid hemorrhage, head trauma, infection (meningitis), tumors, aqueductal stenosis

Differential Dx

- Other causes of dementia
  - Alzheimer's dementia
  - Vascular dementia
  - Infectious dementia
  - Metabolic dementia
- Chronic alcohol abuse
- Parkinson's disease
- Psychiatric disturbances

Epidemiology

- Age > 60
- Males > females

Signs/Symptoms

- Classic triad: Wobbly, wacky, wet
  - Gait disturbance: Wide-based, shuffling steps (apraxia)
  - Dementia
  - Urinary incontinence
- Weakness
- Malaise
- Lethargy

Diagnosis

- Clinical history of classic triad; patients often have a history of CNS insult
- Lumbar puncture shows normal or high-normal CSF pressure
- Characteristic improvement in gait after CSF drainage
- CT/MRI show enlarged ventricles and communicating hydrocephalus; narrowed cerebral sulci

Treatment

- Removal of CSF via lumbar puncture may provide temporary relief
- Ventriculo-peritoneal shunt is the treatment of choice
  - Incontinence is the symptom that shows the most improvement
  - Some patients with other causes of dementia may transiently improve with VP shunting, but these cases will relapse
  - VP shunting is less effective if there has been a long duration of symptoms

Prognosis/Clinical Course

- Gradual onset and progression of symptoms
- Symptoms may be reversible with treatment

132. Huntington's Chorea

Etiology

- A genetic disease characterized by choreaform movements, mental status decline, and personality changes
- Caused by an autosomal dominant mutation in chromosome 4 that results in increased CAG repeats (spontaneous mutations also occur)
- Results in a loss of GABA neurons in the caudate and putamen

Differential Dx

- Neuroacanthocytosis
- Sydenham's chorea
- Various causes of dementia (e.g., Alzheimer's disease, Pick's disease, infectious and metabolic causes)
- Tardive dyskinesia from neuroleptics

Epidemiology

- Typical age of onset is 35–40 years old, but may occur earlier in severe cases—age of onset can be predicted by the number of CAG repeats in chromosome 4 (the more repeats, the earlier the onset of symptoms)

Signs/Symptoms

- Involuntary choreic movements of hands and face
    - Worse with voluntary movement
    - Increased by emotional stimuli
    - Disappears with sleep
- Dementia
    - Memory loss
    - Apathy
- Personality changes
    - Agitation
    - Psychosis
    - Irritability
    - Antisocial behavior
- Brisk reflexes
- Unable to maintain tongue protrusion

Diagnosis

- History and physical exam (especially family history) are the basis for diagnosis
- Lab and CSF studies are normal
- CT/MRI shows cerebral atrophy
- EEG shows diffuse changes
- Diagnosis can be made on the basis of genetic testing; however, careful consideration must be given to screening unaffected family members as there is no way to alter the course of the disease

Treatment

- There is no treatment for the disease
- Initial efforts can be made to control the choreic movements with neuroleptics, haloperidol, reserpine

Prognosis/Clinical Course

- Progressive course
- Eventually, voluntary movements become very difficult and the personality changes lead to the need for institutionalization
- Death occurs about 15 years after the onset of symptoms

133. Parkinson's Disease

Etiology

- Parkinson's disease (idiopathic paralysis agitans) is a progressive, degenerative disease resulting from the loss of dopaminergic neurons in the substantia nigra and other CNS areas
- Characterized by slow movement, rigidity, and resting tremor
- The initial insult in unknown

Differential Dx

- Drug-induced parkinsonism (especially dopamine receptor antagonists—antiemetics, antipsychotics, reserpine)
- Essential tremor
- Normal pressure hydrocephalus
- Mass lesions (tumor, subdural hematoma)
- Infarct
- Wilson's disease
- Diffuse Lewy body disease
- Poisoning (carbon monoxide, methanol, manganese)

Epidemiology

- Very common—affects 1% of Americans over age 50
- Males > females
- Mean age at onset 55 years old, but may vary from 20 to 80 years

Signs/Symptoms

- Classic triad
  - Tremor (resting, "pill-rolling" tremor that decreases with movement)
  - Cogwheel rigidity
  - Bradykinesia
- Positive symptoms include tremor, rigidity, and flexed posture
- Negative symptoms include loss of reflexes, bradykinesia, and freezing
- Masked facies
- Unstable posture
- Difficulties with activities of daily living (e.g., dressing, eating, writing)

Diagnosis

- History and physical examination are generally diagnostic
- Clinical response to therapy with dopamine agonists suggests Parkinson's disease
- Autopsy shows Lewy bodies
- CT is useful to rule out other pathology

Treatment

- Treatment is aimed at increasing the levels of dopamine in the CNS
  - Levadopa plus carbidopa is the most effective drug
  - Levadopa is a precursor of dopamine that easily crosses the blood–brain barrier and is metabolized to dopamine
  - Carbidopa inactivates hepatic enzymes that would otherwise metabolize levadopa before reaching the brain
  - Does not affect the progression of the disease
- Dopamine agonists and anticholinergics
- Bromocriptine
- Amantidine
- Selegiline has no effect on symptoms but apparently slows the progression of the disease
- Thalamotomy and/or deep brain stimulation

Prognosis/Clinical Course

- A progressive disorder without a definitive cure; treatment is lifelong
- Medications have prominent side effects, such as dyskinesia

134. Myasthenia Gravis

Etiology

- An autoimmune disease caused by the development of antibodies to acetylcholine receptors on the post-synaptic neuromuscular junction
- Results in an interference of neuromuscular transmission, leading to an insidious onset of muscular weakness and disability
- Associated with thymic tumors (hyperplasia, thymoma), thyrotoxicosis, D-penicillamine usage, rheumatoid arthritis, SLE

Differential Dx

- Amyotrophic lateral sclerosis
- Guillain-Barré syndrome
- Lambert-Eaton
- Hyperthyroidism
- Botulism
- Poliomyelitis
- Organophosphate poisoning
- Mitochondrial myopathy
- Compressive lesions
- D-penicillamine (temporary reaction)

Epidemiology

- May occur at any age
- HLA associations

Signs/Symptoms

- Weakness
  - Weakness is especially prominent following persistent activity
  - Weakness most often fluctuates, but may be constant
  - Weakness of respiratory musculature results in hypoventilation and respiratory compromise in 10%
  - Ocular muscles are frequently involved (85%), resulting in diplopia and ptosis
  - Difficulty chewing and swallowing
  - Limb weakness
- Fatigability: Better in the morning, worse at the end of the day; improves with rest
- Normal reflexes and sensory function

Diagnosis

- Clinical diagnosis based on history, physical, and anticholinergic challenge test
- Anticholinergic challenge: Administration of edrophonium will improve neuromuscular function in patients with MG
- Blood, urine, and CSF are normal
- EMG: Repetitive nerve stimulation results in decreased muscle responses
- Acetylcholine receptor antibodies are present in most affected patients
- CT of the mediastinum: Rule out thymoma or thymic hyperplasia
- TSH: Rule out hyperthyroidism

Treatment

- Anticholinesterases, such as pyridostigmine, are used as symptomatic treatment
- Steroids, IVIG, immunosuppression, and/or plasmapheresis address the underlying autoimmune disease
- Thymectomy may be curative, but may take months to see an effect
- Avoid aminoglycosides, sedatives, β-blockers, and other medications that may cause or enhance weakness

Prognosis/Clinical Course

- Characterized by remissions and exacerbations of fluctuating weakness, but does not follow a steadily progressive course
- If limited to ocular muscles for >2 years, it rarely extends to other muscles
- With the appropriate use of supportive measures, MG is rarely fatal

135. Multiple Sclerosis

Etiology

- An acquired demyelinating disease of young adults
- Destruction of myelin sheaths results in demyelination and inflammation of CNS white matter; multiple plaques of demyelination of different ages and in different locations are seen (separated by both "time and space")
- Unknown etiology—probably of autoimmune etiology in genetically susceptible persons

Epidemiology

- Peak onset ages 20–40; rarely occurs after 50
- Increasing incidence with increasing latitude: <1/100,000 at the equator; up to 80/100,000 in the northern US and Canada
- Females > males

Differential Dx

- Other demyelinating diseases (i.e., central pontine myelinolysis)
- Structural lesions
- Brain tumor
- Head trauma
- Encephalomyelitis
- Vasculitis
- Vascular diseases
- Chronic infections
- Vitamin B_{12} deficiency resulting in subacute combined degeneration
- Neurosarcoidosis
- Neurosyphilis
- HIV encephalopathy

Signs/Symptoms

- Visual disturbances
- Weakness
- Sensory loss/paresthesias
- Vertigo
- Gait ataxia
- Spasticity
- Posterior column involvement
- Trigeminal neuralgia
- Euphoria/depression
- Incontinence/urinary retention
- Impotence
- Increased reflexes
- Babinski reflex
- Lhermitte sign: Sensation of electricity down the back upon passive flexion of the neck

Diagnosis

- Broken down by history of clinical attacks, MRI lesions, and ancillary tests (i.e., CSF analysis, visual evoked potentials) to determine likelihood of disease: "Clinically definite," "lab supported definite," "clinically probable," or "lab supported probable
- MRI is the most sensitive test; shows multiple white matter abnormalities
- CSF: Oligoclonal bands, increased IgG; protein is normal or slightly increased
- Slowed evoked responses to visual, somatosensory, and other stimuli

Treatment

- There is no cure for MS, but existing therapies often give good results
- Interferon-β and glatiramer reduce relapse frequency and severity
- Corticosteroids are also used to treat relapses
- Symptomatic treatment
  - Physical therapy
  - Prostheses/orthotics
  - Amantadine to reduce fatigue
  - Baclofen, tizanidine, clonidine, and benzodiazepines to reduce spasticity
  - Antidepressants
  - Treat bladder dysfunction
  - Pain relief

Prognosis/Clinical Course

- Course marked by exacerbations and remissions
  - Relapsing remitting: Episodes of acute worsening and recovery
  - 2° progressive: Gradual deterioration with superimposed relapses
  - 1° progressive: Gradual deterioration from onset
  - Progressive relapsing: Gradual deterioration from onset with relapses superimposed
- Deficits that last >6 months usually persist
- No reliable prognostic indicators
- Death from MS itself is rare; may predispose to pneumonia and decubitus ulcer formation, and resulting morbidity and mortality

136. Guillain-Barré Syndrome

Etiology

- An acquired inflammatory disorder of peripheral nerves, characterized by acute onset of progressive weakness in more than one limb
- Many types of GBS exist; most cases are diseases of demyelination
- The attack may be mild, resulting in only ataxia, or severe, with rapid paralysis of bulbar and respiratory muscles
- Frequently follows viral illness, *Campylobacter* infection, surgery, or immunizations

Epidemiology

- Incidence: 1/100,000
- Males = Females
- Incidence gradually increases with age, but may occur at any age

Differential Dx

- Chronic idiopathic demyelinating polyneuropathy
- Hexocarbon use/abuse
- Acute intermittent porphyria
- Structural lesion
- Myasthenia gravis
- Multiple sclerosis
- ALS
- Poliomyelitis
- Botulism
- Diphtheria
- Lyme disease
- HIV
- Heavy metal poisoning

Signs/Symptoms

- Ataxia may be the only complaint in mild cases
- Progressive weakness of extremities
  - Symmetric
  - Ascending: Begins distally and progresses to proximal muscles (respiratory, trunk, cranial muscles)
  - More severe proximally
- Hypoventilation due to weakness of respiratory muscles
- Weakness of muscles innervated by the cranial nerves results in ocular symptoms, swallowing difficulty, etc
- Absence of deep tendon reflexes
- Some patients complain of severe, visceral pain

Diagnosis

- History and physical examination
  - Required: Progressive weakness in more than one limb and areflexia
  - Suggestive: Symmetric weakness, cranial nerve involvement
- CSF: Normal early; may show increased protein with few cells after 1 week
- EMG: Diffuse demyelination and decreased nerve conduction velocities
- Monitor respiratory function: Check tidal volumes and negative inspiratory force
- Rule out Lyme disease and HIV

Treatment

- Emergent hospitalization
- Treatment is primarily supportive
  - Monitor respiratory function
  - Intubation and mechanical ventilation if respiratory muscles are involved
  - Physical therapy
- IVIG or plasmapheresis may decrease severity and duration of disease
- No benefit from steroids for acute GBS but useful in cases of chronic idiopathic demyelinating polyneuropathy

Prognosis/Clinical Course

- Most patients make a full recovery, although it may take several months
- Most severe symptoms appear in the first week, but may progress in severity for up to 3 weeks
- 35% of untreated patients have residual weakness
- 2% recurrence rate

137. Amyotrophic Lateral Sclerosis

Etiology

- ALS (Lou Gehrig's disease) is characterized by progressive weakness due to loss of upper and lower motor neurons
- Both upper and lower neuron motor neurons are affected, due to degeneration of anterior horn motor neurons (LMN) and corticospinal tracts (UMN)
- Involves distal musculature, trunk, and cranial muscles, eventually leading to respiratory failure and death

Epidemiology

- Most common motor neuron disease
- Usually affects patients >40 years old
- Males > Females
- About 10% of cases are familial—both autosomal dominant and recessive forms

Differential Dx

- Cervical spondylitic myelopathy
- Progressive spinal muscular atrophy
- Primary lateral sclerosis
- Multifocal motor neuropathy
- Myasthenia gravis
- Multiple sclerosis
- Vitamin B_{12} deficiency
- Tropical spastic paraplegia
- Poliomyelitis
- Guillain-Barré syndrome
- Syringomyelia
- Hyperthyroidism
- Heavy metal intoxication

Signs/Symptoms

- Weakness, cramping, and aching
- Diffuse fasciculations, including tongue
- Gait problems
- Asymmetric weakness/atrophy of hands
- Dysphagia, hoarseness
- Spares voluntary eye muscles and urinary sphincter
- Upper motor neuron signs
  - Spasticity
  - Hyperreflexia
  - Upward Babinski reflex
- Lower motor neuron signs
  - Flaccid paralysis
  - Areflexia/hyporeflexia
  - Fasciculations
  - Downward Babinski reflex

Diagnosis

- History and physical exam are often diagnostic
- EMG and nerve conduction studies
- CSF may have increased protein content
- Muscle biopsy may be necessary, showing denervation; also useful to exclude primary muscle disease
- Cervical MRI should be performed to rule out cervical spondylosis, a potentially correctable condition
- Creatinine kinase is often normal (as opposed to myopathies, which may have extremely elevated CK)
- Thyroid and parathyroid studies
- 24-hour urine for heavy metals

Treatment

- No effective drug therapy
- Riluzole may prolong survival by 3–6 months
- Supportive care
  - Evaluate for swallowing dysfunction
  - Tracheostomy to prevent aspiration
  - Pulmonary toilet
  - G-tube for feeding
  - Physical therapy
  - Bracing
  - Spasticity is treated with baclofen or diazepam

Prognosis/Clinical Course

- Unrelenting and progressive course, without remissions or relapses
- Median survival 3–4 years
- Cognition is not affected
- Death due to respiratory compromise, pneumonia, DVT, and other complications of immobility
- With tracheostomy and G-tube, patients may be able to live for many years; however, they become severely physically impaired
- Advanced directives should be pursued early in the course of disease

138. Migraine

Etiology

- May be triggered by bright light, stress, diet (e.g., chocolate), trauma, alcohol, OCP, exercise
- Other primary headaches
  - Tension headache: Diffuse, bilateral pain; may last for hours to days; not associated with nausea/vomiting, photophobia, or aura
  - Cluster headache: Severe unilateral pain, generally around eye, temple, or forehead; lasts minutes to hours; usually occurs at night; occurs daily for months, then remits for many months or years

Epidemiology

- Migraines are probably underdiagnosed—some studies show that the majority of headaches are migraine attacks
- Onset often in adolescence/young adulthood

Differential Dx

- Other primary headaches (cluster, tension)
- Subarachnoid hemorrhage
- Trauma
- Hypertensive headache
- Temporal arteritis
- Mass lesion (tumor, subdural hematoma)
- Increased intracranial pressure
- Post-lumbar puncture headache
- Infection (meningitis, sinusitis)
- Drug-rebound headache
- Stroke

Signs/Symptoms

- Common migraine
  - Intense headache—throbbing pain, frontal or temporal, unilateral or bilateral
  - Nausea
  - Photophobia
  - No aura or neurologic deficits
  - May last for a day or longer
- Classic migraine
  - Symptoms of common migraine
  - Preceded by aura that lasts a few minutes (most often visual, such as flashing lights)
  - May have temporary neurologic deficits (hemiplegia, aphasia, sensory deficits, vertigo)

Diagnosis

- Diagnosis is based on history and physical exam—diagnostic tests are useful only in ruling out other causes when necessary
- In patients with severe headache but no history of migraines, persistent headaches, or neurologic findings, more sinister causes of headache should be ruled out
- Serum and CSF studies to rule out infection
- Head CT to rule out subarachnoid hemorrhage or mass (e.g., tumor, subdural hematoma)
- TSH to rule out hyper/hypothyroidism
- EEG
- If recent lumbar puncture or spine procedure, consider lumbar MRI to rule out psuedomeningocele

Treatment

- Identify triggers and modify reversible factors
- Acute attacks
  - Rest in a dark, quiet room
  - Sumatriptan and related serotonin agonists
  - Ergotamines
  - NSAIDs
  - Other analgesics, sedatives, and antiemetics may also be effective
- For patients who experience more than 1 migraine per week, prophylactic medications should be considered
  - β-blockers and/or calcium-channel blockers
  - Tricyclic antidepressants (i.e., amitriptyline)
  - Anticonvulsants (i.e., valproic acid)

Prognosis/Clinical Course

- Most patients can be adequately treated with prophylactic medications
- After a several-month headache-free period, medications can be tapered and sometimes eliminated

139. Syncope

Etiology

- Acute, reversible reduction in cerebral blood flow, resulting in a transient alteration of consciousness
- Most often due to cardiac, cerebrovascular, or autonomic dysfunction
  - Most causes are probably vasovagal in etiology
  - Cardiac causes include arrhythmias, MI, valvular disease, and drug toxicity (e.g., digitalis, quinidine, propranolol, procainamide)
  - Cerebrovascular: Carotid disease, vertebrobasilar insufficiency
- 40% of cases are idiopathic

Differential Dx

- Hypoglycemia
- Anemia
- Anxiety attack
- Seizure

Epidemiology

- 3% of visits to emergency rooms are due to syncope

Signs/Symptoms

- Lightheadedness
- Loss of motor tone
- Transient alteration in consciousness
- Pallor
- Malaise
- Shallow, rapid breathing
- May be related to position (as in orthostatic hypotension) or situation (such as coughing, micturition, defecation)

Diagnosis

- History and physical examination
  - Thorough cardiac, vascular, and neurologic exams
  - BP in lying, sitting, and standing positions
  - Relationship to posture, activity, and precipitating events
  - Medical history and medications
- EKG should be done in most patients
- CBC and chemistries may identify anemia, hypoglycemia, or electrolyte abnormalities as the source of syncope
- Blood and/or urine toxicology screens
- Further cardiovascular testing, as necessary (cardiac enzymes, 24-hour Holter monitor, echocardiogram, exercise testing, invasive cardiac monitoring)
- Neuroimaging: Carotid and/or basilar Doppler ultrasound, MRI +/− angiogram, EEG if seizure disorder is suspected
- Tilt table test may induce vasovagal episode

Treatment

- Treat the underlying disorder

Prognosis/Clinical Course

- Many patients who experience syncope have fall-related injuries
- Prognosis depends on the cause of syncope

140. Seizure

Etiology

- Abnormal neuronal discharge leading to a disturbance of cerebral function
- Epilepsy is a group of disorders that result in recurrent seizures
  - Tonic-clonic (grand mal): LOC, no aura, alternating stiffening/shaking
  - Absence (petit mal): Brief loss of consciousness (5–10 sec) without loss of postural tone; may occur dozens or even hundreds of times per day
  - Simple partial: Seizure activity of a localized area of brain, without LOC
  - Complex partial: Seizure activity primarily of temporal lobe, with impaired consciousness

Epidemiology

- About 10% of U.S. population will experience at least 1 seizure during their lifetime
- About 3% of U.S. population will have epilepsy during their lifetime
- Idiopathic epilepsy accounts for at least 75% of cases
- Petit mal seizures begin in childhood and rarely persist after age 20

Differential Dx

- Common causes of seizure
  - Trauma
  - Infection (meningitis, encephalitis, HIV)
  - Stroke
  - Mass lesions
  - Hypoglycemia
  - Uremia
  - Hyperthermia
  - Electrolyte abnormalities
  - Drug overdose or withdrawal
  - Cerebral ischemia
  - Eclampsia
  - Porphyria
  - Syncope

Signs/Symptoms

- Seizures may be preceded by a sensory or psychic aura
- Lightheadedness
- Visual, olfactory, or gustatory changes
- Focal sensory disturbances, such as paresthesias
- Focal motor disturbances, such as involuntary jerking of the hand or head turning
- Loss or impairment of consciousness
- Stiffening and/or jerking movements
- Post-ictal state may result in confusion, agitation, prolonged alteration of consciousness, or weakness (Todd's paralysis)

Diagnosis

- History and physical examination; recognition of the specific type of seizure; medication/drug exposure
- Evaluate potential systemic causes of seizure: CBC, chemistries, calcium, glucose, ESR, hepatic and renal function tests
- MRI is the preferred imaging modality to detect any underlying cerebral pathology
- CT is less sensitive than MRI but is quicker and cheaper; hemorrhage is best evaluated by CT
- EEG may be diagnostic of epileptiform activity and can classify the specific type of seizure; however, a normal EEG does not exclude seizure as a diagnosis
- Toxicology screen if drug overdose or withdrawal is suspected
- Lumbar puncture if meningitis or encephalitis is suspected

Treatment

- Treat underlying systemic causes, if possible
- Avoid alcohol, medications, and/or other drugs that may provoke seizure activity
- Anticonvulsant medications should be tailored to the type of seizure activity
  - First-time seizures generally do not warrant anticonvulsants unless an underlying, uncorrectable cause is found
  - Valproate (Depakote) is most often used for generalized seizures, including tonic-clonic and absence
  - Phenytoin (Dilantin) or Carbamazepine (Tegretol) for partial seizures
  - Ethosuximide (Zaronin) for absence seizures only

Prognosis/Clinical Course

- Status epilepticus is recurrent, unceasing tonic-clonic seizures
- Less than half of first-time seizures will have a recurrence; however, after a second seizure, nearly 75% will develop epilepsy
- Seizures are generally eliminated or well controlled by adequate anticonvulsant therapy

141. Status Epilepticus

Etiology

- Defined as a single seizure lasting for more than 30 minutes or multiple seizures that occur without fully regaining consciousness between events
- Multiple etiologies exist; the most common patient is someone with a known seizure disorder who has subtherapeutic levels of antiepileptic drugs

Differential Dx

- Causes of status epilepticus:
  - Febrile
  - Stroke
  - Epilepsy
  - Tumor
  - Trauma
  - Infection
  - Metabolic derangement
  - Alcohol withdrawal
  - Anoxia

Epidemiology

- Most common at extremes of age (children under age 5 and adults over age 60), but may occur at any age
- 100,000 cases/year in the US
- 10% of patients with epilepsy will present with status epilepticus
- 50% do not have a history of epilepsy

Signs/Symptoms

- Convulsions: Tonic-clonic seizures are the most common; other types of seizures are also possible

Diagnosis

- Workup should include:
  - Complete history and physical exam
  - Serum chemistries, drug levels, toxicology screen
  - CT/MRI of the brain
  - Lumbar puncture if imaging studies are negative
  - Brain biopsy may be needed for lesions seen on CT/MRI

Treatment

- Treatment of the seizure should be started before waiting for any of the diagnostic tests to return—eliminate seizure activity, then treat the underlying condition
- IV phenytoin and/or benzodiazepines
- Thiamine should be administered first in alcoholics
- Glucose if hypoglycemic
- Naloxone if drug overdose is possible
- If not responsive to above measures, phenobarbital or high-dose benzodiazepines may be used
- Intubation may be necessary
- Identify and treat the underlying condition

Prognosis/Clinical Course

- Prognosis is related to the underlying condition
- Death occurs in 2-3% of children and 7-10% of adults
- Prolonged seizures can lead to permanent brain damage
- Release of catecholamines during seizures may trigger fatal cardiac arrhythmias

142. Temporal Arteritis

Etiology

- An inflammatory condition of unknown cause that affects all layers of the wall of extracranial arteries, most often the temporal artery
- The classic picture of temporal arteritis is an elderly patient complaining of a new onset of headache (especially unilateral) and/or visual loss
- Untreated, it can lead to blindness
- One of three entities that are a part of giant-cell arteritis: Polymyalgia rheumatica, aortic arch syndrome, and temporal arteritis

Differential Dx

- Migraine
- Structural lesion
- Increased intracranial pressure
- Trigeminal neuralgia
- Other causes of headache

Epidemiology

- Primarily occurs in patients > age 50
- Females > males

Signs/Symptoms

- Unilateral temporal or diffuse headache
- Fever
- Malaise
- Arthralgia
- Weight loss
- Jaw/tongue claudications
- Sudden, temporary loss of vision (amaurosis fugax) often precedes permanent blindness
- Temporal or scalp pain/tenderness
- Indurated temporal artery
- Pale optic disk

Diagnosis

- History and physical exam
- CBC may show leukocytosis and/or anemia
- Elevated ESR (often > 80 mm/hour)
- Biopsy of superficial temporal artery is diagnostic

Treatment

- Responds well to high-dose corticosteroids
  - Prednisone daily; titer to a dose that keeps the ESR normal
  - Methotrexate is also effective
  - To prevent blindness, treatment should be initiated before biopsy if temporal arteritis is suspected
  - Maintain treatment for 1–2 years

Prognosis/Clinical Course

- Generally adequately controlled with steroids
- Untreated, it can lead to blindness: 50% will lose sight in one or both eyes
- Once blindness occurs, it is often permanent; however, if therapy is started after unilateral vision loss, the other eye is protected

143. Bacterial Meningitis

Etiology

- A serious infection of the CNS that can be caused by various organisms
- Etiology is related to the patient's age and immune status
  - Postsurgical, trauma: *Staphylococcus aureus,* gram-negative bacilli
  - Neonate: Group B strep, *Listeria, E. coli*
  - Alcoholic: *Streptococcus pneumoniae*
  - Infant/child: *S. pneumoniae, Neisseria meningitidis, Haemophilus influenzae*
  - Adult/older children: *S. pneumoniae, N. meningitidis, Listeria*
  - Immunocompromised: Adult organisms plus *Cryptococcus neoformans, Mycobacterium tuberculosis,* HIV aseptic meningitis

Differential Dx

- Migraine
- Subarachnoid hemorrhage
- Aseptic meningitis
- Carcinomatous meningitis
- Other infections
- Mass lesions
- Other causes of increased intracranial pressure

Epidemiology

- Age-specific, as describe above
- Host immunologic status also plays a role
- Those with recurrent meningitis need to be evaluated for CSF fistula, dermal sinus, or post-traumatic CSF leakage

Signs/Symptoms

- Change in mental status
- Fever (may be absent in early stages)
- Emesis
- Headache
- Tachycardia
- Hypotension
- Rash
- Stiff neck
- Kernig sign: With patient in supine position with hip and knee flexed to 90°, further extension of knee causes neck and hamstring pain
- Brudzinski sign: Flexing the neck of a supine patient results in reflexive hip and knee flexion
- Focal neurologic deficits

Diagnosis

- History and physical exam
- Positive Kernig and Brudzinski signs (not sensitive)
- CBC: Leukocytosis may be present
- CSF: Certain diagnoses rest on isolation of the organism from the CSF
  - Increased opening pressure (20–50 cm H_2O)
  - Cloudy appearance
  - Cell count elevated (1000–5000)
  - Increased protein
  - Decreased glucose (ratio of CSF to serum glucose ≤ 0.4)
  - Organisms may be seen on gram stain
  - Check CSF cryptococcal antigen for *Cryptococcus*
  - Acid-fast bacilli smear and culture if *M. tuberculosis* is suspected

Treatment

- Because of the severity of the disease, begin empiric treatment immediately; narrow the antibiotic choice when further information is available
- Empiric treatment with a 3rd generation cephalosporin is usually recommended, perhaps with the addition of ampicillin to cover *Listeria;* vancomycin may be added if penicillin- or cephalosporin-resistant pneumococcus is suspected
- Host factors may influence the choice of antibiotics
- Treat dehydration aggressively
- Anticonvulsants may be required to treat seizures
- Treat contacts of patients with meningococcal meningitis with rifampin prophylactically

Prognosis/Clinical Course

- Overall mortality is now as low as 10%; however, if untreated, mortality can reach 90%
- Course may be complicated by DIC or concurrent infections
- CNS sequelae are rare if treated; they include hydrocephalous, deafness, seizures, blindness, and cranial nerve palsies

144. Coma

Etiology

- A state of altered consciousness due to damage of the cerebral hemispheres and/or brainstem; patient does not follow verbal commands, does not speak, and does not open eyes to pain—a GCS score of ≤8
- Comatose patients are unresponsive to all stimuli; distinguish from lethargy (patient responds to voice commands) and stupor (patient responds to pain)
- Structural coma: Due to mass lesions, vascular infarcts, hemorrhage
- Metabolic coma: Due to endocrine, electrolyte imbalances, seizures
- Psychogenic coma due to catatonia, conversion disorder, etc.

Epidemiology

- Epidemiology is related to the underlying condition

Differential Dx

- Hypoxia
- Ischemia
- Hypoglycemia
- Metabolic derangements
- Failure of other organs (pituitary, liver, renal)
- Trauma
- Infection
- Drugs (e.g., antibiotics, barbiturates, phenytoin, benzodiazepines)
- Hemorrhage
- Seizure
- Psychiatric disturbance
- Malingering

Signs/Symptoms

- Inability to respond to commands and painful stimuli
- Abnormal respirations
- Pupillary and extraocular muscle abnormalities (i.e., small pinpoint pupils, large unreactive pupils, unilateral fixed pupil, lack of horizontal eye movement)
  – Decreased/absent/asymmetric pupil reactivity suggests a structural cause
- Motor abnormalities
  – Decorticate/flexor posturing
  – Decerebrate/extensor posturing
  – Tremor, asterixis, myoclonus, seizures
- Symptoms of underlying cause: Sudden headache (subarachnoid hemorrhage), fever and neck stiffness (meningitis), and others

Diagnosis

- History and physical examination
- CT/MRI to identify structural lesions
- Lumbar puncture to determine infection, bleeding; must rule out increased intracranial pressure before LP to avoid increasing the risk of herniation
- EEG
- Toxicology screen for drugs and medications
- Chemistries and glucose
- Tests of organ dysfunction
  – EKG and cardiac enzymes
  – Chest X-ray
  – Arterial blood gas
  – Liver function tests
  – Coagulation studies
  – BUN/creatinine and ammonia levels
  – Thyroid function tests

Treatment

- Airway, Breathing, and Circulation
- STAT laboratory and imaging studies
- Manage increased intracranial pressure and/or brain herniation by elevation of the head, hyperventilation, mannitol, and/or steroids
- If cause is unknown, administer glucose, thiamine, and naloxone
- Correct electrolyte and acid–base disturbances as necessary
- Antiepileptics and benzodiazepines as necessary to treat seizures
- Treat underlying pathologies (e.g., antibiotics for meningitis and other infections, surgical intervention as necessary for mass lesions and hemorrhage)

Prognosis/Clinical Course

- The prognosis depends on the underlying cause of the coma

145. Neurofibromatosis

Etiology

- Genetic diseases with autosomal dominant transmission
- The two forms of neurofibromatosis differ in etiology and presentation
  - NF-1 (von Recklinghausen's disease; peripheral NF) is due to a defect on chromosome 17; may present with only cutaneous lesions; may present with unilateral acoustic neuroma (tumor of cranial nerve VIII)
  - NF-2 (central NF) is due to a defect on chromosome 22; presents with bilateral acoustic neuromas and other benign tumors by early 20s

Differential Dx

- Albright's syndrome
- Posterior fossa tumors (meningioma, cholesteatoma)
- Metastatic brain cancer

Epidemiology

- Up to 50% of cases are due to new mutations
- Males = females
- NF-1 is one of the most common genetic disorders (1/3000)

Signs/Symptoms

- NF-1
  - Café-au-lait spots: Freckle-like macules; occur mostly on trunk
  - Axillary and/or inguinal freckles
  - Lisch nodules: Pigmented nodules on iris of eye
  - Neurofibromas: Benign tumors of Schwann cells; may be felt as nodules along peripheral nerves
  - Skeletal and spinal deformities
  - Symptoms of acoustic neuroma
- NF-2
  - Symptoms of acoustic neuromas, meningiomas, and other growths
  - Hearing loss   – Gait ataxia
  - Vertigo   – Facial pain
  - Tinnitus   – Headache

Diagnosis

- Audiometry may show sensorineural hearing loss
- CSF studies: Elevated protein
- MRI may visualize posterior fossa tumor(s)
- Diagnosis of NF-1 requires 2 or more of the following:
  - 6 café-au-lait spots
  - Axillary or inguinal freckling
  - 2 neurofibromas or 1 plexiform neurofibroma
  - First-degree relative with NF-1
  - Lisch nodules
  - Bone lesion
- Diagnosis of NF-2
  - Bilateral cranial nerve VIII tumor
  - First-degree relative with NF-2 and a unilateral acoustic neuroma
  - First-degree relative with NF-2 plus 2 of the following: Glioma, meningioma, schwannoma, neurofibroma, or juvenile posterior subcapsular lenticular opacity

Treatment

- There is no cure for neurofibromatosis; treatment is based on managing symptoms and associated tumors
- Treat tumors with surgery or radiation
- Patients are often mentally handicapped and require special education or speech therapy

Prognosis/Clinical Course

- Families with NF should undergo genetic counseling, as there is no cure for the disease

Hematologic Disease

ERICA LINDEN, MD

146. Iron-Deficiency Anemia

Etiology

- Most commonly due to poor iron intake; other causes include menstrual blood loss, states of rapid growth (i.e., adolescence), blood donation, blood loss (GI bleed, Hodgkin's disease, excessive menses), pregnancy, and malabsorption (gastrectomy, sprue, inflammatory bowel disease)
- Iron is absorbed in the proximal small intestine, stored as ferritin, bound to transferrin in the blood, and transported to bone marrow for incorporation into RBCs

Epidemiology

- Much more common in females due to menstruation—1/3 of the female U.S. population has *no* iron stores
- Vegetarians are at particular risk due to poor oral intake of iron and high phosphate intake (which inhibits iron uptake)
- Pregnancy, due to increased utilization and expanded blood volume
- Males with iron-deficiency anemia: Assume GI bleeding

Differential Dx

- Thalassemia or defective hemoglobin synthesis
- Chronic inflammatory disease with inadequate supply of iron
- Myelodysplastic syndrome
- Aplastic anemia
- Anemia of chronic disease
  - Renal disease— ↓ production or release of erythropoeitin
  - Hypometabolic states (protein malnutrition, endocrine deficiency—i.e., hypothyroidism)
  - Marrow damage

Signs/Symptoms

- Fatigue, weakness, malaise
- Palpitations
- Pallor
- Decreased exercise tolerance, SOB
- Severe iron deficiency
  - Mouth soreness (cheilosis)
  - Difficulty swallowing
  - Spooning/curling of nails (koilonychia)
- May lead to high-output heart failure

Diagnosis

- Decreased serum iron: <30 μg/dL (normal: 50–150)
- Increased transferrin iron binding capacity (TIBC): >360 (normal: 300–360)
- Decreased ferritin: <15 (normal: 50–150 male; 15–50 female)
- Decreased transferrin saturation: <10% (normal: 25–50%)
- Contrast with anemia of chronic disease, characterized by increased ferritin, decreased TIBC, increased transferrin saturation
- Bone marrow examination: Decreased sideroblasts (developing erythroblasts with iron deposits)
- Peripheral smear: Microcytic, hypochromic anemia; anisocytosis; poikilocytosis; may have increased platelets
- Workup should also include diet history, menstrual history, and family history (rule out thalassemia and other causes)

Treatment

- Treat underlying cause
  - Iron supplementation if poor intake
  - Stop blood loss
  - Treat malabsorption
- Iron supplementation
  - Oral: Ferrous sulfate 325 mg po TID between meals; extended-release preparations
  - Parenteral: If unable to tolerate oral iron or in severe iron deficiency—IM or IV iron dextran injection (must give test dose and watch for allergic symptoms)
- Be sure to properly diagnose iron-deficiency anemia rather than hemoglobinopathy or ineffective erythropoiesis due to the possibility of creating an iron overload state

Prognosis/Clinical Course

- Stages
  - Iron store depletion: Decreased marrow iron stores, decreased serum ferritin, increased TIBC
  - Iron-deficient erythropoiesis: Decreased serum iron, decreased iron saturation
  - Iron-deficiency anemia: Microcytic, hypochromic anemia with anisocytosis/poikilocytosis
- Clinical course can be benign if the iron deficiency is corrected or severe if heart failure ensues in patients with poor cardiac reserve

147. Megaloblastic Anemia

Etiology

- Deficiency of vitamin B_{12} or folate results in impaired DNA synthesis; cell division is therefore slowed despite normal cytoplasmic development, leading to large, megaloblastic RBCs
- Vitamin B_{12} deficiency may be due to poor dietary intake of vitamin B_{12}, pernicious anemia (autoimmune destruction of parietal cells), ileal disease or resection resulting in malabsorption of vitamin B_{12}, tropical sprue, fish tapeworm (*Diphyllobothrium latum*)
- Folate deficiency: Most common in alcoholics; many iatrogenic causes

Epidemiology

- Vitamin B_{12} deficiency: More common in pure vegetarians and patients with pernicious anemia
- Folate deficiency: Alcoholics, malnutrition, iatrogenic
- Pernicious anemia: Elderly females; associated with autoimmune diseases (Graves' disease, thyroiditis, adrenal insufficiency)

Differential Dx

- Iatrogenic: Cytotoxic drugs (i.e., 6-MP, 5-FU), anticonvulsants, folate inhibitors (trimethoprim, methotrexate)
- Myelodysplastic syndrome or hematologic malignancy
- Chronic hemolytic anemia
- Pregnancy
- Liver disease
- Hypothyroidism
- Zollinger-Ellison syndrome
- Pancreatitis

Signs/Symptoms

- Anemia: Pallor, fatigue, weakness, decreased exercise tolerance
- Vitamin B_{12} deficiency
  - Symptoms of anemia and, rarely, thrombocytopenia (purpura)
  - Beefy, red, smooth tongue
  - Anorexia and weight loss
  - Neurologic symptoms: Numbness, paresthesias, ataxia, sphincter disturbances, positive Romberg and Babinski signs
- Folate deficiency
  - Diarrhea
  - Cheilosis
  - Glossitis
  - Signs of malnutrition

Diagnosis

- CBC: Anemia (hemoglobin <12 g/dL); MCV >110 (if MCV is between 100 and 110, consider hemolysis, liver damage, alcoholism, hypothyroidism, or aplastic anemia)
- Peripheral smear: Anisocytosis, poikilocytosis, nucleated RBCs, hypersegmented WBCs, misshaped platelets
- Bone marrow biopsy/aspiration: Hypercellular marrow with decreased myeloid-to-erythroid precursor ratio; decreased megakaryocytes
- Vitamin B_{12} level <100 pg/mL (normal 200–900)
- Folate level <4 ng/mL (normal 6–20) or decreased RBC folate
- Pernicious anemia: Anti-parietal cell antibodies in 90% of cases; anti-intrinsic factor antibodies in 10%
- Schilling test will distinguish nutritional or absorptive vitamin B_{12} deficiency from pernicious anemia

Treatment

- Determine specific etiology
- Must rule out vitamin B_{12} deficiency before treating with folate, as neurologic symptoms will not be corrected by folate
- Vitamin B_{12} deficiency: Vitamin B_{12} 1000 μg/day IM × 7 days
- Folate deficiency: Folate 1 mg po QD
- Pernicious anemia: Treat with intramuscular vitamin B_{12} supplementation and glucocorticoids
- Treat bacterial overgrowth with antibiotics (tetracycline or ampicillin)

Prognosis/Clinical Course

- Nutritional deficiency can be easily treated with supplementation; however, the underlying cause should be clearly identified (i.e., increased cell turnover due to malignancy, iatrogenic cause, bacterial overgrowth)
- Neurologic damage from vitamin B_{12} deficiency may be reversible if detected early
- Pernicious anemia is associated with an increased risk of gastric cancer; monitor these patients regularly

148. Hemolytic Anemia

Etiology

- Premature RBC destruction marked by excessive reticulocytosis
- RBC destruction may be extravascular (due to premature removal from circulation by liver or spleen) or intravascular (due to disruption of RBC membranes during circulation)
- Inherited hemolytic anemias may be due to RBC membrane defects (i.e., hereditary spherocytosis), RBC enzyme defects (i.e., G6PD deficiency), or hemoglobinopathies (i.e., sickle cell disease)
- Acquired forms may be immune or non-immune related

Epidemiology

- Inherited hemolytic anemias are rare; often associated with family history of anemia, jaundice, early cholecystitis, or need for splenectomy
- Acquired hemolytic anemias often occur in otherwise sick patients (often secondary to malignancy, infection, or drugs)

Differential Dx

- Hypersplenism (e.g., lymphoma, infiltrative diseases, splenomegaly due to cirrhosis)
- Immunologic causes (warm-reactive IgG antibodies, cold-reactive IgM antibodies, drug-dependent antibodies)
- Traumatic (prosthetic valves, TTP, HUS, DIC)
- Paroxysmal nocturnal hemoglobinuria
- Hemoglobinopathies
- G6PD deficiency
- Hexokinase deficiency
- Hereditary spherocytosis

Signs/Symptoms

- Anemia: Fatigue, pallor, poor exercise tolerance
- Hemolytic symptoms: Jaundice/icterus, hemoglobinuria (red-brown urine), splenomegaly
- Unique symptoms depending on etiology
  - G6PD: Hemolytic crises in response to oxidative stresses, such as fava beans, antimalarials, sulfonamides, vitamin K
  - Symptoms of sickle cell anemia
  - Hypersplenism: Marked splenomegaly with stigmata of underlying disease
  - Paroxysmal nocturnal hemoglobinuria: 10–15% have aplastic anemia, venous thromboses, hemolytic anemia

Diagnosis

- CBC with peripheral smear shows anemia and abnormal RBC morphology
  - Spherocytes: Round RBCs without central pallor (HS)
  - Target cells: Increased surface area:volume ratio (thalassemia, sickle cell disease)
  - Acanthocytes: Multiple spines on membrane (liver disease)
  - Heinz bodies: Precipitated hemoglobin in cytoplasm
  - Sickled RBCs in sickle cell disease
- Reticulocyte count $3\times$ normal (normal 2–4%)
- Elevated unconjugated bilirubin (4–5 mg/dL), LDH, and plasma hemoglobin
- Decreased/absent haptoglobin
- Urine: Elevated hemoglobin and hemosiderin
- Coombs and indirect Coombs tests

Treatment

- Often splenectomy is required to halt hemolytic process, especially in inherited RBC membrane disorders
  - Indications for splenectomy include hereditary spherocytosis, elliptocytosis, sickle cell disease, hypersplenism, TTP, and patients who fail steroids for immunologic hemolytic anemias
  - If splenectomy is planned, administer prophylactic pneumococcal vaccine and folate supplementation
- Treat specific causes (see also Sickle Cell Disease)
  - RBC enzyme defects: Avoid oxidative stresses
  - Warm-antibody hemolysis: Glucocorticoids/IVIG, splenectomy, cytotoxic therapy
  - Cold-antibody hemolysis: Cytotoxic therapy
  - Trauma-related: Plasmapheresis, steroids, antiplatelet agents, splenectomy
  - Drug-related: Eliminate offending drug (e.g., PCN)
  - PNH: Bone marrow transplant

Prognosis/Clinical Course

- Inherited membrane disorders worsen during stress/infection
- RBC enzyme defects worsen during oxidative stresses
- Hypersplenism: Splenectomy may be dangerous in patients with cirrhosis
- Cold-antibody hemolysis: Often self-limited
- Drug-related disease remits with removal of the offending agent in most cases
- PNH: May progress to acute myelogenous leukemia without a marrow transplant

149. Sickle Cell Disease

Etiology

- Inherited disorder resulting in production of defective hemoglobin
- Defect in position 6 of β-globin gene, causing glutamic acid to be substituted by valine; the defective hemoglobin has diminished solubility in the deoxygenated form, resulting in sickle-shaped RBCs that have difficulty traversing the microvasculature
- Results in occlusions and infarcts of the spleen, brain, kidney, lung, and other organs
- Spleen removes these abnormal cells, resulting in hemolytic anemia

Differential Dx

- Acquired hemoglobinopathies (methemoglobin, sulfhemoglobin, carboxyhemoglobin)
- Thalassemia
- Iron-deficiency anemia
- Bone marrow disease (leukemia)
- Other inherited hemoglobinopathies

Epidemiology

- Common where malaria is endemic
- Very common in African American populations (nearly 10% are heterozygous for sickle trait; about 0.3% are homozygous)
- Homozygotes have sickle cell disease; heterozygotes are carriers

Signs/Symptoms

- Anemia: pallor, fatigue, decreased exercise tolerance
- Rheologic manifestations (due to microvascular occlusion)
  - Dacrylitis (swelling of fingers)
  - Leg ulcers
  - Priapism
  - Pulmonary, cerebral, and splenic emboli, resulting in pulmonary HTN, strokes, autosplenectomy
  - Retinal vessel obstruction; blindness
  - Aseptic necrosis
- Hemolysis: Jaundice, gallstones, cholecystitis
- Crises: Skeletal pain, fever, massive pooling of RBCs (acute fall in Hb), jaundice

Diagnosis

- CBC with peripheral smear
  - Microcytic, hypochromic anemia
  - Sickled cells due to crystallization of defective hemoglobin
- Elevated reticulocyte count
- Hemoglobin electrophoresis is diagnostic: Shows elevated HbS (100% HbS in sickle cell disease; 50% in carriers)
- Hemolytic anemia with elevated bilirubin
- Bone scan to document infarcts during painful crises
- Blood cultures and urine cultures to rule out infection during crises
- CXR if patient is dyspneic (to rule out acute chest syndrome)

Treatment

- Symptomatic support
  - Avoid triggers: Infection, fever, hypoxia, dehydration, low O_2 tension (i.e., high altitude)
  - Folic acid supplementation
  - Haemophilus influenzae and pneumococcus vaccines
  - Penicillin prophylaxis to prevent pneumococcal sepsis (until age 6)
- Leg ulcers/painful crises: Bed rest, skin grafts, hydration, analgesics
- Transfusions as needed
- Antisickling agents: Hydroxyurea will increase production of fetal hemoglobin, therefore increasing O_2 delivery
- Allogenic bone marrow transplant
- Broad-spectrum antibiotics in infections

Prognosis/Clinical Course

- Microvascular occlusion of various organs due to stiff, sickled RBCs results in crises
  - Painful crisis (most common): Skeletal pain and fever
  - Sequestration crisis: Acute fall in hemoglobin, pooling in spleen/liver
  - Hemolytic crisis: Jaundice, fall in hemoglobin
  - Acute chest syndrome: Fever, chest pain, dyspnea, pulmonary infiltration; may be fatal (consider ICU admission)
- Survival depends on mean number of crises per year
  - 3 + crises/year: Average life expectancy ~35
  - 1 crisis/year: Average life expectancy 50 years

150. Thalassemia

Etiology

- Genetic disorder resulting in decreased amounts of functional hemoglobin
- Mature adult hemoglobin (HbA) is a tetramer of two α and two β chains ($\alpha_2\beta_2$); if this ratio is aberrant, the resulting Hb precipitates in the RBC and the RBC is consumed by the spleen, resulting in a hemolytic anemia
- α-Thalassemia: Deletion of α-globin gene(s) results in an excess of β-globin chains; deletion of all 4 α genes is incompatible with life; deletion of 3 α genes results in α-thalassemia; deletion of 1–2 α genes is carrier state only
- β-Thalassemia: Defective β-globin gene(s) results in an excess of α chains

Differential Dx

- Iron-deficiency anemia
- Hemoglobinopathies (i.e., sickle cell disease)
- Acquired hemoglobinopathy (methemoglobin, sulfhemoglobin, carboxyhemoglobin)
- Hemolytic anemias
- Erythroleukemia (M6)
- Myelodysplastic syndromes

Epidemiology

- Especially common where malaria is endemic
- Thalassemias are the most common genetic disorder worldwide
- Up to 15% of Mediterranean and Southeast Asian populations are affected
- 15% of blacks are silent carriers of α-thalassemia

Signs/Symptoms

- Anemia: Pallor, fatigue, decreased exercise tolerance
- α-Thalassemia
  - Deletion of all 4 α genes: In utero death from hydrops fetalis
  - Deletion of 3 α genes (HbH disease): Severe anemia with signs of hemolysis
  - Deletion of 2 α genes: Mild anemia
  - Deletion of 1 α gene: Silent carrier
- β-Thalassemia major: Severe anemia and bone changes; chipmunk face; frontal bossing; copper-colored skin; hemolysis (jaundice/icterus, hepatosplenomegaly)
- β-Thalassemia minor: Microcytic anemia

Diagnosis

- CBC with peripheral smear
  - Anemia: Severity depends on loss of appropriate globin chains
  - Microcytosis: MCV <80; often <70
  - Hypochromia: Pale-appearing RBCs
  - Abnormal cells: Heinz bodies (RBC inclusions), target cells
- Hemoglobin electrophoresis is diagnostic
  - Normal: 97% HbA ($\alpha_2\beta_2$); 3% HbF ($\alpha_2\gamma_2$) or HbA$_2$ ($\alpha_2\delta_2$)
  - α-Thalassemia: Decreased HbA, with increasing percentage of HbH (β_4), depending on severity
  - β-Thalassemia: Absent or diminished HbA, replaced by HbF or HbA$_2$

Treatment

- Patients should receive supportive therapy for anemia and genetic counseling; antenatal testing is available
- Transfusions as needed
- Splenectomy if increasing need for transfusions or if clinical signs of hemolysis (vaccinate with pneumococcal vaccine before splenectomy)
- β-Thalassemia
  - Folic acid supplementation
  - Bone marrow transplant

Prognosis/Clinical Course

- Patients are often initially wrongly treated for iron-deficiency anemia to the point of iron overload
- α-Thalassemia carriers: Benign diseases; genetic counseling should be offered
- α-Thalassemia disease (HbH disease): Severe hemolysis may occur; splenectomy should be offered
- Hydrops fetalis: Death in utero
- β-Thalassemia major: Severe anemia with fatal course (by age 30) unless bone marrow transplant is performed
- β-Thalassemia minor: Mild anemia, generally asymptomatic

151. Hemophilia

Etiology

- Inherited disorder resulting in deficient or defective coagulation factors
- Hemophilia A is most common: Deficiency of coagulation Factor VIII
- Hemophilia B (Christmas disease): Deficiency of coagulation Factor IX
- Both have X-linked patterns of inheritance
- Hemophilia A and B are clinically indistinguishable
- Von Willebrand's disease is a deficiency of von Willebrand factor, which stabilizes Factor VIII

Differential Dx

- Hemophilia A (Factor VIII deficiency)
- Hemophilia B (Factor IX deficiency)
- Von Willebrand's disease
- Acquired coagulation disorder: DIC, liver disease, vitamin K deficiency
- Factor XI deficiency
- Factor XII deficiency

Epidemiology

- Rare
- Hemophilia A: 1:10,000 males
- Hemophilia B: 1:100,000 males
- Females may be affected, but extremely rarely

Signs/Symptoms

- Delayed bleeding after trauma/surgery
  - Affected patients can still form a platelet plug, but they are unable to stabilize it
  - Delayed bleeding into closed spaces may result in compartment syndrome or venous congestion and may be mistaken for a mass/tumor
- Hemarthrosis: Blood in synovial joint following trauma
- Oropharyngeal bleeding may require intubation
- CNS bleeds may occur without trauma
- Hematuria

Diagnosis

- Prolonged PTT
- PT, platelet count, and bleeding time are usually normal
- Assay of Factor VIII or IX
- Restriction fragment length polymorphism (RFLP) analysis for Factor VIII deficiency
- Mixing studies: Add normal (control) serum to patient's serum until hemostasis is achieved; this corrective effect of control serum is expressed as a percentage

Treatment

- Prevent trauma
- Avoid aspirin and other antiplatelet drugs
- Treat bleeding episodes by supplementing coagulation factors
  - Factor VIII or IX concentrates (monoclonal purified factors or recombinant factors eliminate risk of HIV and hepatitis C transmission)
  - Fresh frozen plasma or cryoprecipitate
  - Prothrombin protein complex (activated coagulation factors) for hemophilia A only—risk of thrombosis if used in hemophilia B

Prognosis/Clinical Course

- Patients generally present at a young age, often at birth (presents as cephalohematoma or excessive bleeding at circumcision)
- Complications of therapy are common, including transfusion-related infections and chronic liver disease
- Newer treatments, which include recombinant factors, prevent these devastating side effects
- Following factor infusion, patients may develop Factor VIII inhibitor, an IgG molecule that inactivates Factor VIII; these patients can be treated with prothrombin protein complexes
- Genetic counseling may be offered to families

152. Von Willebrand's Disease

Etiology

- The absence of von Willebrand's factor (VWF) results in a failure to form a primary platelet plug
- Type I: Autosomal dominant; deficiency of VWF
- Type II: Autosomal dominant; defective VWF
- Type III: Autosomal recessive; complete absence of VWF
- Acquired defects (often iatrogenic) are much more common than inherited defects

Epidemiology

- VWD is the most common inherited bleeding disorder
- Affects 1 in 800 individuals

Differential Dx

- Thrombocytopenia
- Platelet adhesion disorder (VWD, uremia)
- Platelet aggregation disorder (Glanzmann's thrombasthenia, afibrinogenemia, drugs)
- Granule-release disorders (Chediak-Higashi syndrome, aspirin, NSAIDs, uremia)
- Damage to endothelium (DIC, HUS, TTP, HSP)
- Abnormal subendothelial matrix (Marfan's, scurvy, Ehlers-Danlos)
- Abnormal vessels (angiodysplasia)

Signs/Symptoms

- Delayed bleeding
- Superficial bleeding due to failure to form platelet plug
  - Skin: Petechiae, purpura, easy bruising
  - Mucus membranes: Oropharyngeal bleeding, epistaxis, GI bleeding
  - Genitourinary bleeding: Menorrhagia

Diagnosis

- Prolonged bleeding time
- Von Willebrand's factor assays
  - VWF antigen immunoassay
  - VWF ristoceitin cofactor assay
  - Factor VIII assay
- Flow-cytometry measurement of membrane glycoproteins
- Electron microscopy assessment of platelet granules

Treatment

- Administer Factor VIII concentrates (e.g., preoperatively)
- DDAVP: A synthetic analog of ADH; induces release of VWF
- If drug-induced, discontinue offending agent (e.g., aspirin)
- Uremia: Dialysis often corrects bleeding diathesis

Prognosis/Clinical Course

- Types I and II VWD are subclinical diseases; they become an issue in trauma or surgery
- Type III VWD is problematic during menses or any minor trauma

153. Thrombocytopenia

Etiology

- Decreased platelet count; may be due to decreased marrow production, increased splenic sequestration, or accelerated destruction of platelets
  - Immune platelet destruction: Idiopathic thrombocytopenic purpura (ITP), infection, drugs (i.e., heparin)
  - Non-immune platelet destruction: Abnormal vessels (i.e., vasculitis), fibrin thrombus (DIC, TTP, HUS), intravascular prostheses

Epidemiology

- Acute ITP: More common in children; generally follows viral exanthem or upper respiratory infection
- Chronic ITP: More common in adults; affects more females than males; ages 20–40

Differential Dx

- Impaired production of platelets
  - Marrow aplasia or fibrosis
  - Marrow infiltration by metastases (especially breast, prostate, lung, thyroid)
  - Cytotoxic drugs
  - Thrombocytopenia absent radius syndrome
- Splenic sequestration
  - Portal hypertension
  - Myeloproliferative disorder
  - Leukemia/lymphoma
  - Gaucher's disease
- Accelerated destruction of platelets
  - See Etiology

Signs/Symptoms

- Superficial bleeding
  - Skin: Easy bruising, petechiae
  - Mucous membranes: Epistaxis
  - Genitourinary: Menorrhagia
- Splenomegaly (in cases of splenic sequestration)

Diagnosis

- CBC: Decreased platelet count
- Bone marrow exam is generally required unless the etiology of thrombocytopenia is certain (e.g., a child with a rapid decrease in platelets after viral illness, suggesting ITP); marrow shows decreased megakaryocytes in cases of decreased platelet production
- History of viral illness/URI (in cases of ITP)
- History of drug administration, especially heparin, chemotherapy (e.g., alkylating agents), antibiotics (penicillin, sulfonamides), antiretrovirals (e.g., AZT), thiazides
- For ITP, can measure platelet-associated IgG (rarely done)
- Obtain ANA in cases of chronic ITP
- Peripheral blood smear: Rule out pseudothrombocytopenia (platelets "clump" together)
- Check coagulation studies: PT/PTT, fibrinogen, D-dimer; rule out DIC

Treatment

- TTP/HUS: Plasmapheresis is treatment of choice
- ITP
  - Steroids, IVIG, and/or AntiRhD (winRho)
  - Splenectomy
  - Cytotoxic drugs are controversial (azathioprine, danazol)
  - Do not transfuse unless clinically necessary
- DIC: Treat underlying cause
- Stop offending drug if secondary to medication
- For all other causes of thrombocytopenia, treatment is based on platelet count and clinical scenario
  - <20,000/μL: Transfuse platelets due to risk of intracranial bleed
  - <50,000/μL plus active bleeding: Transfuse

Prognosis/Clinical Course

- Acute ITP is self-limited
  - 60% recover in 4–6 weeks
  - >90% recover in 3–6 months
- Chronic ITP follows an indolent, chronic course
  - 50% will normalize on high-dose steroids; however, platelets counts will fall once again upon withdrawal of steroids
  - Most cases (60%) respond to splenectomy; however, thrombocytopenia may recur with accessory spleen

154. Disseminated Intravascular Coagulation

Etiology

- DIC (also known as consumptive coagulopathy) is an explosive, life-threatening bleeding disorder in which coagulation factors are haphazardly activated and degraded simultaneously
- The resultant clinical picture involves bleeding as well as thrombosis
- The trigger is a diffuse endothelial cell injury or release of tissue factors, such as obstetric complications (amniotic fluid embolus, abruption, retained dead fetus), hemolysis, malignancy, trauma, infection/sepsis, acute pancreatitis, or ARDS

Differential Dx

- See Etiology
- Disseminated endothelial cell injury
- Hemolytic-uremic syndrome
- Thrombotic thrombocytopenic purpura

Epidemiology

- Most patients are acutely ill (often in ICU)

Signs/Symptoms

- Bleeding phenomena
  - Skin/mucous membrane bleeding
  - Hemorrhage from surgical scars, puncture sites, IV sites
- Thrombotic phenomena
  - Gangrenous digits, genitalia, and nose
  - Peripheral acrocyanosis

Diagnosis

- CBC: Thrombocytopenia; fragmented RBCs (schistocytes)
- Increased PT and PTT
- Increased fibrin degradation products or fibrin split products
- Increased D-dimer
- Decreased fibrinogen correlates with more bleeding
- Seek underlying cause (e.g., via blood cultures)

Treatment

- Reverse underlying cause
  - Treat infection, deliver baby if abruption, or other appropriate measures
- Control major symptoms (either bleeding or thrombosis)
  - Bleeding: Fresh frozen plasma, platelets, and/or heparin
  - Thrombosis: IV heparin

Prognosis/Clinical Course

- DIC is a progressive and fatal process
- Treatment is supportive until the underlying cause can be reversed

155. Hypercoagulable States

Etiology

- Inherited
  - Defective inhibition of coagulation factors: Factor V Leiden, protein C or S deficiency, antithrombin III deficiency, prothrombin gene mutation
  - Impaired clot lysis: Dysfibrinogenemia, plasminogen deficiency, tissue plasminogen activator (TPA) deficiency
  - Others, such as homocysteinuria
- Acquired: SLE, malignancy (Trousseau's syndrome), myeloproliferative disorder, TTP, estrogen treatment, hyperlipidemia, diabetes, polycythemia

Differential Dx

- Inherited versus acquired hypercoagulable states (see Etiology)
- Pregnancy
- Obesity
- Postoperative
- Immobilization
- Old age
- Nephrotic syndrome
- CHF

Epidemiology

- Family history of thrombotic events (stroke, MI, pulmonary embolism, DVT, sudden death)
- 25% of familial hypercoagulability is due to Factor V Leiden (a single point mutation (arg → gln) at position 506 of the Factor V gene)
- Prothrombin gene mutation accounts for nearly 20% of familial cases

Signs/Symptoms

- Recurrent DVTs: Unilateral leg swelling, calf pain, Homan's sign (pain/tightness on dorsiflexion of foot)
- Recurrent pulmonary emboli: SOB, fever, pleuritic chest pain, obstructive shock, sudden death; may result in pulmonary HTN with eventual right heart failure (cor pulmonale)

Diagnosis

- DVT: Assessed by Doppler ultrasound
- Pulmonary embolism
  - CXR may show wedge-shaped infarct(s)
  - V/Q perfusion scan may show V/Q mismatch
  - Helical CT: Large obstructive lesions
  - Pulmonary angiogram is diagnostic
- SLE: Anticardiolipin antibodies and lupus anticoagulant
- Factor V Leiden mutation
- Prothrombin gene mutation
- Homocysteine levels
- Protein C and S levels
- Antithrombin III levels
- Rule out occult malignancy

Treatment

- Seek and treat underlying causes
- Treat DVT/PE: Heparin initially followed by oral anticoagulation for 3 or more months (see DVT and/or Pulmonary Embolism)
- Some inherited hypercoagulable states require lifelong anticoagulation
- Family screening is recommended

Prognosis/Clinical Course

- Likelihood of recurrence determines need for long-term anticoagulation, for example:
  - Homozygous Factor V mutation: Recommended lifelong anticoagulation after initial episode of hypercoagulability
  - Heterozygous Factor V mutation, protein C and S deficiency, and prothrombin gene mutation have lower risk of recurrence: Consider lifelong anticoagulation after second episode
  - Antithrombin III deficiency has high likelihood of recurrence: Lifelong anticoagulation is recommended

156. Hodgkin's Disease

Etiology

- Malignancy of lymphoid tissue characterized by presence of Reed-Sternberg (RS) cell in appropriate cellular background
- HD behaves in a characteristic way—contiguous spread from lymph node to lymph node, with a central distribution of affected nodes (mediastinum, neck, etc)
- Role of Epstein-Barr virus is suspected

Differential Dx

- Non-Hodgkin's lymphoma
- Viral infection (EBV, CMV, HIV, adenitis)
- Bacterial infection (*Bartonella*, TB)
- Fungal infection (histoplasmosis)
- Parasitic infection (toxoplasmosis)
- Sarcoidosis
- Occult malignancy: Lung, breast, GI cancer

Epidemiology

- 7500 new cases per year
- Bimodal distribution of peak incidence: Young adults (ages 15–35) and adults > age 50
- More prevalent in males, especially young-onset HD
- Risk in monozygotic twins increases nearly 100-fold

Signs/Symptoms

- Majority of patients are asymptomatic
- Localized lymphadenopathy
  - Central structures: Mediastinum, neck/supraclavicular
  - Firm, freely moveable, nontender
  - 70% present with superficial lymph node enlargement
  - May be detected on routine CXR
- Constitutional symptoms (B symptoms)
  - Fever >38°C (100.3°F)
  - Night sweats
  - Weight loss >10% in 6 months
- Nonspecific symptoms: Rash, cough, chest pain, SOB, bone pain, GI discomfort, fatigue, malaise, pruritis
- May have disulfuram-like reaction (flushing with alcohol ingestion)

Diagnosis

- Gold standard: Lymph node biopsy demonstrating RS cells (large cell with bilobed/multilobed nucleus with prominent nucleoli) in appropriate cellular background
- Flow cytometry: CD15+ and CD30+ on RS cell
- Staging evaluation after pathologic diagnosis
  - Physical exam with emphasis on lymph nodes, spleen size
  - Presence of B symptoms
  - Labs: CBC, LFTs, renal function tests, uric acid, ESR
  - Chest X-ray
  - CT of thorax, abdomen, and pelvis to document lymphadenopathy
  - Bilateral bone marrow biopsy/aspiration to assess for marrow involvement
  - Lymphangiograms have generally been replaced by gallium scans, MRI, and PET scans

Treatment

- Depends on staging
  - Stage I: 1 lymphatic structure involved
  - Stage II: >1 lymphatic structure involved, on same side of diaphragm
  - Stage III: Lymphatic involvement on both sides of diaphragm
  - Stage IV: Disseminated/marrow involvement
  - B = presence of B symptoms; E = extralymphatic spread
- Localized disease (stages I–II): Radiation therapy
- Advanced disease (stages IIB–IV): Chemotherapy
  - Standard therapy is ABVD (adriamycin, bleomycin, vincristine, dacarbazine)
  - Salvage therapy for recurrence: MOPP (mechlorethamine, vincristine, procarbazine, prednisone)
- Consider autologous bone marrow transplant

Prognosis/Clinical Course

- Four types of HD
  - Nodular sclerosis: Most common; more common in females prognosis
  - Mixed cellularity: 2nd most common prognosis
  - Lymphocyte predominant: Uncommon; best prognosis
  - Lymphocyte depleted: Least common; poorest prognosis
- HD is a curable disease (85% curable with treatment)
- Post-treatment complications: Patients may develop myelodysplasia or acute myelogenous leukemia 10–15 years following treatment

157. Non-Hodgkin's Lymphoma

Etiology

- NHL is a malignancy of lymphoid cells that reside in lymphoid tissues (in contrast to leukemias, where malignant lymphoid cells reside in marrow)
- 90% of NHL are of B-cell origin
- Most common type of NHL is follicular lymphoma (accounts for 50%)
- Indolent NHL: Small lymphocytic lymphoma (SLL), marginal zone/MALToma, *Mycosis fungoides* (cutaneous T-cell lymphoma)
- Aggressive NHL: Adult T-cell lymphoma (HTLV-associated), Burkitt's lymphoma, large cell, mantle cell, and others

Epidemiology

- 45,000 new cases per year
- Sixth most common cause of cancer-related death
- May be associated with Down's syndrome
- Other risk factors include Epstein-Barr virus, HTLV-1, *Helicobacter pylori* (MALToma), and chronic immunosuppression

Differential Dx

- Hodgkin's disease
- Viral infection (EBV, CMV, HIV)
- Bacterial infection (*Bartonella,* TB)
- Fungal infection (histoplasmosis)
- Parasitic infection (toxoplasmosis)
- Sarcoidosis
- Occult malignancy

Signs/Symptoms

- Localized, persistent lymphadenopathy
  - Painless
  - >1 cm for 4 weeks
  - In contrast to Hodgkin's disease, tends to be peripheral (axillary, epitrochlear, abdominal)
  - Noncontiguous spread
- Majority of cases are asymptomatic
- Constitutional symptoms (B symptoms)
  - Fever >38°C (100.3°F)
  - Night sweats
  - Weight loss >10% in 6 months
- Nonspecific symptoms: Fatigue, malaise, pruritis
- Symptoms of localized compression: Cough, chest discomfort, GI discomfort

Diagnosis

- Lymph node biopsy with pathology, flow cytometry, and cytogenetics
- Staging workup
  - Physical exam (lymph node, spleen, liver size)
  - Document B symptoms
  - Labs: CBC, LFTs, LDH, renal function tests, uric acid, calcium, serum protein electrophoresis, β_2 microglobulin
  - Chest X-ray
  - CT—TAP (thorax, abdomen, pelvis)
  - Bilateral bone marrow biopsy
- Consider gallium scan/MRI/PET scan

Treatment

- Most indolent lymphomas present with advanced disease
- Treatment is mostly determined by histology
- Treatment of aggressive histologies consists of combination chemotherapy, generally CHOP (cyclophosphamide, adriamycin, vincristine, prednisone)
- Observation only is common in asymptomatic patients with indolent histologies
- Single-agent chemotherapy in SLL/CLL (chlorambucil/cyclophosphamide)
- MALToma: Treat *H. pylori* infection
- Salvage treatment: Allograft bone marrow transplant, HLA-matched

Prognosis/Clinical Course

- Staging is same as in Hodgkin's disease
- Long natural history: Nodes may wax and wane, noncontiguous spread
- Prognosis primarily depends on the patient's response to treatment
- Other prognostic factors include performance status, proliferative index, high β_2 microglobulin, high LDH, age, and specific chromosomal abnormalities

158. Acute Leukemia

Etiology

- Malignancy of pluripotent hematopoietic stem cells of bone marrow
- Acute lymphoblastic leukemia (ALL): Lymphoid origin (80% B-cell origin); classified L_1–L_3
- Acute myeloid leukemia (AML): Myeloid origin; classified M_0–M_7
- May be due to chromosome abnormalities (Down's syndrome, trisomy 13), chromatin fragility (Fanconi's anemia, Bloom syndrome, ataxia-telangectasia), chemicals (benzene, smoking), X-ray treatment, drugs (alkylating agents)

Differential Dx

- Aplastic anemia
- Myeloproliferative or myelodysplastic disorder
- Infection (HIV, EBV, TB)
- Inflammatory disorders
- Leukemoid reaction
- Other malignancies (Hodgkin's disease, NHL, metastatic disease)

Epidemiology

- ALL: Majority of cases in children; peak ages 3–5; 10% of acute leukemia in adults; affects more males than females
- AML: Incidence increases with age, peak > age 60; affects more males than females; affects more whites than blacks

Signs/Symptoms

- Symptoms reflect cell line depression (anemia, thrombocytopenia, leukopenia)
  - Anemia-related: Fatigue, pallor, palpitations
  - Thrombocytopenia-related: Poor hemostasis (epistaxis, bleeding, bruising)
  - Leukopenia-related: Infections, fever
- Lymphadenopathy, hepatosplenomegaly
- Gingival hypertrophy/skin infiltration with leukemic cells (chloroma)
- Bone pain
- Nonspecific symptoms: Fatigue (the presenting symptom in 50% of cases), fever, weakness, anorexia/weight loss

Diagnosis

- History and physical examination
- CBC
  - WBC usually >15,000 (>100,000 in 10–20%), but may be below 5,000 (25% of patients)
  - Platelets usually <100,000
  - Normocytic, normochromic anemia
- Bone marrow biopsy/aspirate
  - >30% blasts in either peripheral blood or bone marrow
  - Blast: ↑ Nuclear:cytoplasmic ratio, prominent nucleoli, scant cytoplasm, hypogranulated (reflects immaturity)
- Labs: LFTs, renal function tests, LDH, calcium, uric acid, lysozyme, phosphorus, PT/PTT
- Chest X-ray, EKG and evaluation of LV ejection fraction
- Blood type/HLA typing for possible treatment
- Lumbar puncture in symptomatic AML patients and all ALL patients (ALL can spread intrathecally to CNS)

Treatment

- Acute leukemias are treated with chemotherapy, with the goal of treatment being complete remission
- Induction: Reduce tumor burden to $<10^9$ cells
  - ALL: Anthracycline, vincristine, prednisone
  - AML: Anthracycline, cytarabine
- Consolidation: Eradicate residual leukemia
  - ALL: High-dose cell-cycle specific
  - AML: Anthracycline, cytarabine
- Maintenance: Maintain complete remission
  - ALL: Methotrexate, 6-MP, vincristine, prednisone
  - AML: No maintenance therapy
- Prophylaxis: Prevent leukemic infiltration (usually CNS)—X-ray treatment or intrathecal methotrexate
- Bone marrow transplant

Prognosis/Clinical Course

- Untreated disease is uniformly fatal
- DIC may occur (in M_3 AML)
- Prognostic factors
  - Most important: Attainment of complete remission by examination of peripheral blood and bone marrow—absence of blasts, blood neutrophil count >1500, platelet count >100,000
  - Age: Older patients have a poorer prognosis
  - Performance status
  - Specific leukemia markers (i.e., Philadelphia chromosome in ALL—poorer prognosis)
  - Duration of pretreatment symptoms
- 40% of ALL patients achieve complete remission; 3-year survival is 45%
- 65–75% of AML patients achieve complete remission

159. Chronic Lymphocytic Leukemia

Etiology

- A lymphoid malignancy of mature B cells
- Patients are often asymptomatic
- No known inciting agents
- The most common adult leukemia
- Small lymphocytic lymphoma (SLL) is the lymphoma presentation of CLL

Differential Dx

- Reactive lymphocytosis
- Viral infection (EBV)
- Prolymphocytic leukemia (aggressive transformation of CLL)
- Large granulocytic leukemia
- Hairy cell leukemia
- Splenic lymphoma
- NHL with leukemic phase

Epidemiology

- Median age = 60 years
- Males > females
- Especially prevalent in Russian/Eastern European Jews

Signs/Symptoms

- Asymptomatic in half of patients
- Lymphadenopathy, hepatosplenomegaly
- Frequent infections with opsonized organisms (staphylococci, streptococci)
- Anemia: Pallor, fatigue
- Thrombocytopenia: Bleeding, bruising
- Constitutional symptoms are uncommon—if present, may suggest transformation to a more aggressive form of leukemia or lymphoma

Diagnosis

- CBC: Increased WBCs with lymphocytosis (70–90%)
- Bone marrow biopsy/aspirate: >30% lymphocytes; presence of CD 19, 20, 5, or 23 on flow cytometry
- Associated with autoimmune hemolytic anemia and thrombocytopenia

Treatment

- Supportive care with IVIG and splenectomy
- Treatment: Alkylating agents (chlorambucil, cyclophosphamide, prednisone for autoimmune complications); combination chemotherapy has not been proven to yield clear benefit
- Indications for treatment
  - Symptomatic lymphadenopathy
  - Cytopenia due to disease progression or autoimmune phenomena
  - Systemic symptoms
- High-dose chemotherapy and bone marrow transplant treatments are being investigated

Prognosis/Clinical Course

- May be asymptomatic and have a very long natural history
- Survival depends on staging
  - Stage 0: Lymphocytosis only (12-year survival)
  - Stage I: Lymphocytosis and adenopathy (9-year survival)
  - Stage II: Lymphocytosis and splenomegaly (7-year survival)
  - Stage III: Anemia (1- to 2-year survival)
  - Stage IV: Thrombocytopenia (1- to 2-year survival)

160. Multiple Myeloma

Etiology

- Malignancy of terminal differentiated B cells or plasma cells
- Unknown etiology; related to radiation exposure and/or chronic antigenic stimulation
- Symptoms result from the tumor, products of the tumor cells, and the host response
- Direct tumor infiltration of bone results in lytic bone lesions, pathologic fractures (spinal cord compression may result from vertebral lesions), and hypercalcemia

Differential Dx

- MGUS (monoclonal gammopathy of uncertain significance)—25% of cases will progress to multiple myeloma
- Solitary plasmacytoma
- Waldenstrom's macroglobulinemia
- Heavy chain disease

Epidemiology

- Increased incidence with increasing age
- Peak age = 68 years
- Males > females
- Blacks > whites

Signs/Symptoms

- Bone pain is the most common complaint
  - Localized pain may indicate pathologic fracture
  - Usually back/ribs
  - Vertebral collapse may result in spinal cord compression
- Recurrent pneumonia and pyelonephritis
- Anemia: Pallor, fatigue, palpitations
- Neurologic symptoms
  - Hypercalcemia: Lethargy, weakness, confusion, depression
  - Hyperviscosity: HA, fatigue, visual disturbance, retinopathy
  - Peripheral nerve infiltration: Carpal tunnel syndrome, polyneuropathies
- Splenomegaly/adenopathy uncommon

Diagnosis

- Classic triad
  - Marrow plasmacytosis (>10%)
  - Lytic bone lesions
  - Serum or urine M protein spike (monoclonal) on protein electrophoresis in gamma region
- Diagnostic workup
  - CBC
  - Bone marrow biopsy/aspirate
  - Serum and urine protein electrophoresis
  - Quantitative immunoglobins
  - Labs: Renal function tests, chemistries, calcium, uric acid, alkaline phosphatase, β_2 microglobulin, LDH
  - Urine tests: 24-hour urine for protein, Bence-Jones protein (light chains)
  - Chest X-ray and bone radiographs

Treatment

- Localized plasmacytomas and pathologic fractures/cord compression treated with radiation therapy
- Myeloma treatment
  - Chemotherapy to stop progression of disease: Alkylating agent (melphalan) plus prednisone; other therapies include IFN-α, arsenic, and thalidomide
  - Bisphosphanates for bony lesions
  - Renal protective measures: Fluids, allopurinol, avoid IV dye
  - Treat infections as necessary
  - Plasmapheresis for hyperviscosity
  - Bone marrow transplant for chemoresponsive disease to prolong remission

Prognosis/Clinical Course

- 10% of patients have an indolent course with slow progression over many years
- 15% die within 3 months of diagnosis; 15% die per year thereafter
- Stage I (mean survival = 5 years)
  - Hb >10 g/dL
  - Serum Ca <12 mg/dL
  - Normal bone X-ray or solitary lesion
  - Low M component (in urine or blood)
- Stage II (mean survival = 4.5 years): Patients not fitting into Stages I or III
- Stage III (mean survival = 1–2 years)
  - Hb <8.5 g/dL
  - Serum Ca >12 mg/dL
  - Advanced lytic bone lesions
  - High M component
- Renal failure in 25% due to hypercalcemia, amyloid, infiltration by myeloma cells

161. Myelodysplastic Syndromes

Etiology

- Ineffective hematopoiesis is characterized by pancytopenia, a low reticulocyte count, and abnormal hematopoietic cell features
- Two endpoints of disease: Acute leukemia or myelofibrosis
- Pathogenesis: Acquired deficiency of stem cells due to:
  - Genetic: Down's syndrome, Fanconi's anemia, von Recklinghausen's disease
  - Chemicals: Alkylating agents, benzene
  - May be secondary to treatment (i.e., chemotherapy for aplastic anemia, X-ray treatments)

Differential Dx

- Aplastic anemia
- Vitamin deficiencies (B_{12}, folate, B_6)
- Paroxysmal nocturnal hemoglobinuria
- Aleukemic acute leukemia
- Acute and chronic myelofibrosis
- Cirrhosis

Epidemiology

- 3000 new cases per year
- Most common in 70–80 year-olds

Signs/Symptoms

- Often asymptomatic
- Most symptoms attributable to anemia (weakness, fatigue, palpitations, HA, dizziness, irritability)
- Excessive bleeding due to thrombocytopenia
- Hepatosplenomegaly (uncommon)

Diagnosis

- Primarily diagnosed on CBC: Cytopenia in 1 or more lineages
- Peripheral smear
  - Anisocytosis (size difference in RBCs)
  - RBC abnormalities
  - Hypolobulated, hypogranular PMNs
  - Increased monocytosis
  - Increased platelet size
- Decreased reticulocyte count
- Bone marrow biopsy/aspirate show similar abnormalities as peripheral smear
- Cytogenetics: Deletions in 7, 8, or 5q

Treatment

- Supportive therapy
  - RBC transfusion
  - Erythropoietin
  - Platelet transfusion
  - G-CSF and GM-CSF
  - Vitamin treatment
- Allogenic bone marrow transplant may be curative
  - 60% of transplants fail due to complications/ recurrence
- High-dose chemotherapy

Prognosis/Clinical Course

- Course depends on the severity of the disease and number of blasts
- Can be a chronic condition requiring transfusions
- Progresses to AML in 10% of cases

162. Myeloproliferative Disorders

Etiology

- Disorder of multipotent hematopoietic progenitor stem cells, resulting in overproduction of blood cells
- Classified based on the predominant abnormal clone
  - Polycythemia vera (PV): Increased RBCs
  - Essential thrombocytosis (ET): Elevated (and abnormal) platelets
  - Chronic myelogenous leukemia (CML): Increased WBCs (presence of Philadelphia chromosome)
  - Idiopathic myelofibrosis (IM): All cell lines decreased

Epidemiology

- Affects adults aged 40–60

Differential Dx

- PV: Hypoxia (smoker's polycythemia), Gaisbock syndrome, renal disease, hepatic disease, paraneoplastic syndromes (pheochromocytoma, renal cell cancer, hepatoma), exogenous androgens
- ET: Sepsis, splenectomy, inflammatory conditions
- CML: Leukemoid reaction, chronic neutrophilic leukemia, acute leukemia
- IM: Aplastic anemia, metastatic cancer, infection, SLE, aleukemic leukemia

Signs/Symptoms

- Most patients are asymptomatic
- PV: Intra-abdominal venous thrombosis, massive splenomegaly, pruritis, vertigo, tinnitus, HA, visual disturbance, HTN, digital ischemia
- ET: Signs of hemorrhage (abnormal platelets) and thrombosis (too many platelets), microvascular occlusion, mild splenomegaly
- CML: Constitutional symptoms (fatigue, weight loss, malaise), splenomegaly, LUQ pain/mass, frequent infxns, early satiety, bleeding/thrombosis, leukostasis and vaso-oclusive syndromes (CVA, MI, venous thrombosis)
- IM: Hepatosplenomegaly, symptoms of anemia/thrombocytopenia/neutropenia

Diagnosis

- CBC is the key to diagnosis, as most patients are initially asymptomatic
- Bone marrow biopsy/aspirate is required to rule out acute leukemia
- PV: Increased RBC mass; normal O_2 saturation; splenomegaly
- ET: Platelets $> 600 \times 10^9$ on 2 occasions with normal RBC mass; marrow fibrosis; splenomegaly; absence of Philadelphia chromosome
- CML: t(9,22) bcr-abl translocation; presence of Philadelphia chromosome; increased WBCs (basophils, eosinophils, PMNs, and monocytes all increased); leukocyte alkaline phosphatase (LAP) usually decreased
- IM: Anemia, thrombocytopenia, teardrop cells, nucleated RBCs; dry tap; splenomegaly; autoimmune abnormalities (positive Coombs test, rheumatoid factor, ANA)

Treatment

- PV: Phlebotomy, PUVA for pruritis, chemotherapy (alkylating agents, anagrelide, IFN-α)
- ET: Hydroxyurea, anagrelide to decrease platelets, low-dose aspirin
- CML: New treatment is bcr-abl tyrosine kinase inhibitor—STI571 (Gleevec), IFN-α, combination chemotherapy, splenectomy
- IM: Allogenic bone marrow transplant, allopurinol to decrease uric acid, hydroxyurea for organomegaly, IFN-α

Prognosis/Clinical Course

- PV: May be indolent or lead to myelofibrosis/leukemia
- ET: Rarely progresses to acute leukemia; always poses a risk of thrombosis; younger patients (<40 years) may not need treatment
- CML: Median survival is 4 years; three stages of disease:
  - Chronic phase (<5% blasts)
  - Accelerated phase: Hepatosplenomegaly with progressive anemia and thrombocytopenia (<30% blasts)
  - Blast crisis: Essentially acute myelogenous leukemia—short survival (>30% blasts)
- IM: Median survival is 5 years; predisposed to lung infections

Reproductive Disease

ELLEN SMITH, MD, FACP

163. Sexually Transmitted Diseases

Etiology

- Herpes: Herpes simplex virus
- Syphilis: *Treponema pallidum*
- Chancroid: *Haemophilus ducreyi*
- Lymphogranuloma venereum: *Chlamydia trachomatis*
- Granuloma inguinale: *Calymmatobacterium granulomatis*
- Condyloma acuminata: Human papillomavirus (venereal warts)
- Gonorrhea: *Neisseria gonorrhoeae*
- Vaginitis: *Trichomonas vaginalis*
- Cervicitis/urethritis: *N. gonorrhoeae, Chlamydia,* ureaplasma

Differential Dx

- HIV
- PID
- Ectopic pregnancy
- Tuberculosis involving lymph nodes
- Lymphomas
- Poor hygiene
- Diverticulitis
- Viral skin infections
- Other STDs
- Candidiasis
- UTI

Epidemiology

- Incidence of STDs has decreased in homosexuals but the prevalence persists due to heterosexual transmission
- The most common associated coinfection is HIV
- Unprotected sex, promiscuity, and low socioeconomic status are risk factors

Signs/Symptoms

- *Painful* genital sores: Herpes, chancroid
- *Painless* genital sores: Syphilis, condyloma acuminata, granuloma inguinale, lymphogranuloma venereum
- Herpes: Painful vesicles; itching and burning; may present with fever, HA
- Lymphogranuloma venereum: Fever, malaise, bilateral tender inguinal adenopathy (may fistulize and form abscess)
- Chancroid: Painful, deep ulcer with exudate (suppurative in 60% of cases); followed in 1–2 weeks by painful local lymphadenitis
- Vaginitis/urethritis: Purulent discharge with pubic pain and/or dysuria

Diagnosis

- Herpes: Clinical identification of its characteristic ulcer, Tzank smear, tissue culture or serology
- Syphilis: RPR, VDRL
- Chancroid: Generally diagnosed by the appropriate clinical picture with negative herpes and syphilis workup
- Lymphogranuloma venereum: Complement fixation
- Granuloma inguinale: Scraping with Wright's and Giemsa stains that show Donovan bodies
- Urethritis/cervicitis: *N. gonorrhoeae* culture and *Chlamydia* test
- HIV screening in any patient with STD
- HPV: Females should undergo regular Pap smears to rule out cervical dysplasia and cancer; anal smear of homosexual men to rule out anal-rectal cancers

Treatment

- Herpes: Acyclovir for severe cases; prophylactic treatment with acyclovir only for >5 episodes per year; topical treatment is not effective
- Syphilis, gonorrhea, *Chlamydia:* See separate entries
- Chancroid: Ceftriaxone IM once or azithromycin po once
- *Trichomonas vaginalis:* Metronidazole × 7 days
- Lymphogranuloma inguinale: Tetracycline or doxycycline × 21 days
- HPV: Destroy or excise warts
- Counseling for safe-sex practices

Prognosis/Clinical Course

- Excellent prognosis with treatment with the exception of tertiary syphilis and HIV
- Herpes recurrence (due to HSV being dormant in nerve root ganglia); infection is usually much more severe and extensive in immunocompromised hosts
- Chancroid treatment is generally effective if appropriately diagnosed
- LGV can result in chronic lymphangitis, scarring, and genital distortion due to fibrosis if not fully treated
- Test for and treat for other STDs when any STD is found
- Encourage partner to be tested and treated to prevent reinfection(s) between partners

164. STDs: Gonorrhea and Chlamydia

Etiology

- Bacterial infection with:
  - *Chlamydia trachomatis:* Obligate intracellular pathogen
  - *Neisseria gonorrhoeae:* Gram-negative intracellular diplococcus

Differential Dx

- Vaginitis
- Appendicitis
- Gastroenteritis
- Pregnancy (with or without complications)
- Tubo-ovarian abscess
- Other STDs
- Nongonococcal urethritis
- Reiter's syndrome (urethritis)
- Mittleschmerz

Epidemiology

- *Chlamydia* is the most commonly reported STD in US—incidence 200 per 100,000 but as high as 20% in some populations
- 600,000 cases of gonorrhea per year in US
- Less frequent when barrier contraception is used
- Be sure to test and treat partners if possible
- Report to Health Department as per state guidelines

Signs/Symptoms

- Majority of cases are asymptomatic
- Vaginal discharge: Mucopurulent discharge from cervix or urethra
- Urethral discharge, often purulent
- Dysuria, urgency, frequency
- Pelvic pain, dyspareunia, cervical motion tenderness if pelvic inflammatory disease (PID) develops
- Upper-right quadrant pain can be seen in gonorrhea with development of Fitz-Hugh-Curtis syndrome (perihepatitis)

Diagnosis

- Mucopurulent cervical or urethral specimens
- Positive culture testing on cervical or urethral specimens
- Direct fluorescent antibody or enzyme immunoassay for *Chlamydia*
- Ligase chain reaction (LCR) or polymerase chain reaction (PCR) on cervical, urethral, or urine specimens
- LCR and PCR DNA amplification techniques are now the gold standard for diagnosing both gonorrhea and *Chlamydia*
- PID is diagnosed with these assays as well as cervical motion tenderness, lower abdominal tenderness, and adnexal tenderness, fever, leukocytosis, and Gram stain
- Screening for *Chlamydia* and *N. gonorrhoeae* is recommended in all sexually active women (and possibly men) younger than age 25 and for older sexually active women (and possibly men) with multiple partners, inadequate barrier protection, and/or a history of multiple STDs

Treatment

- Coinfection is so common that nearly all cases should be treated for both *Chlamydia* and gonorrhea
- *Chlamydia*
  - Doxycycline × 7 days
  - Azithromycin × 1 dose (if pregnant or noncompliant)
  - Erythromycin × 7 days (if pregnant)
- Gonorrhea
  - Ciprofloxacin × 1 dose
  - Ceftriaxone IM × 1 dose (if pregnant)
  - Cefixime × 1 dose (if pregnant)
- PID
  - Ofloxacin × 14 days
  - Metronidazole × 14 days

Prognosis/Clinical Course

- Many asymptomatic cases, which may result in propagation of an infection to the patient's sexual partners
- Prognosis is good if treated early, but worse if treated later or if PID develops
- PID increases the likelihood of infertility, ectopic pregnancy, and chronic pelvic pain
- Asymptomatic, untreated cases may cause scarring of fallopian tubes, resulting in infertility and/or ectopic pregnancy
- Treat for other STDs when any STD is found (consider HIV, hepatitis B and C, syphilis)
- Treat partner to prevent reinfection back and forth between partners

165. STDs: Syphilis

Etiology

- A systemic disease caused by *Treponema pallidum*
- Disease begins after incubation of 2–6 weeks
- First manifestation is a primary skin lesion (chancre) with regional enlarged lymph nodes
- Secondary bacteremic period follows weeks to months after chancre: Mucocutaneous rash, lymphadenopathy, fever, and systemic disease
- Tertiary stage may include CNS, vascular, skin, and skeletal lesions
- Latent syphilis: Positive serologies without clinical manifestations

Epidemiology

- Most common method of transmission is sexual contact, then transfusions and perinatal infection
- Incidence in homosexual and bisexual populations has decreased secondary to scares of HIV epidemic
- Increasing incidence in African Americans

Differential Dx

- Chancroid
- Lymphogranuloma venereum
- Herpes simplex
- Malignancy
- HIV
- Gonorrhea
- Pityriasis rosea (similar to rash of 2° syphilis)
- Viral syndrome
- Peripheral vascular disease (similar to CV symptoms of 3° syphilis)
- Meningitis (similar to neurosyphilis)

Signs/Symptoms

- 1°: *Painless* ulcer (chancre) occurs at site of inoculation (bacterial infection of ulcer may cause pain)
- 2°: Maculopapular rash on palms and soles, mucus membrane lesions (condyloma lata); nontender adenopathy; fever, weight loss, fatigue, sore throat
- 3°: Gummas—subcutaneous, ulcerative lesions of skin (also possible in bone, heart, CNS); neurosyphilis involves meningeal signs, paresis, tabes dorsalis (degeneration of posterior columns of spinal cord, resulting in Argyll Robertson pupil—does not react to light but does accommodate, and hypotonia); CV—aortic aneurysm, aortic regurgitation

Diagnosis

- Serologic tests: Generally positive in 1° syphilis; always positive in 2° syphilis; nearly always positive in 3° syphilis
  - VDRL (Venereal Disease Research Laboratory) or RPR (Rapid Plasma Reagin) are cheap and quick but less sensitive; false-positives may occur in young females, in pregnancy, and in patients with SLE, mononucleosis, and endocarditis; always confirm with FTA-ABS
  - FTA-ABS (Fluorescent Treponemal Antibody test—ABSorbed) is more sensitive and specific
  - No diagnostic test will detect primary syphilis with certainty (sensitivity only 75–85%); therefore, a negative test does not exclude primary syphilis and must be repeated in 4–6 weeks
- Dark-field microscopy of skin lesion or lymph node aspirate
- CSF examination if suspicious of neurosyphilis: Pleocytosis with increased protein

Treatment

- 1°, 2°, or early latent syphilis (<1 year)
  - Penicillin IM in 1 dose *or*
  - Oral doxycycline × two weeks in penicillin allergy
- 3° (with normal CSF) or late latent syphilis (>1 year)
  - Penicillin IM weekly × 3 doses *or*
  - Oral doxycycline × 4 weeks
- Neurosyphilis: IV penicillin for 10–14 days
- Consider more aggressive treatment in HIV-infected patients

Prognosis/Clinical Course

- Recovery in all stages is excellent
- Sequelae of secondary syphilis (aortitis) or tertiary syphilis (tabes dorsalis, neuropathy, or paresis) may not recover and may need other supportive therapy
- RPR should be a part of health maintenance exams for all patients at risk for STDs
- Test all patients with syphilis for other STDs, including HIV infection
- VDRL or RPR is used to monitor response to treatment; it should become negative (or at least have a fourfold decrease) within a year in most cases; any subsequent fourfold increase should be considered a recurrence or reinfection and treatment should be repeated

166. STDs: Human Papillomavirus

Etiology

- The vast majority of cases of cervical dysplasia and cancer are due to infection by human papillomavirus
  - Types 6, 11, and 35 have a low dysplasia potential—more likely to cause warts or low-grade squamous intraepithelial lesion (LGSIL)
  - Types 16, 18, 35, and others have a higher dysplasia potential—more likely to cause high-grade squamous intraepithelial lesion (HGSIL), carcinoma in situ (CIS), and invasive carcinoma

Differential Dx

- Vigorous intercourse
- Vaginal infection/vaginitis
- Introduction of objects into vagina
- Spotting, often due to irregular OCP use
- DUB
- PCOS

Epidemiology

- With the widespread use of Pap smears, the incidence of cervical cancer has decreased significantly; still very high incidence in poor areas without access to Pap smears
- Tobacco abuse and OCP use increase risk
- Early sexual activity, unprotected sex, and multiple sexual partners increase the risk of being exposed to HPV

Signs/Symptoms

- Most patients with cervical dysplasia are asymptomatic
- Less commonly, patients present with:
  - Post-coital vaginal bleeding
  - Vaginal discharge
  - Irregular vaginal bleeding (spotting)
  - Vaginal pain
  - Bloody, malodorous discharge (late presentation)
- Cervical exam
  - Unexplained cervical friability
  - Cervical nodules or thickening

Diagnosis

- Identified by Pap smear screening in most cases
- Colposcopy with endocervical sampling and biopsy give a definitive diagnosis to guide treatment
- Colposcopy with immediate LEEP (see Treatment) is indicated for patients who are very unlikely to follow up for definitive treatment

Treatment

- Pap smear result of ASCUS (atypical squamous cells of unknown significance) should be repeated; if it persists, proceed to colposcopy
- All abnormal Pap smears (LGSIL/HGSIL/CIS/cancer) require colposcopy
- Treatment is based on post-colposcopy findings: May include frequent repeat Pap smears; discontinuation of smoking; removal of atypical areas of the cervix via loop electrosurgical excision procedure (LEEP), laser therapy, or hysterectomy
- All glandular abnormalities (atypical glands of unknown significance—AGUS, glandular atypia) require colposcopy and adequate endometrial evaluation

Prognosis/Clinical Course

- ASCUS frequently returns to normal; 10% of cases progress to low- or high-grade SIL
- LGSIL may also return to normal, remain as LGSIL, or progress to high-grade SIL (20%); close follow-up is required
- HGSIL should be treated because it progresses to cancer in about 25% of cases
- CIS and cancer often have a good outcome if treated early, but may result in significant mortality and morbidity
- HIV infection increases the risk of a rapid transition to dysplasia or cancer

167. Breast Cancer

Etiology

- Risk factors: Previous breast cancer, family history, BRCA gene mutations, increased estrogens (early menarche, late menopause, nulliparity, OCP use, hormone replacement therapy, obesity)
- Most affected patients have no risk factors

Epidemiology

- Most common cancer in women; 1 in 8 women will develop it; nearly 4% will die of it; second most common cause of cancer death (#1 is lung cancer)
- Incidence increasing, but mortality has remained stable
- Median age = mid-50s; increasing risk with age

Differential Dx

- Cyst
- Fibroadenoma
- Fibrocystic change
- Breast abscess
- Breast cancer
  - Tubular (most favorable)
  - Colloid/mucinous
  - Papillary
  - Medullary
  - Invasive lobular
  - Invasive ductal
  - Inflammatory (worst prognosis)

Signs/Symptoms

- Asymptomatic breast mass is most common complaint
- Breast pain, if present, suggests less likely to be cancer
- Bloody discharge (ominous sign)
- Unilateral discharge (especially in intraductal cancer)
- Asymmetry of breasts
- Skin changes and dimpling of skin
- Nipple retraction
- Lymphadenopathy—axillary, supra/infraclavicular
- Benign masses tend to be mobile, soft, and cystic

Diagnosis

- PE: Look for symmetry, skin changes, nipple retraction, drainage, enlarged nodes
- Mammography: Annual over age 40; sooner if symptomatic; 20% false-negative, so a normal test does not rule out cancer
- Ultrasound: For symptomatic patients with normal mammogram; distinguishes between solid or cystic lesion
- MRI: To evaluate questionable lesions on mammogram
- Fine-needle aspiration: Will drain lesion if it is cystic; if solid, FNA is used to extract cells for cytologic exam
- Core-needle biopsy for large lesion (may soon replace FNA)
- Excisional biopsy is the definitive test—may be curative if full lesion is removed
- If positive biopsy, node sample must be done
- CXR/chest CT: Evaluate thoracic bone and lung metastases
- LFTs, U/S, and CT of liver: Evaluate liver metastases
- Bone scan/alk phos/calcium level: Evaluate bone mets

Treatment

- Observe for 1–2 cycles if lump appears physiologic (young patients)
- Breast conservation surgery: Lumpectomy, axillary lymphadenectomy, and postoperative radiation have equivalent survival to mastectomy
- Modified radical mastectomy
- Adjuvant therapy if lymph nodes are positive for cancer cells
  - Tamoxifen for 2–5 years if estrogen/progesterone receptors are present on tumor cells (as effective as chemotherapy in post-menopausal women)
  - Multidrug chemotherapy for 4–6 months
  - Radiation for local treatment
  - Ovarian ablation in premenopausal patients

Prognosis/Clinical Course

- Criteria for inoperability: Extensive edema of breast/arm, satellite nodules, inflammatory carcinoma, parasternal tumor, supraclavicular or distant metastases
- Prognosis correlated with size of tumor and number of positive nodes
- If nodes negative, 70% do not recur and no adjuvant therapy needed
- Follow-up: Monitor for recurrence (5 × baseline risk in contralateral breast)
  - Monthly self-breast exams
  - Regular physical examinations
  - Yearly mammograms
- Recurrence within 2 yrs has poor prognosis
- Must rule out mets: Most common are bone (back pain), brain (seizures, headache), lung (SOB, cough), and liver

168. Leiomyoma (Fibroids)

Etiology

- Benign smooth muscle tumor

Differential Dx

- Ovarian cyst
- Ovarian carcinoma
- Tubo-ovarian abscess
- Endometriosis
- Endometrial carcinoma
- Adenomyosis
- Myometrial hypertrophy
- Leiomyosarcoma
- PID
- Cervical cancer
- Pregnancy

Epidemiology

- 20–25% of reproductive age women
- 3–4 times more common in black women

Signs/Symptoms

- Often asymptomatic
- Symptoms
  – Hypermenorrhea
  – Metrorrhagia
  – Dysmenorrhea
  – Pain
  – Pressure
  – Urinary frequency and urgency
  – Dyspareunia
  – Infertility
  – Spontaneous abortion
- Firm, irregular uterine mass

Diagnosis

- Complete history and physical examination
- Bimanual examination with direct palpation
- β-HCG to rule out pregnancy
- Pap smear and endometrial biopsy
- Ultrasound is often diagnostic
- Hysterosalpingography for definitive diagnosis
- CBC to rule out anemia if heavy bleeding

Treatment

- Treatment depends on patient's age, parity, pregnancy status, and desire for future fertility
- Majority do not require treatment—follow with periodic examinations, Pap smear, and ultrasound
- Depo-Provera to induce amenorrhea if bleeding is heavy
- GnRH agonist to limit growth
- Myomectomy
- Hysterectomy (especially if severe anemia or severe symptoms and fertility is no longer desired)

Prognosis/Clinical Course

- Increase in size with estrogen therapy and during pregnancy
- Decrease in size and often disappear after menopause
- Removal of the leiomyoma should be considered when it grows larger than a 12- to 14-week pregnant uterus

169. Dysfunctional Uterine Bleeding

Etiology

- Bleeding caused by factors other than pelvic anatomic abnormalities, pregnancy, bleeding disorders, endocrine disorders, or medications
- Due to hormonal changes and other aspects of the reproductive system that are not easily quantifiable
- Anovulatory cycles associated with menarche and menopause are common causes of DUB

Differential Dx

- Hyper/hypothyroidism
- Pregnancy (or ectopic)
- Endometrial fibroid, hyperplasia, or cancer
- Cervical inflammation, infection, polyp, or trauma
- Atrophic vaginitis
- Vaginal trauma
- Ovarian cyst
- PCOS
- Bleeding diathesis (coagulopathy, von Willebrand's disease, leukemia, thrombocytopenia, hepatic disease)
- Meds (warfarin, OCP, forms of progesterone)
- Anovulatory cycles

Epidemiology

- DUB is the most common form of irregular vaginal bleeding

Signs/Symptoms

- Menorrhagia: Prolonged and/or excessive, yet regular, bleeding
- Metrorrhagia: Irregular and more frequent than normal bleeding, but with a regular amount of flow
- Menometrorrhagia: Prolonged and/or excessive bleeding at frequent, irregular intervals
- Polymenorrhea: Regular and more frequent than every 21 days
- Oligomenorrhea: Bleeding < every 35 days and at least once every six months; also used to describe lighter than normal flow
- Amenorrhea: No bleeding for 6+ months
- Intermenstrual bleeding: Between periods
- Postmenopausal bleeding: Bleeding at least one year after menopause

Diagnosis

- DUB is a diagnosis of exclusion; one must adequately exclude all possible diagnoses
- History and physical may reveal the etiology
- Urine or serum pregnancy test to rule out pregnancy
- TSH and CBC
- Cervical cultures
- Coagulation studies (PT/PTT/INR)
- Pelvic ultrasound is indicated for all patients who have any pelvic abnormality, who are too large to examine adequately, and/or to measure endometrial thickness; hysteroscopy may also be considered
- Endometrial biopsy in all cases of postmenopausal bleeding, as well as obese or diabetic patients who have a higher baseline risk of endometrial cancer

Treatment

- Treat underlying cause if possible
- Progesterone challenge test (progesterone 10 mg QD for 10 days) is recommended to temporarily stop excessive bleeding or bring on bleeding in a patient who is oligomenorrheic—but only after pregnancy has been excluded; if successful, repeat challenges every one to three months will often effectively regulate flow
- Oral contraceptives will regulate flow in patients who need simultaneous contraception or have polycystic ovarian syndrome; may also benefit patients who have stress-related DUB
- Hormone replacement therapy (HRT) may regulate flow in perimenopausal women, but must not be used until pathology has been effectively ruled out

Prognosis/Clinical Course

- The prognosis of DUB is generally excellent, as long as a complete evaluation to rule out significant pathology is performed prior to making the diagnosis
- Several courses of therapy may be needed to fully manage the bleeding; this issue should be discussed with the patient prior to embarking on a treatment course
- Atrophic vaginitis is the most common cause of postmenopausal vaginal bleeding; however, all cases of postmenopausal bleeding must be worked up for endometrial cancer

170. Endometriosis

Etiology

- The presence of functioning endometrial tissue outside the uterus
- Most common areas of ectopic endometrial tissue are ovaries, but may occur anywhere in body (e.g., eye, lung)
- Endometrioma: Area of endometriosis large enough to be a tumor
- Chocolate cyst: An endometrioma that is filled with old blood, often resembling tar or chocolate
- Cause not definitively proven; theories include retrograde menstruation and coelemic theory (normal cells change into endometrial cells)

Epidemiology

- Incidence and risk factors are not accurately identified
- Apparent risk factors include family history, polymenorrhea or menorrhagia, multiple pregnancies, and prolonged oral contraceptive use

Differential Dx

- PID
- UTI
- Ovarian cyst
- Ovarian/uterine cancer
- Ovarian torsion
- Scarring from prior surgery or PID
- Vaginismus
- Vaginitis
- Vaginal foreign body
- Vaginal trauma
- Amenorrhea
- Endometrioma
- Appendicitis

Signs/Symptoms

- Triad of cyclic pelvic pain, dyspareunia (deep), and infertility
- May be asymptomatic
- Dysmenorrhea is common, but not specific for endometriosis
- Abnormal menses
- Dysuria or hematuria, especially with menses
- Constipation, diarrhea, bowel frequency, and/or painful defecation
- Rare before menarche or after menopause
- Suprapubic tenderness
- Painful nodules of uterosacral ligaments
- Fixed uterus, especially retroverted
- Induration of cul-de-sac

Diagnosis

- Complete history and physical examination
- Laparoscopy is the gold standard for diagnosis
- Urinalysis
- β-HCG
- Ultrasound

Treatment

- Treatment depends on the level of symptoms and desire for present and future fertility
- NSAIDs used perimenstrually for symptom relief (ibuprofen for 2–3 days premenstrual and continued through menses)
- Oral contraceptives
- Danazol and GnRH agonists (leuprolide)
- Laparoscopic ablation of ectopic endometrial tissue
- Total abdominal hysterectomy (TAH) with or without bilateral salpingo-oophorectomy (BSO) may be needed if pain is severe and childbearing is no longer desired

Prognosis/Clinical Course

- Acyclic OCPs can reduce dysmenorrhea by creating an oligomenorrheic state
- Recurrence is common for most medical therapies (about 50%) without definitive surgical treatment
- Menopause is curative in most cases
- Fertility is increased by approximately 12% in women who have surgical treatment of their endometriosis; if this is unsuccessful, typical infertility treatments such as clomiphene citrate or leuprolide can increase the potential for fertility
- Successful conception occurs in approximately 60% of treated patients with advanced endometriosis and infertility

171. Ovarian Cysts and Tumors

Etiology

- Functional ovarian cysts are due to normal hormonal cycling
- 80% of ovarian tumors are benign; ovarian cysts are the most common cause of ovarian enlargement in menstruating women
- Malignant transformation of ovarian tissue may be due to chronic uninterrupted ovulation (nulliparity, delayed childbearing, late menopause; conversely, OCPs are protective because they suppress ovulation)
- Account for 25% of all gynecologic malignancies but 50% of gynecologic cancer deaths

Epidemiology

- Lifetime risk of ovarian cancer in the US is 1.4 per 100 women (fifth most common cancer in females)
- Risk of ovarian cancer increases with familial ovarian cancer syndrome, breast-ovarian cancer syndrome, or hereditary nonpolyposis colorectal cancer syndrome

Differential Dx

- Ovarian cyst
- Ectopic pregnancy
- Ovarian neoplasm (benign or malignant)
  - Germ cell (15%)
  - Epithelial (80%)
  - Sex cord stromal tumors (5%)
  - Metastases (5%)
- Ovarian torsion
- Endometrioma
- Leiomyoma/sarcoma
- Tubo-ovarian abscess
- Hydrosalpinx
- Appendicitis
- Appendiceal abscess
- Pelvic kidney

Signs/Symptoms

- Asymptomatic pelvic mass (approximately 30%)
- Pressure or pain in lateral pelvic region (>50%)
- Dysmenorrhea
- Irregular menses
- Nausea/vomiting and other GI complaints
- Urinary complaints
- Endocrine abnormalities
- Precocious puberty

Diagnosis

- Adnexal masses are often found incidentally on routine history and physical examination of women; pay special attention to menstrual, sexual, and pregnancy history as well as any family history of ovarian or other gynecologic cancers
- Pregnancy test (urine or serum)
- Pelvic ultrasound is often diagnostic
- Some authors suggest CA-125 tumor marker evaluation
- Solid lesions and complex cysts require:
  - CT scan (or MRI) of pelvis and abdomen
  - Referral to gynecology or gynecologic oncology for laparoscopy or laparotomy
- If cancer, look for metastases

Treatment

- Simple cysts <3 cm are followed clinically or with ultrasound
- Simple cysts ≥3 cm and <5 cm are followed in one to two cycles with a repeat ultrasound
- Noncyclic oral contraceptives should be given to patients with simple cysts, unless there are contraindications to this treatment
- Simple cysts >5 cm should be referred to a gynecologist for excision; an increase in pain or size requires reevaluation
- Complex and solid cysts should be referred to a gynecologist or gynecologic oncologist
- Ovarian cancers may be treated with hysterectomy, simple excision, and/or chemotherapy

Prognosis/Clinical Course

- Simple cysts are virtually always benign
- Cysts >5 cm have a minimally higher malignancy potential, but it is still very low
- Ovarian tumors have varied outcomes depending on whether they are benign or malignant, and their grade and stage
- Screen for ovarian cancer for women with a relative with ovarian cancer or other risk factors
  - Genetic evaluation (BRCA1 and 2)
  - Screening with CA-125, α-fetoprotein, lactate dehydrogenase, or β-HCG
  - Pelvic ultrasound
- 5-year survival for ovarian cancer is <30%
- Bowel metastases may result in bowel obstruction (carcinomatous ileus)
- Ascites may result from peritoneal spread

172. Polycystic Ovarian Syndrome*

Etiology

*Previously called Stein-Leventhal syndrome
- Androgen excess, possibly due to excess LH stimulation of ovaries

Epidemiology

- Affects 5% of reproductive-aged women; may constitute the most common endocrinopathy in this age group
- Associated with obesity

Differential Dx

- Androgen-producing tumors of the ovary or adrenal gland
- Human gonadotropin-producing tumors outside the reproductive tract
- Hyper/hypothyroidism
- Prolactinemia
- Prolactinoma
- Cushing's syndrome
- Hyperthecosis
- Acquired or congenital adrenal hyperplasia
- Familial hirsutism (common in certain ethnic groups)

Signs/Symptoms

- HAIR-AN
  - Hyperandrogenism (hirsutism)
  - Insulin resistance (obesity, glucose intolerance)
  - Acanthosis nigricans (velvety, raised, hyperpigmented skin lesions on back of neck, axilla, and genitalia)
- Menstrual irregularities: Often oligomenorrhea or amenorrhea; may be anovulatory
- Decreased fertility or infertility
- Obesity
- Hyperlipidemia is common
- Enlarged ovaries

Diagnosis

- Diagnosis based on clinical syndrome, as evaluated by comprehensive history and physical examination
- Diagnosis depends on hyperandrogenism, either clinical or biochemical, and the exclusion of other diseases
- The isolated finding of polycystic ovaries is very common (occurring in 16–25% of the normal population); it is therefore not useful diagnostically
- Must rule out other causes of hirsutism and/or obesity, such as thyroid disease; do at least TSH, DHEA-S, and free testosterone levels
- Glucose, Hb_{A1c}, insulin levels, FSH and LH (LH:FSH ratio >2.5)
- Ultrasound of ovaries is not generally part of the diagnostic workup; shows enlarged ovaries with numerous cysts with characteristic "pearl necklace" appearance (ring-like cysts on the ovaries)

Treatment

- Oral contraceptives to regulate menstrual cycle
- Spironolactone to decrease hirsutism
- Eflornithine (Vaniqa) topical cream: Decreases hirsutism
- Clomiphine citrate: Induces ovulation
- Pioglitazone (Actos): Increases insulin sensitivity and regulates menstrual cycle
- Metformin (Glucophage): Increases insulin sensitivity, regulates menses, induces weight loss, and decreases acanthosis nigricans
- Weight loss: Increases insulin sensitivity, regulates menses, and decreases lipids

Prognosis/Clinical Course

- OCPs very effectively regulate menses in women not desiring pregnancy; monthly progesterone challenges are also an option for women who do not need contraception; both decrease the risk of endometrial cancer
- Clomiphene induces ovulation in about 75%
- Pioglitazone and metformin may decrease the risk of subsequent diabetes; metformin often leads to weight loss
- Prognosis for fertility, decreased hirsutism, and decreased glucose intolerance is better if weight loss is achieved
- Treatment may result in increased fertility, so adequate contraception should be instituted as necessary
- Increased risk of endometrial cancer due to estrogen excess

173. Vaginal Discharge

Etiology

- Generally results from either an STD (*Trichomonas vaginalis, Neisseria gonorrhoeae/Chlamydia trachomatis,* or bacterial vaginosis—often *Gardnerella vaginalis*), alteration of normal vaginal flora (*Candida albicans* overgrowth), or inflammatory response (atrophic vaginitis)

Epidemiology

- *Trichomonas, N. gonorrhoeae,* and *Chlamydia* are very common causes of STDs
- *Candida* more common with recent antibiotic use, poorly controlled diabetes, and pregnancy
- Atrophic vaginitis is common in postmenopausal women, especially those not on hormone replacement

Differential Dx

- Normal physiologic discharge
- Foreign body vaginitis (i.e., tampon left in too long)
- Irritant/allergic vaginitis
- Cervicitis
- Cervical dysplasia, cancer, or polyps
- Vaginal or vulvar trauma
- Vaginal or vulvar cancer
- Increased discharge associated with pregnancy

Signs/Symptoms

- All may be asymptomatic
- Increased discharge volume
- Change in odor, consistency, or color of discharge
- *Trichomonas:* "Strawberry cervix"
- Gonorrhea/*Chlamydia:* May be associated with pelvic pain, dysmenorrhea, dyspareunia
- BV: Characteristic fishy odor
- *Candida:* Intense pruritis; raw, inflamed, erythematous introitus
- Atrophic vaginitis: Poor coital lubrication with or without dyspareunia; dysuria due to atrophic urethral tissue

Diagnosis

- History and physical examination are crucial
- Wet mount with KOH prep:

	pH	Discharge	Odor	Wet Mount
Trich	>4.5	Yellow-green, copious	Present	Motile, flagellated
BV	>4.5	White-gray	Fishy	Clue cells
Candida	<4.5	White, curd-like	None	Pseudo–hyphae
Gonorrhea/ *Chlamydia*		Mucopurulent	Varies	PMNs
Atrophic vag		Absent, pale cervix	None	Few epithelial cells

Treatment

- *Trichomonas:* Metronidazole 2 g po once or 500 mg BID × 7 days (no alcohol with metronidazole)
  – Intravaginal clotrimazole if pregnant or unable to use metronidazole
- Gonorrhea/*Chlamydia:* See STDS: Gonorrhea and Chlamydia
- BV: Metronidazole 2 g po once or 500 mg BID × 7 days
- *Candida:* Clotrimazole 1% cream intravaginally QD × 5–7 days or fluconazole 150 mg po once
- Atrophic vaginitis: Topical or oral hormone replacement if appropriate

Prognosis/Clinical Course

- *Trichomonas:* Treat partner to prevent reinfection
- BV: Increased risk of premature labor, premature rupture of membranes, chorioamnionitis, and PID; no evidence that treating partner affects outcome
- *Candida:* If recurs after appropriate treatment, consider underlying diabetes, HIV, antibiotic usage
- Atrophic vaginitis: Treatment with either hormonal or lubricant therapy is usually successful
- Test for and treat other STDs when any STD is found; consider HIV, hepatitis B and C, syphilis testing

Etiology

- Multiple medical causes of infertility, in both males and females
  - Thyroid abnormalities and other endocrinopathies
  - Anovulatory cycles (PCOS, luteal-phase defects)
  - Endometriosis
  - Fibroids (leiomyoma) or uterine polyps
  - Premature menopause
  - Scarring from PID or prior abdominal surgery
  - Testicular atrophy (mumps) or scarring

Epidemiology

- Occurs in about 1 in 6 couples
- 50% female factors, 40% male factors, 10% unknown
- More common in women over age 35

Differential Dx

Signs/Symptoms

- Infertility is usually asymptomatic
- Certain symptoms suggest specific diagnoses:
  - Fatigue, weight gain, slowed return of reflexes: Hypothyroidism
  - Dyspareunia: Endometriosis, pelvic scarring, ovarian cysts
  - Pelvic fullness: Fibroids, endometriosis
  - Obesity, hirsutism, oligomenorrhea: PCOS with anovulatory cycles
  - Painful testicles: Prior injury or scarring
  - Painful ejaculation: Infection, prostatitis
  - Undescended testicle(s)

Diagnosis

- Classically defined as failure to achieve pregnancy after one year of unprotected intercourse
- Complete history and physical exam for both partners
- Verify appropriate sexual intercourse frequency/technique
- Review menstrual history for regularity of timing and flow
- Irregular frequency (oligomenorrhea or amenorrhea) suggests anovulatory cycles
- TSH, prolactin to rule out hyper/hypothyroidism, prolactinoma
- Record, chart, and review 3 cycles of basal body temperature
- Endometrial biopsy
- Cervical mucus anti-sperm antibodies
- Hysterosalpingogram to investigate uterine cavity and fallopian tubes
- Semen analysis
- Women >age 35: Estradiol and FSH on day 3 of cycle and progesterone on day 21 of cycle

Treatment

- Basal body temperature review: Recommend intercourse days to correlate with increased temperature
- Ovulation testing with intercourse on day of ovulation or next day (assesses for LH surge)
- Correction of other factors (e.g., treat hypothyroidism)
- Weight loss in PCOS patients
- Avoid elevated temperature of testicles (avoid hot baths, use boxer shorts, and so on)
- Clomiphene citrate from days 3–7 or 5–9 of cycle
- Referral to gynecologist for endometriosis treatment with Lupron, removal/burning of fibroids, repair of tubal scarring, in vitro fertilization, or other remedies

Prognosis/Clinical Course

- Prognosis depends on cause of infertility
- Better prognostic factors
  - Correctable causes
  - Hypothyroidism
  - Successful prior conception
- Moderate prognostic factors
  - History of appendectomy or abdominal surgery without evidence of peritonitis
- Poorer prognostic factors
  - Unknown cause after workup
  - Female age >35
  - Tubal scarring/testicular scarring
  - Undescended testicles
  - Aspermia or abnormal semen analysis
  - Prior peritonitis
- Consider emotional toll of infertility on couples

175. Incontinence

Etiology

- Stress incontinence: Inadequate bladder neck/sphincter tone, resulting in urine leakage during coughing, exercise, or valsalva maneuver
- Urge incontinence: Due to spontaneous bladder contractions
  - Distinguish central neurologic disorders vs. local bladder disorders
- Detrusor muscle instability
- Overflow incontinence: Overdistension of bladder due to outlet obstruction
- UTI may cause temporary incontinence
- Medications: Diuretics, anticholinergics, antihistamines, α-blockers

Epidemiology

- Females > males, especially females > age 60
- Affects 60% of institutionalized men and women
- Multifactorial causes
- Fewer than 5% of affected patients initiate a discussion of incontinence with their physician

Differential Dx

- Atrophic urethritis
- Decreased sphincter tone (i.e., after multiple births)
- UTI
- Prostatitis/BPH/cancer
- Urethritis
- Medication side effects
- Urologic/pelvic trauma
- Prior urologic/gynecologic surgery
- Multiple sclerosis
- Neurologic/spinal cord problems
- Diabetes/neuropathy
- Bladder cancer
- Cystocele

Signs/Symptoms

- Inability to hold urine
- Urinary frequency or urgency
- Lack of awareness of impending incontinence
- Straining
- Irregular stream intensity or caliber
- Small or larger quantities of urine with incontinence episodes
- Dysuria may be present
- Hematuria may be present
- May be associated with valsalva or exercise
- Perineal/genital paresthesia suggests neurologic cause

Diagnosis

- Ask patients about incontinence, particularly the elderly
- Comprehensive history and physical examination, with particular attention to neurologic, urologic, abdominal/back/spine, and genital evaluation
- Urinalysis, culture and sensitivity, cytology
- Post-void residual (catheterization of patient for residual volume after voiding—normal is less than 100 cc)
- Serum creatinine to evaluate renal function
- Glucose (diabetes) and calcium (bone metastases from prostate cancer) levels
- Ultrasound of kidneys, bladder, and pelvis, if indicated
- Voiding cystourethrogram (VCUG)
- Urodynamic testing

Treatment

- Goals of treatment: Preserve renal function, optimize quality of life, and treat/prevent infections
- Kegel exercises, physical therapy
- Timed voiding/volume restriction
- Treat UTI if present (see the Urinary Tract Infection entry)
- Neurologic/spinal cord dysfunction: Treat/optimize primary cause, catheterize regularly to prevent bladder distention, or use timed voiding
- Decrease bladder contractility/improve detrusor muscle instability
  - Oxybutynin (Ditropan) or extended release (Ditropan XL)
  - Tolterodine (Detrol)
  - Imipramine pamoate (Tofranil)
- Estrogen replacement for urethral atrophy
- Surgical options if all other treatments are unsuccessful

Prognosis/Clinical Course

- Good prognosis for acute UTI
- Good prognosis if offending medications can be discontinued

176. Hematuria

Etiology

- A symptom or sign, not a final diagnosis
- May be gross (visible to eye) or microscopic
- Excessive anticoagulation can contribute to hematuria, but does not preclude a full workup

Differential Dx

- Hereditary (Alport syndrome)
- Cystitis/UTI
- Pyelonephritis
- Trauma/instrumentation/catheterization
- IgA nephropathy
- Bladder/prostate cancer
- Prostatitis/BPH
- Epididymitis
- Nephrolithiasis
- Extreme exercise
- Urethritis
- Urethral stricture
- Urethral carbuncle
- Analgesic nephropathy
- Sickle cell disease
- Bleeding diathesis/coagulopathy

Epidemiology

- Very common
- Underlying malignancy in about 10% of cases

Signs/Symptoms

- Often no other symptoms
- Dysuria in UTI, BPH, prostatitis, or urethritis
- Flank pain in pyelonephritis or nephrolithiasis
- Fever in infections or malignancies
- Menstrual irregularities may be present
- Perineal and/or pelvic pain may be present

Diagnosis

- Thorough history and physical examination
- Microscopic or gross blood in the urine
- Urinalysis: 2–3 RBC per high-power field is normal; presence of bacteria, WBC, or elevated levels of RBCs are abnormal
- Urine culture and sensitivity
- Creatinine to assess renal function
- CBC, PT/PTT/INR to evaluate for bleeding diathesis
- Spiral CT and strain urine if renal calculus is suspected
- Pelvic exam to rule out vaginal source of bleeding
- Consider referral to urologist
- Renal ultrasound or intravenous pyelogram if anatomical abnormality is suspected

Treatment

- Treat primary cause

Prognosis/Clinical Course

- Close follow-up is necessary in older patients due to high risk of underlying malignancy (i.e., bladder, prostate)

177. Urinary Tract Infection

Etiology

- Lower UTI: Cystitis
- Upper UTI: Pyelonephritis
- Community-acquired organisms include *E. coli* (#1 cause), *Staphylococcus saprophyticus* (#2), *Proteus, Klebsiella,* and *Enterococcus*
- Catheter-associated infections due to *Pseudomonas, Klebsiella, E. coli, Proteus, Serratia,* and *Candida* (in immunocompromised patients)
- Increased risk in pregnancy, diabetes, recent antibiotic use, immunosuppression, and anatomical abnormalities (BPH, vesicoureteral reflux)

Epidemiology

- Community-acquired
  - Increased incidence with sexual activity
  - Much higher incidence in women due to short urethra
  - Increased incidence in pregnancy
- Catheter-acquired
  - Risk increases 3–5% per day

Differential Dx

- Asymptomatic bacteriuria
- Appendicitis
- PID
- Pregnancy
- Nephrolithiasis
- Diverticulosis
- Urinary incontinence
- Vaginitis/vaginosis
- Bladder cancer
- Renal cysts
- Renal cell carcinoma
- Tubo-ovarian abscess
- Vaginal foreign body
- Prostatitis

Signs/Symptoms

- Lower UTI
  - Frequency, urgency
  - Dysuria
  - Hematuria
  - Nausea/vomiting
  - Abdominal pain
  - Suprapubic tenderness
  - Change in odor of urine
  - Urinary retention
- Upper UTI/pyelonephritis
  - All lower UTI signs/symptoms
  - Fever/chills
  - Flank pain
  - Change in color of urine
- Urosepsis: Hypotension, fever, mental status changes

Diagnosis

- History and physical, with pelvic exam if indicated
- Pregnancy test, if indicated
- Urinalysis: >5–8 leukocytes, bacteriuria, elevated leukocyte esterase, hematuria (WBC casts suggest pyelonephritis)
  - Pyuria without bacteriuria denotes atypical infection, such as TB, *Candida, Mycoplasma,* or *Chlamydia*
- Clean-catch urine culture is diagnostic (obtain cultures before beginning antibiotics)
  - <1000 CFUs: Negative culture
  - 1000–100,000 CFUs: Contaminated culture—reevaluate
  - >100,000 CFUs: Positive culture
  - Always request sensitivities of cultured organisms as antibiotic resistance is rampant
- Gram stain
- CBC: Leukocytosis
- Always look for bacteremic or embolic sources of infection (kidney abscess, lung abscess, endocarditis, prosthesis infection)

Treatment

- Simple lower UTI
  - TMP-SMX or quinolone for 3 days
  - In pregnancy: Amoxicillin × 7 days or nitrofurantoin
  - If comorbidities exist, treat for 10 days
- Complicated UTI (severe illness or pyelonephritis)
  - IV ampicillin plus gentamycin, IV ampicillin plus sulbactam, IV quinolone, or IV 3rd generation cephalosporin
- If nosocomial infection, include antipseudomonal antibiotic
- Phenazopyridine is excellent for short-term urinary anesthesia to decrease irritant symptoms
- If catheter-associated, change catheter

Prognosis/Clinical Course

- Excellent prognosis for uncomplicated infections
- Higher morbidity and mortality with nosocomial and complicated UTIs and urosepsis
- Males <50 with more than one episode of UTI should be evaluated for structural abnormalities, such as vesicoureteral reflux

178. Epididymitis

Etiology

- A common clinical condition—inflammation of the epididymis
- Usually caused by sexually transmitted organisms in sexually active men under age 35 (except children), especially *Neisseria gonorrhoeae* and *Chlamydia trachomatis*
- Usually caused by common urinary pathogens in men older than 35, especially *E. coli* and *Enterobacter*
- Often spreads from the urethra or prostate

Epidemiology

- Fairly common
- More common after urinary instrumentation/surgery
- Amiodarone-induced epididymitis (noninfectious) is possible

Differential Dx

- Testicular trauma
- Testicular cancer
- Testicular torsion
- Inguinal hernia
- Amiodarone-induced epididymitis (noninfectious)
- UTI
- Prostatitis
- Hydrocele
- Post-vasectomy epididymal congestion
- Orchitis

Signs/Symptoms

- Diffuse groin or perineal pain
- Fever, chills, and sweats
- Urethral discharge
- Dysuria, hematuria, and/or frequency
- Very painful epididymis, sometimes with fullness or swelling
- Gentle testicular elevation often decreases pain (Prehn's sign)
- Acute unilateral testicular pain and swelling is suggestive of testicular torsion or trauma

Diagnosis

- Clinical diagnosis via exam of testicles and epididymis—do not miss more serious conditions, such as testicular torsion or testicular cancer
    - Absence of testicular masses
    - Absence of inguinal hernia
    - Elevated testicle or irregularly positioned testicle is more consistent with testicular torsion; if torsion is considered, a STAT testicular ultrasound, Doppler flow study, or radionuclide scan of the testicle is indicated
- Urethral gram stain
- Urinalysis and culture: Pyuria and bacteriuria
- *N. gonorrhoeae/Chlamydia* culture to rule out urethritis
- CBC: Leukocytosis

Treatment

- Adequate pain control, usually with NSAIDs
- Antibiotics
    - Age <35 or sexually transmitted: Treat for *N. gonorrhoeae* and *Chlamydia* infection (ceftriaxone IM once and doxycycline × 10 days)
    - Age >35:TMP-SMX × 10–14 days or ciprofloxacin × 10–14 days
- Testicular support and elevation

Prognosis/Clinical Course

- Epididymitis is generally successfully treated
- Long-term sequelae can include chronic pain, testicular infarction, abscess formation, and infertility
- Pain may last from days to weeks
- If pain increases after treatment starts, it is important to reconsider alternative diagnoses
- Older men with epididymitis must be evaluated for obstructive urinary problems such as BPH and urethral stricture
- Sexual partners should be examined and treated

179. Erectile Dysfunction

Etiology

- The inability to achieve and maintain erection sufficient to perform satisfactory sexual activity
- May be situational (specific times, places, partner)
- Most commonly vascular in origin
  - Arterial atherosclerosis (diabetes): Decreased blood flow to penis
  - Venous leaks: Decreased amount of blood remaining in penis during erection

Differential Dx

- Vascular (diabetes, atherosclerosis)
- Drug and/or alcohol use
- Hormonal abnormalities (thyroid dysfunction)
- Kidney/liver disease
- Medications, including herbal and OTC drugs
- Pelvic/perineal/testicular surgery or trauma
- Neurologic (stroke, seizures, multiple sclerosis)
- Anxiety/depression

Epidemiology

- Affects 20–30 million men in the US
- Affects >30% of men who are 40–70 years of age
- Categorized as organic, non-organic/psychogenic, or mixed

Signs/Symptoms

- Inability to obtain or maintain an adequate erection
- May occur "sometimes" or "always"
- If adequate morning erection, consider non-organic causes

Diagnosis

- Focused history and physical examination, with attention to medications/drugs, smoking, diabetes, HTN, atherosclerosis, psychosocial issues, and sexual/relationship issues
- CBC
- Routine chemistry profile (renal/hepatic/glucose)
- Thyroid-stimulating hormone
- Free testosterone, LH/FSH, prolactin
- Urinalysis
- Screen for depression
- DHEA-S
- Urology referral
- Assess other possible vascular disease: Coronary artery disease, peripheral vascular disease

Treatment

- Treat underlying disorders such as stress and depression, cardiac disease, liver or kidney diseases, thyroid disease; adjust causative medications; avoid alcohol and drugs
- Behavioral therapy/support
- Sildenafil (Viagra) 1 hour precoital
  - Be sure patient is not taking any nitroglycerin products
- Vacuum constriction of penis
- Penile prostaglandin injections
- Penile prosthesis
- Penile surgery
  - Rigid, semi rigid, and/or malleable rod
  - Inflatable device
  - Vascular reconstruction

Prognosis/Clinical Course

- Generally fairly good prognosis if overall condition allows adequate energy and stamina for normal sexual relations and reasonable psychiatric health
- May need to approach erectile dysfunction from many different angles
- Always consider underlying cause of erectile dysfunction and treat aggressively
- Significant chronic conditions (medical and psychiatric) will often worsen the prognosis
- Clinical course is variable

180. Prostate Disorders—BPH

Etiology

- Benign prostatic hypertrophy is an enlargement of the prostate not caused by cancer, infection, or other pathologic processes

Differential Dx

- Prostate cancer
- Prostatitis
- Prostatic swelling seen after excessive alcohol consumption
- Urethral stricture
- UTI/cystitis
- Medication side effects (e.g., anticholinergics)
- Bladder or other urinary system tumor
- Renal calculus
- Neurogenic bladder

Epidemiology

- Most common benign tumor in men
- About 50% of patients over 50 have BPH, about 60% of patients over 60, and so on

Signs/Symptoms

- May be asymptomatic
- Urinary hesitancy (cannot start)
- Urinary urgency (cannot wait)
- Nocturia
- Sensation of incomplete emptying
- Poor urinary stream quality (weak or narrow stream)
- Urinary dribbling
- Dysuria
- Rectal examination reveals an enlarged prostate, without nodules or tenderness

Diagnosis

- History of clinical symptoms most important; often found incidentally
- Consider using the American Urologic Association Symptom Index, a series of 7 questions with graded answers that assess common BPH symptoms
- Rectal examination
- Urinalysis should be normal (secondary infection may cause pyuria or hematuria)
- Prostate-specific antigen (PSA) test
- Creatinine
- Ultrasound is not indicated; however, if done for other reasons, it will reveal an enlarged prostate, bladder distention, and high post-void residual volume
- If incomplete emptying is considered, perform a post-void residual catheterization to determine the degree of incomplete emptying

Treatment

- The goal of treatment is to improve the quality of symptoms for the patient (e.g., manage nocturia so patient can have adequate sleep) and avoid future problems
- Medical therapy
  - α-adrenergic blocking agents, including doxazosin, tamsulosin, and terazosin
  - 5-α reductase enzyme inhibitor agents (finasteride)
  - Saw palmetto (not FDA-approved) has an unknown mechanism of action, but has been shown to be effective
- Surgical
  - Transurethral resection of the prostate (TURP)
  - Prostatectomy (rarely necessary for isolated BPH)
  - Balloon dilatation of the prostate

Prognosis/Clinical Course

- BPH usually progresses with age, but symptoms can often be managed with either medical or surgical therapy
- Dosages of medical therapeutics usually need to be adjusted upward as treatment progresses
- Choice of medical therapy is often influenced more by the patient's comorbid conditions and the side-effect profile of each medication rather than the effectiveness of the medication (all of which are similar at appropriate doses)
- Avoid other medications that will worsen symptoms (i.e., anticholinergics)

181. Prostate Disorders—Prostatitis

Etiology

- Inflammation without identification of causative organism is the most common cause of prostatitis
- *E. coli* causes 80% of cases of acute and chronic bacterial prostatitis; other infectious organisms include *Pseudomonas aeruginosa, Neisseria gonorrhoeae, Klebsiella pneumoniae, Proteus mirabilis,* streptococcus, *Enterococcus,* and *Staphylococcus aureus*

Epidemiology

- Chronic bacterial prostatitis is more common in older men than acute bacterial prostatitis
- Nonbacterial prostatitis and prostatodynia are much more common than acute or chronic bacterial prostatitis

Differential Dx

- BPH
- Prostate cancer
- Prostatodynia
- Urethral stricture
- Bladder cancer
- Urinary tract infection
- Pyelonephritis
- Urosepsis
- Urethritis
- Epididymitis
- Renal colic
- Perirectal abscess

Signs/Symptoms

- Acute bacterial prostatitis
  - Acute febrile illness, chills, myalgias, arthralgias
  - Rectal, perineal, or low back pain
  - Dysuria, urgency, and frequency
- Chronic bacterial prostatitis
  - Subacute or chronic symptoms; may be asymptomatic
  - Rectal, perineal, or low back pain
  - Dysuria, urgency, and frequency
- Nonbacterial prostatitis/prostatodynia
  - Rectal or perineal pain
  - Dysuria, urgency, hesitancy, nocturia, weak urinary stream, painful ejaculation, postejaculatory pain, and hematospermia

Diagnosis

- Acute bacterial prostatitis
  - Urinalysis shows WBCs
  - Culture should show offending organism (consider *N. gonorrhoeae* and *Chlamydia* culture)
  - Avoid rectal exam due to possible bacteremic spread
- Chronic bacterial prostatitis
  - Rectal exam reveals boggy and tender prostate
  - Urinalysis shows WBCs
  - Culture should show offending organism, especially after prostatic massage
- Nonbacterial prostatitis
  - Rectal exam reveals tender prostate
  - Urinalysis shows WBCs, but culture is negative
- Prostatodynia
  - Rectal exam reveals a tender prostate
  - Urinalysis and culture are both normal

Treatment

- Acute bacterial prostatitis: Treat for 4–6 weeks
  - Fluoroquinolones
  - Doxycycline or ampicillin
  - Trimethoprim-sulfamethoxazole
- Chronic bacterial prostatitis: Treat for 3 or more months
  - Fluoroquinolones
  - Doxycycline
  - Cephalexin
- Nonbacterial prostatitis and prostatodynia
  - Tetracycline, doxycycline, or erythromycin is often used for 6–12 weeks, even though no bacterial source is identified
  - α_1-Adrenergic blocking agents, such as terazosin
  - NSAIDs

Prognosis/Clinical Course

- Acute bacterial prostatitis
  - Generally successful treatment if full course of antibiotics is taken; if not, chronic bacterial prostatitis or prostatic abscess may occur
  - Avoid rectal exam, which may induce bacteremia
- Chronic bacterial prostatitis
  - Variable effectiveness of treatment, probably due to poor penetration of antibiotics into the non-inflamed prostate
- Nonbacterial prostatitis and prostatodynia
  - Both are difficult to cure; symptom improvement occurs in about 1/2 of patients
  - Treatment should be continued for a minimum of 6 weeks

182. Prostate Disorders—Cancer

Etiology

- Nearly 100% are adenocarcinomas
- Prostate cancer is a very controversial subject, primarily because of the effectiveness of screening. While many men develop prostate cancer, few suffer any direct morbidity or mortality. Unfortunately, we cannot determine which men will live with their disease without problems and which will develop symptoms or suffer adverse outcomes. Additionally, the treatments may induce significant morbidity and mortality, such as impotence, urinary incontinence, and infection.

Epidemiology

- Most frequent new cancer diagnosis in men
- Second only to lung cancer as a cause of cancer death in men
- Approximately 1 in 10 men will develop prostate cancer
- Many men die *with* prostate cancer rather than *from* prostate cancer
- Blacks > whites

Differential Dx

- Benign prostatic nodule
- Benign prostatic hypertrophy
- Prostatitis
- UTI
- Pelvic mass/lymphoma (unilateral lymphedema)
- Urethral stricture
- Neurogenic bladder

Signs/Symptoms

- Often asymptomatic
- Urinary symptoms
- Urgency, hesitancy
- Poor stream
- Hematuria
- Hard prostate nodule on digital rectal exam
- Unilateral lymphedema
- Weight loss
- Back pain with spinal metastases

Diagnosis

- Screening is controversial because there is no conclusive evidence of improved outcomes with screening
- Consider screening beginning at age 40 in African-Americans and those with a positive family history
- Consider screening others at age 50
- Screening methods
  - Digital rectal examination (DRE)
  - Prostate-specific antigen (PSA)
- Biopsy of prostate mass is diagnostic
- Bone pain, elevated alkaline phosphatase, or hypercalcemia may indicate bone metastases

Treatment

- Referral to urologist for definitive diagnosis, staging, and treatment
- Prostatectomy
- Radiation therapy (external beam or brachytherapy)
- Hormonal therapy
- Observation with regular PSA, exam, and ultrasound
- Effective treatment of pain: NSAIDs and/or narcotic analgesics
- Androgen ablation and chemotherapy for metastases

Prognosis/Clinical Course

- Prognosis depends on grade and stage
- Two systems are used
  - Gleason score (histology)
  - TNM (tumor, nodes, metastases)
- Five-year survival rates
  - Well differentiated: Nearly 100%
  - Poorly differentiated: <70%
- Side effects of treatment
  - Postoperative infection
  - Erectile dysfunction
  - Urinary incontinence
  - Retrograde ejaculation
  - Bowel problems
  - Radiation proctitis

183. Testicular Cancer

Etiology

- Germ cell in origin
  - Seminoma
  - Embryonal cell carcinoma
  - Teratoma
  - Choriocarcinoma
  - Many are of mixed origin

Differential Dx

- Testicular torsion
- Testicular trauma
- Benign testicular mass (cord lipoma, fibrous pseudotumor, adenomatoid tumor, epididymal cystadenoma, testicular cysts)
- Epididymitis
- Epididymal tumor
- Diffuse edema from cardiac/lymphatic disease
- Testicular/scrotal infection
- Torsion of appendix epididymis
- Hydrocele/spermatocele

Epidemiology

- Leading cause of solid tumors in men aged 20–34 years
- Incidence approximately 3/1000
- Incidence increases up to 20-fold in men with undescended testes (cryptorchidism) or orrhipexy (surgically descended testes)
- Rare in blacks

Signs/Symptoms

- Asymptomatic scrotal mass is the most common presentation
- A normal testicle feels like a hard boiled egg without the shell
- Lymphadenopathy (retroperitoneal, mediastinal, supraclavicular) may indicate metastatic disease
- Pulmonary symptoms may indicate metastases to lungs
- A painful scrotal mass may occur with incidental testicular trauma (higher propensity for a tumor to bleed—Lance Armstrong was diagnosed in this fashion)

Diagnosis

- History and physical examination, with attention toward lymphatic and GU system
- Transillumination if a hydrocele or spermaocele is suspected; however, a reactive hydrocele can occur secondary to testicular carcinoma
- Scrotal ultrasound
- CXR for metastases
- Tumor markers: α-Fetoprotein (AFP), quantitative β-HCG (human chorionic gonadotrophin), LDH
- Urgent urologic consult for definitive diagnosis, staging, and treatment
- CT scan and node examination for staging
- Do not delay diagnosis or misdiagnose as epididymitis

Treatment

- Emergent evaluation by a urologist
- Surgery: Radical orchiectomy (surgical removal of testis)
- Chemotherapy for advanced disease or metastases
- Radiation therapy
- Close follow-up to detect recurrences

Prognosis/Clinical Course

- Early disease (Stage A) is nearly 100% curable
- Stages B and C have 5-year survival rates greater than 90%
- Treatment success decreases with delays in diagnosis and/or treatment

Dermatologic Disease

ERNEST WIGGINS, MD

184. Acne Vulgaris

Etiology

- Disease of the pilosebaceous follicles
- Follicular hyperkeratinization forms plug in the sebaceous duct, causing blockage of duct and retention of sebum
  - Blockage of duct → rupture of follicle → inflammatory reaction
  - Retention of sebum → ideal media for growth of *Propionibacterium acnes* → provokes inflammatory reaction
- Testosterone stimulates production of sebum; estrogen suppresses sebum (thus, OCP is protective)

Differential Dx

- Acne rosacea
- Acne fulminans
- Polycystic ovarian syndrome
- Erythema infectiosum
- Hidradenitis suppurativa
- Pyoderma faciale
- Steroid acne

Epidemiology

- Up to 85% of adolescent population is affected
- 10–20% of adults are affected
- May begin as early as 6 years old with increase at puberty
- Family history may help predict severity

Signs/Symptoms

- Closed comedo (whitehead)
- Open comedo (blackhead)
- Inflammatory lesions
- Affects areas with increased concentration of sebaceous glands: face, neck, chest, and back
- Chronic lesions may produce scarring and hyperpigmentation
- May be pruritic

Diagnosis

- Clinical
- Comedones are the hallmark
- Increased serum DHEA-S levels
- Acne stages
  - Type 1: Comedonal, with no scarring
  - Type 2: Papular, mild/minimal scarring
  - Type 3: Pustular, moderate scarring
  - Type 4: Nodulocystic, severe scarring

Treatment

- Topical retinoids, benzoyl peroxide, and antibiotics
- Oral contraceptive pills for women
- Spironolactone (acts as anti-androgen)
- Oral antibiotics for inflammatory acne
  - Tetracycline 500 mg po BID
  - Erythromycin 500 mg po BID
  - Ampicillin 500 mg po BID
  - Many other choices
- Oral isotretinoin (Accutane)
- Surgical comedo extraction
- Dietary changes: Avoid foods that exacerbate condition

Prognosis/Clinical Course

- Isotretinoin is a teratogen; must screen for pregnancy and warn patient of risks of conception while using this drug
- Dry skin is a complication of many acne drugs
- Cyst formation, pigmentary changes, and scarring of skin may occur

185. Blistering Disorders

Etiology

- Autoimmune diseases causing loss of cell–cell adhesion in epidermis
- Pemphigus vulgaris: IgG antibody against desmoglein adhesion molecule; results in intraepidermal blistering; affects younger patients
- Bullous pemphigoid: Autoantibody against basement membrane glycoproteins; results in subepidermal blistering; affects elderly patients

Differential Dx

- Erythema multiforme
- Stevens-Johnson syndrome
- HSV (impetigo herpitiformis)
- Apthae
- Lichen planus
- Pyoderma
- Bullous impetigo
- Porphyria cutanea tarda

Epidemiology

- Pemphigus: Most common in middle-aged patients with HLA-DR4 phenotype
- Bullous pemphigoid: Especially in elderly

Signs/Symptoms

- Pemphigus
  - Easily ruptured, painful bullae; starts within oral cavity and extends to skin, scalp, face, and chest
  - Nikolsky sign: Top layer of bullae easily sloughs off
- Pemphigoid
  - Involves flexural areas (axilla, groin); widespread eruption common
  - Hard-tense bullae, +/− oral lesions
  - Pruritic

Diagnosis

- Pemphigus
  - Skin biopsy
  - Immunofluorescence will demonstrate IgG deposits between cells
- Pemphigoid
  - Biopsy: Deposits of IgG in basement membrane between dermis and epidermis; increased eosinophils in dermis

Treatment

- Corticosteroids
- Azothioprine and cyclophosphamide
- Local wound care to decrease risk of secondary infection

Prognosis/Clinical Course

- Pemphigus: Mortality rate of 5% with treatment; prognosis is poorer in advanced age, widespread disease, or increasing steroid dose
- Pemphigoid: Chronic disease; not life-threatening

186. Burns

Etiology

- Causes damage to skin barrier and induces systemic immunosuppression (decreased T_h cells and Ig levels with increased T_s cell levels)—this predisposes to infection (*Staphylococcus, Streptococcus, Pseudomonas*)
- Post-burn fluid shift: Increase in fluid flow to burned and normal tissue due to endothelial damage, vasoactive substances, and other mediators
- First-degree burn (superficial): Sunburn
- Second-degree burn (partial thickness): Scalding or chemical burn
- Third-degree burn (full thickness): Flame burns

Differential Dx

- Thermal burns
- Electrical burns
- Chemical burns
- Scalded skin syndrome
- Self-inflicted burns
- Abuse patterns

Epidemiology

- Over 2 million cases per year with 70,000 admissions (20,000 to burn units)
- Most burns are hot liquid scalds seen in children

Signs/Symptoms

- First-degree (superficial): Painful erythema; dry skin without blistering; minimal or no edema
- Second-degree (partial thickness): Moistened blisters; mottled gray or erythematous; extremely painful
- Third-degree (full thickness): Eschar formation; leathery or waxy appearance; dry, painless, white pearly and darkened lesions; hair easily removed; visible thrombosed vessels are pathognomonic
- Signs of infected burn wound: Conversion of partial-thickness burn to full-thickness; ↑ amounts of erythema or edema at margins; sudden separation of eschar from underlying tissue; fever; purulent drainage

Diagnosis

- History and physical exam are the basis of diagnosis
- Infection diagnosed by wound culture or biopsy demonstrating $>10^5$ organisms
- Size of burn in adults is estimated by "Rule of 9's" (for second- and third-degree burns)
  - Dorsal truck = 18%
  - Ventral trunk = 18%
  - Each arm = 9%
  - Each leg = 18%
  - Perineum = 1%
  - Head/neck = 9%

Treatment

- Immediate management: ABCDE's of trauma resuscitation (Airway, Breathing, Circulation, Disability, Exposure)
- Fluid maintenance and nutrition are important due to massive fluid shifts (burn edema) and increased metabolic demands of stressed state
  - Parkland formula (for initial 24 hours): 4 mL of crystalloid/kg/% body surface area burned
  - Monitor by urine output >0.5 cc/kg/hour
- Local wound care
  - Topical agents to decrease infectious burden on tissue: Silver sulfadiazene, silver nitrate, mafenide
  - Surgical excision of eschars with skin grafting may be necessary
  - Tetanus prophylaxis
  - Pain control with analgesics, including narcotics
  - Keep small burns in cool water until pain subsides

Prognosis/Clinical Course

- First-degree burns tend to be uncomplicated and heal within 5–7 days
- Second-degree burns generally heal in 3–4 weeks, unless deep invasion or superimposed infection occurs
- All burned skin is at increased risk of sunburn for 1 year and may also show pigmentary changes
- Complications: Local infection (most important complication to avoid), pneumonia, pulmonary emboli, UTI, endocarditis, suppurative thrombophlebitis
- Patients should be admitted to a specialized burn unit if they present with smoke inhalation, electrical burns, >20% of body surface involved, or second-degree burns to the hands, feet, face, or perineum

187. Cutaneous Fungal Infections

Etiology

- Dermatophyte infections (tineas) are fungal infections of nonviable keratinized structures (hair, nails, stratum corneum)
  – May be transmitted from contact with soil, animals, or humans
- Yeast infections include candidiasis and pityriasis versicolor (also known as tinea versicolor—but not truly a dermatophyte)
- Candidiasis
  – Vaginal: White curdlike discharge
  – Oral (thrush): White plaques on oral and buccal mucosa
  – Cutaneous: Nail infections, hair follicle infections

Epidemiology

- Presents in people of all ages and races
- Especially in immunocompromised states, diabetes, antibiotic use, and steroid use
- Genetic predisposition to dermatophyte infection

Differential Dx

- Psoriasis
- Lupus
- Seborrheic dermatitis
- Secondary syphilis
- Impetigo
- Lichen planus
- Pityriasis rosea
- Eczema
- Erythrasma
- Intertrigo
- Contact dermatitis
- Vitiligo

Signs/Symptoms

- Tinea pedis (athlete's foot): Pruritic, scaly, pink rash along sides of feet, soles, and between toes; may affect hand also
- Tinea cruris (jock itch): Pruritic, annular erythematous lesion on inner thigh and groin (does not affect scrotum)
- Tinea corporis (ringworm): Affects torso, extremities; asymptomatic or pruritic; may present as papular, pustular, vesicular, scaly, or eczematous rash
- Tinea capitis (ringworm of scalp): Asymptomatic patches of hair loss
- Pityriasis versicolor: Asymptomatic maculopapular scales on upper trunk; precipitated by heat (converts yeast to hyphae)

Diagnosis

- Tinea infections
  – Clinical appearance and history
  – Microscopic examination with KOH prep reveals branching hyphae
  – Fungal culture if necessary; however, diagnosis is specific to location of infection rather than specific organism
  – Tinea capitis may fluoresce green under a Wood's lamp
- Tinea versicolor
  – KOH examination shows short hyphae and round spores ("spaghetti and meatball" appearance)
  – Orange-gold fluorescence under Wood's lamp
- Candidiasis
  – Clinical appearance
  – KOH examination: Yeast and pseudomycelia
  – Isolated and grown in lab using Sabouraud's agar

Treatment

- Tinea infections
  – Selenium sulfide shampoo in scalp/hair involvement
  – Topical antifungals
  – Low-potency steroid creams if severe pruritis or inflammation
  – Systemic antifungals if necessary
  – Tinea capitis must be treated systemically with griseofulvin $\times$ 6–8 weeks or other oral antifungals
- Pityriasis versicolor
  – Selenium sulfide lotion
  – Topical antifungals
  – Oral ketoconazole
- Candidiasis
  – Topical and oral antifungals

Prognosis/Clinical Course

- Systemic *Candida* infection may occur, resulting in meningitis, endocarditis, or lung infections—seen especially in immunosuppressed patients or with broad-spectrum antimicrobial use

188. Cutaneous Parasitic Infections

Etiology

- Pediculosis (lice): Spread by physical contact or fomites
- Scabies: Infestation by *Sarcoptes scabiei* mite by personal contact or fomites; burrow into stratum corneum of skin and lay eggs

Differential Dx

- Seborrheic dermatitis
- Atopic dermatitis
- Lichen simplex
- Eczema
- Pyoderma
- Dermatitis herpetiformis
- Flea bites
- Insect bites
- Folliculitis
- Cutaneous larva migrans

Epidemiology

- Pediculosis capitis: School-aged children and adults with poor hygiene; rare in African Americans
- Scabies: Seen in poor, disease-prone areas with minimal hygiene; rare in blacks; occurs in epidemics

Signs/Symptoms

- Pediculosis capitis (head lice): Pruritis; eggs (nits) found on hair shafts; erythematous papules; excoriations
- Pediculosis corporis (body lice): Pruritic, reddish, crusting papules
- Pediculosis pubis (pubic lice or "crabs"): May affect genital area, legs, buttocks, or face; blue macules with severe infection
- Scabies: Reddish, crusting papules; present on genitals, buttocks, wrists/hands/fingers, axillae, or umbilicus; burrows appear as black dotted lines (2–15 mm long); intensely pruritic, especially at night

Diagnosis

- Pediculosis
  - History
  - Identification of eggs on hair or body
- Scabies
  - History
  - Microscopic identification of mites and ova within skin scrapings

Treatment

- Pediculosis
  - Proper hygiene; clean linen and clothing
  - Corticosteroid creams and antihistamines to relieve pruritis
  - Permethrin or Lindane shampoos × 5–10 minutes
  - Treat all members of household
  - Nit removal with fine-toothed comb
- Scabies
  - Proper hygiene; clean linen and clothing
  - Permethrin cream 5% from neck to toes
  - Topical corticosteroids and antihistamines for pruritis
  - Treat all members of household

Prognosis/Clinical Course

- Pediculosis: Highly contagious via personal contact, sharing of clothes, linen, sexual contact
- Scabies: Can persist for months to years—the classic "7-year itch"
- Secondary bacterial infection (impetigo) may occur

189. Dermatitis

Etiology

- Allergic contact dermatitis: Type IV hypersensitivity reaction; common antigens include poison ivy, cosmetics, perfumes, rubber, and detergents; generally presents in childhood; nonallergic contact dermatitis may be caused by skin irritants
- Atopic: An allergic, pruritic dermatitis induced by specific triggers (Type I hypersensitivity); patients have a personal or family history of asthma or hay fever; secondary bacterial infections common
- Seborrheic dermatitis: Benign neoplasm of epidermis

Epidemiology

- Contact: Very common; prevalence of 5–20% in the US
- Atopic: Increased incidence in U.S. urban areas; family history positive in 70% of cases; 10% of all children have some form; onset usually in first years of life
- Seborrheic: Generally in adults over 45; presentation in a child or adolescent should be investigated thoroughly for other possibilities

Differential Dx

- Eczema
- Candidiasis
- Tinea infections
- Lichen simplex chronicus
- Lichen simplex
- Varicella
- Impetigo
- Folliculitis
- Lice
- Measles
- Scabies
- Urticaria
- Dry skin
- Warts
- Photodermatitis
- Herpes zoster
- Herpes simplex
- Lentigo
- Actinic keratosis
- Malignancy

Signs/Symptoms

- Contact dermatitis: Initial erythema followed by intensely pruritic, papulovesicular rash; bullae, lymphadenopathy, and fever may be present; blistering, crusting, lichinification, scaling; location and shape of affected area suggests the specific allergen
- Atopic: Intense pruritis with erythema, edematous papules, crusting, and excoriation; skin becomes chronically dry, hyperkeratotic, and lichenified; may result in exfoliation
- Seborrheic: Asymptomatic unless irritated; slightly elevated, colored lesions; range in color from white to yellow to red/brown/black; rough, greasy texture; mainly on scalp, face, and back

Diagnosis

- Clinical examination
- Patch testing
- Allergy testing is indicated in patients with food allergies or with severe reactions to airborne allergens such as asthma rhinitis
- Histologic examination may be indicated if uncertainty exists

Treatment

- First step: Avoidance of exposure
- Topical steroids or Burow's solution (vinegar and water)
- Antihistamines: diphenhydramine, loratadine, cetirizine
- Severe disease is treated with oral or IM steroids
- Atopic dermatitis
  - Steroids, Burow's solution, antihistamines
  - Keeping skin moisturized is essential: Prevent excessive bathing, use moisturizing creams, well-ventilated surroundings
  - Oral antibiotics for secondary bacterial infections
  - Tricyclic antidepressants may alleviate pruritis
- Seborrheic: Only irritated lesions need to be treated
  - Cryotherapy with liquid nitrogen to remove lesions
  - No effective topical medications

Prognosis/Clinical Course

- Contact dermatitis: Natural course is 2–3 weeks and will resolve spontaneously if the offending agent is removed
- Atopic: A chronic condition; cannot be cured
- Seborrheic: A benign, progressive disorder; new cutaneous growths must be checked regularly for the possibility of malignancy

190. Folliculitis

Etiology

- Inflammation of hair follicles
- Usually due to *Staphylococcus aureus;* also *Pseudomonas* (hot tub folliculitis), *Candida,* and others; trauma, friction, and irritants may play a role
- Furuncle (boil) occurs when the infection extends deep into a follicle, producing a perifollicular abscess
- Carbuncles result from infection of several connecting follicles with subcutaneous abscess formation
- Bacteremia may occur with secondary seeding of organs

Differential Dx

- Pseudofolliculitis
- Viral exanthem
- Varicella
- Psoriasis
- Acne vulgaris
- Insect bite
- Impetigo
- Drug reaction
- Hydradenitis suppurativa
- Epidermal inclusion cyst

Epidemiology

- May occur at any age
- Often seen with seborrheic dermatitis and acne vulgaris
- Furuncles and carbuncles more common in patients with diabetes, malnutrition, steroid treatment, and immunosuppression

Signs/Symptoms

- Occurs in hair-bearing areas such as face, scalp, extremities, and axillae
- Light-colored pustules and papules with erythematous surroundings and a hair at the center; often pruritic and/or painful
- Furuncles appear as firm, tender, erythematous nodules; 1–5 cm; becomes fluctuant within hours to days; leaves a permanent scar
- Carbuncles most common in head, neck, and thighs; painful; may be in excess of 10 cm; will drain from multiple follicular sites within a few days
- Lymphadenopathy, fever, malaise
- Secondary bacterial seeding may result in signs of endocarditis, osteomyelitis, brain abscess, liver abscess

Diagnosis

- Clinical presentation
- Culture for identification of bacterial organism and sensitivities to antibiotics
- Biopsy, if necessary

Treatment

- Wash area well; avoid friction and tight clothing; warm compresses
- Topical benzoyl peroxide, antibiotics, or steroid cream
- Oral antibiotics
  - Cephalexin or erythromycin × 7–14 days
  - Ciprofloxacin if *Pseudomonas* is suspected
- Recurrent episodes should be treated with long-term antibiotics
- Incision and drainage for furuncles

Prognosis/Clinical Course

- Treat to prevent spread, scarring, and seeding of organs
- Be particularly cautious with lesions in central face due to risk of septic cavernous sinus thrombosis

191. Hyperpigmentary Disorders

Etiology

- Pityriasis rosea (PR): Noncontagious, pruritic, salmon-colored patch of skin
- Café-au-lait: Benign hyperplasia of basal cell melanocytes
- Nevi ("moles"): Asymptomatic neoplasms composed of nevus cells derived from melanocytes; may be acquired, congenital, or dysplastic; rarely become malignant (larger lesions are more likely to be malignant)
- Seborrheic keratosis (SK): Proliferation of epidermal keratinocytes; not malignant; very common
- Others: Freckles, lentigines, melasma, solar lentigo

Differential Dx

- PR: Secondary syphilis, viral exanthem, drug eruption
- Café-au-lait: Tinea infections, freckles
- Nevi: Melanoma
- SK: Psoriasis, dermatofibroma, nevi, melanoma

Epidemiology

Signs/Symptoms

- PR: Begins with solitary lesion on trunk or extremities called "Herald patch," followed 1–2 weeks later by erythematous, maculopapular rash resembling Christmas tree; often pruritic
- Café-au-lait: Asymptomatic, tan macules; 0.5–20 cm; sharp margins
- Acquired nevus: Small, flat, brown lesion with sharp margins
- Congenital nevus: Brown, raised lesion; sharp margins; irregular surface; has hair
- Dysplastic nevus: Red/brown lesion with irregular borders and irregular pigmentation on trunk, extremities
- Seborrheic keratosis: Dark yellow-black warty lesions; most common on back, face, scalp, chest; may be pruritic

Diagnosis

- Diagnosis is based on history and clinical examination
- Pathological examination may be useful in classifying the specific form of nevus; excision and pathology examination are indicated only if clinical suspicion of malignant changes exists
- Test for syphilis may be indicated if pityriasis rosea is suspected

Treatment

- PR: Self-limiting; symptomatic relief with antihistamines, antipruritics, and ultraviolet light
- Café-au-lait: No treatment necessary; various lasers may be used to eliminate lesions for cosmetic reasons
- Nevi: Surgical excision if suspicious for melanoma or for cosmetic reasons; dysplastic nevi respond to tretinoin cream
- Seborrheic keratosis: Remove, freeze, or curettage if becomes irritated or inflamed or for cosmetic reasons

Prognosis/Clinical Course

- Six or more café-au-lait spots likely indicate neurofibromatosis (von Recklinghausen's disease)
- PR: Spontaneous remission within three months
- Sign of Leser-Trelat: Huge increase in number or size of seborrheic keratoses within several months—evaluate for internal malignancy

192. Hypopigmentary Disorders

Etiology

- Vitiligo: Acquired loss of melanocytes in skin and hair; possibly of autoimmune origin; may be seen in conjunction with other autoimmune disorders; may occur spontaneously after severe stress or trauma
- Albinism: Congenital disorder of melanin production; absence or abnormality of tyrosinase enzyme

Differential Dx

- Pityriasis alba
- Leukoderma
- Pigmented nevi
- Tinea versicolor
- Piebaldism (partial congenital albinism)
- Guttate hypomelanosis
- Halo nevus

Epidemiology

- Vitiligo: Primarily occurs in darkly pigmented patients; 50% of cases begin in patients < age 20; positive family history in 25–50%; occurs in 1% of people worldwide
- Albinism: Occurs in 1:20,000 people

Signs/Symptoms

- Vitiligo
  - Sharply demarcated nonscaling macular patches of hypopigmentation
  - Symmetrical distribution
  - Common on face and dorsum of hands
  - More obvious in summer
- Albinism
  - Translucent iris
  - Pale skin and hair over entire body; tan skin in blacks
  - Nystagmus, photophobia, visual defects

Diagnosis

- History and physical exam
- Skin biopsy if necessary to confirm diagnosis
- Consider associated autoimmune disorders in patients with vitiligo

Treatment

- Vitiligo
  - Protection from sun
  - Cosmetics
  - Dyes and sunless tanning solutions
  - Topical psoralen or tincture of methoxsalen over affected areas may reverse depigmentation
  - Oral steroids may be effective
- Albinism
  - No curative treatment
  - Protect eyes and skin from sun
  - Annual full-body skin exam

Prognosis/Clinical Course

- Vitiligo: Rapidly progressive, although 10% of patients have spontaneous repigmentation
- Albinism: Annual full-body skin exam to check for malignant lesions

193. Psoriasis

Etiology

- Psoriasis is a chronic disease of epidermal hyperproliferation resulting in immature cells
- Psoriatic epithelial cells have a cell cycle one-tenth as long as normal cells and they take just 1–2 days to migrate to the skin surface from deeper layers to be exfoliated (versus nearly 30 days in normal cells); these cells do not adequately mature, so even minor trauma, inflammation, mild sunburn, and humidity can precipitate lesions

Epidemiology

- Extremely common, affecting 1–2% of the population
- 50–75% of patients have a positive family history
- Psoriatic arthritis is associated with HLA-B27

Differential Dx

- Eczema
- Tinea infections
- Seborrheic dermatitis
- Lichen planus
- Pityriasis rubra pilaris
- Pityriasis rosea
- Onychomycosis
- Fungal infections
- Cutaneous T-cell lymphoma
- Drug reactions

Signs/Symptoms

- Silvery scaly lesions
- Erythematous, sharply demarcated papules and plaques
- Symmetric distribution
- Small to large, droplike/guttate lesions
- Involves extensor surfaces—knees, elbows; also scalp, back, nails, genitalia
- Pruritis may or may not be present
- Pinpoint bleeding when scales are removed due to dilated dermal capillaries
- Nails: Pitted, separated from nail bed
- Psoriatic arthritis: Seronegative arthritis; often begins in DIP joints; swelling of fingers occurs ("sausage digits"); flares and remissions coincide with skin lesions

Diagnosis

- History and physical examination
- Skin biopsy, if necessary, is the gold standard
- KOH test and fungal cultures to distinguish it from fungal infection
- X-ray in psoriatic arthritis shows "pencil-in-cup" deformity of digits

Treatment

- Emollients and ointments
- Corticosteroid ointments or intralesion steroids during flare-ups
- Shampoos for scalp lesions
- Calcipotriol cream (vitamin D analog)
- Anthralin or tar preparations
- Phototherapy: UVA, UVB, or PUVA (UVA plus oral 8-methoxypsoralen)
- Oral/IM methotrexate for severe disease
- Oral etretinate

Prognosis/Clinical Course

- A chronic disease that waxes and wanes over one's lifetime
- Exacerbations may be caused by stress, trauma, respiratory infections, steroid withdrawal, and medications (including lithium, iodine, digoxin, β-blockers, clonidine, and antimalarials)
- Flare-ups tend to occur during winter months
- Koebner phenomenon: Trauma to normal skin can induce local disease
- Guttate psoriasis: Patients without history of psoriasis suddenly develop hundreds of small, red, scaly papules; often following streptococcal infection; once it remits, it usually does not recur
- Emotional consequences of the disease are often much greater than the physical aspects

194. Skin Cancer

Etiology

- Malignant melanoma: Neoplasm of melanocytes
  - Superficial spreading: Most common; best prognosis; back/legs
  - Nodular sclerosing: Rapid growth, often fatal
  - Lentigo maligna: Sun-exposed areas; mostly in the elderly
  - Acral lentiginous: Palms, soles, nail beds; occurs in blacks
- Basal cell carcinoma: Malignancy of epidermal basal cells; slow growth; rare metastases but local ulceration
- Squamous cell carcinoma: May occur in burn scars; local invasion but rare metastases

Epidemiology

- The most common overall cancer worldwide
- Basal cell carcinoma is the most common type of skin cancer, followed by squamous cell carcinoma
- Risk factors include sun exposure, light skin, X-ray or radium burns, arsenic ingestion, family history, and xeroderma pigmentosum

Differential Dx

- Dysplastic nevi
- Keratoacanthoma
- Actinic keratosis
- Verruca vulgaris
- Subungual hematoma
- Seborrheic keratosis
- Benign mole/nevus
- Pigmented epithelioma
- Pseudoepitheliomatous hyperplasia
- Blue nevi
- Dermatofibromas
- Venous lakes
- Pyogenic granulomas
- Warts

Signs/Symptoms

- Melanoma: Solitary lesion, most frequently on back or other sun-exposed areas; flat or raised macule/nodule; satellite pigmentation (due to local metastases) and erythema; ulceration and bleeding; may arise in skin, mucous membranes, CNS, or eyes
- Basal cell: Papule or nodular lesion with central erosion, classic "rodent ulcer"; may have stippled ulceration, waxy pearly edges, and telangectasias; 90% on head and neck
- Squamous cell: Small, hard, reddened, conical nodule +/− ulceration; seen in areas of sun exposure, classically around the mouth/lips, face, and ears; rapidly growing lesion

Diagnosis

- History and physical examination—"A, B, C, D, E"
  - Asymmetric shape: Suggests malignancy
  - Border: Irregular or "smudged" borders suggest malignancy
  - Color: Malignant lesions have non-uniform coloring
  - Diameter: Malignancies tend to be >5 mm
  - Enlargement: Malignant lesions tend to change in size and/or shape
- Malignant lesions may be ulcerated and/or bleeding
- Biopsy is diagnostic
  - Punch biopsy for basal or squamous cell carcinoma
  - Melanoma: Must fully excise lesion for biopsy (do not do punch biopsy)

Treatment

- Gold standard is surgical excision with 1–2 cm margins
  - Mohs' surgery (microscopic excision) for basal cell and squamous cell cancers in cosmetically sensitive areas
- Lymph node dissection if evidence of nodal disease
- Chemotherapy, interferon-β, or interleukin-2 for metastases

Prognosis/Clinical Course

- Metastatic disease to skin and/or internal organs is the most feared complication of melanoma
- Local tissue destruction and cosmetic issues are the most common complications of basal and squamous cell carcinomas
- Five-year follow-up is required
- Staging for melanoma: Breslow's classification of tumor thickness

<0.76 mm	99% 5-year survival
0.76–1.49	85%
1.5–2.49	84%
2.5–3.99	70%
>4	44%
Metastases	<10%

- Staging may also take into account level of invasion (Clark's classification)

195. Skin Lesions in Systemic Disease

Etiology

- Erythema nodosum: Due to *Mycoplasma*/*Chlamydia* infections, sulfonamides, OCPs, autoimmune disorders, pregnancy (50% idiopathic)
- Acanthosis nigricans: Occurs in diabetes mellitus, insulin resistance, malignancy, and other chronic diseases
- Hemochromatosis: A genetic disease in which excessive uptake of iron from gut leads to accumulation of iron in the liver, pancreas, brain, skin, and other organs
- Xanthoma: Hyperlipidemia results in fatty deposits in the skin
- Dermatomyositis: See Poly/Dermatomyositis

Epidemiology

- Hemochromatosis: Peak incidence in fifth decade; genetic link to HLA-A3, -B14, and -B7
- Dermatomyositis: Peak incidence in decades 5–6; women are two times as likely as men to develop it

Differential Dx

- EN: Weber-Christian panniculitis, deep venous thrombosis, cellulitis/erysipelas
- DM: Polymyositis and other connective tissue diseases

Signs/Symptoms

- Erythema nodosum: Classically located on lower extremities; erythematous, tender nodules; arthralgias/pain; fever
- Acanthosis nigricans: Dark pigmented plaques of a velvety texture over flexor and intertriginous surfaces and neck
- Hemochromatosis: Bronzed skin; hepatic cirrhosis and associated esophageal varices; diabetes mellitus; arthropathy; heart failure; pituitary dysfunction
- Xanthoma: Yellowish nodules on face, eyes, extensor surfaces, Achilles tendon
- Dermatomyositis: Proximal muscle weakness with classic heliotropic (violet) rash on eyelids and erythematous rash over dorsum of hands; Gottren's papules (violet lesions) on knuckles

Diagnosis

- Erythema nodosum: Histologic evidence of septal panniculitis; findings associated with etiologic agent
- Acanthosis nigricans: Evaluate for underlying disease; consider fasting blood glucose, TSH, DHEA-S, testosterone; evaluate for malignancy
- Hemochromatosis: Increased transferrin saturation and ferritin levels; elevated LFTs; liver biopsy is diagnostic
- Xanthoma: Lipid panel; TSH; liver and kidney function tests; blood glucose
- Dermatomyositis: Heliotropic rash is pathognomonic; elevated CPK and CK; muscle biopsy shows inflammatory changes near blood vessels; EMG shows polyphasic potentials and fibrillations

Treatment

- Erythema nodosum: Treat underlying cause; NSAIDs for pain
- Acanthosis nigricans: Treat underlying cause
- Hemochromatosis: Weekly phlebotomy to rid body of excess iron stores
- Xanthoma: Reduce hyperlipidemia; surgical excision of nodules may be necessary
- Dermatomyositis: Corticosteroids and antimalarials (i.e., hydroxychloroquine)

Prognosis/Clinical Course

- Erythema nodosum: Resolves once underlying cause is treated; may spontaneously remit within 8 weeks
- Acanthosis nigricans: Prognosis based on underlying disease
- Hemochromatosis: Prognosis based on underlying disease
- Xanthoma: Prognosis based on underlying disease
- Dermatomyositis: Increased risk of malignancy (breast, lung, ovaries, stomach)
  - Poor prognosis if muscle weakness lasts more than 4 months or dysphagia, pulmonary disease, or malignancy develops

196. Urticaria (Hives)

Etiology

- Most cases are immunologically mediated: Type I IgE hypersensitivity causes histamine release from mast cells → local vasodilation, edema, and inflammatory response → wheal and erythema
- Causes include drugs (aspirin, penicillin, morphine, sulfonamides); infections; insect bites; foods and food additives (nuts, fish, egg, milk); systemic disease; direct contact with various irritants; and idiopathic sources

Epidemiology

- Occurs in up to 25% of the overall population
- Family/personal history of atopy may be present

Differential Dx

- Contact dermatitis
- Lymphangitis
- Atopic dermatitis
- Mastocytosis
- Angioedema
- Hepatitis B
- Insect bite
- Erythema multiforme
- Dermatitis herpetiformis
- Bullous pemphigoid
- Vasculitis
- Cellulitis

Signs/Symptoms

- Pruritis
- Reddish, round/oval swellings with pale center and erythematous halo
- Dermatographism: Transient wheal produced by pressure on skin

Diagnosis

- History and physical examination
- Labs: CBC, eosinophil count, ESR, LFTs, urinalysis, hepatitis screen, C_1-esterase inhibitor, complement level, IgE antibodies
- Skin biopsy if lesions persist more than 48 hours
- Cultures/stool cultures to rule out infection
- Elimination diet to pinpoint suspicious foods

Treatment

- Avoid allergen exposure
- Antihistamines are first-line treatment
- Antipruritic lotions and cool compresses for symptomatic relief
- Corticosteroids if necessary; only for short course
- Subcutaneous epinephrine
- Calcium-channel blockers, colchicine, sulfasalazine, dapsone, or danazol may help in some cases
- Beware of anaphylaxis; intubation may be necessary

Prognosis/Clinical Course

- Acute onset, self-limiting
- Most cases remit within 24 hours
- Chronic form may persist beyond 6 weeks
- Some cases may be lifelong
- May be aggravated by heat, fever, alcohol, exercise, or emotional stress

197. Verrucae (Warts)

Etiology

- Benign, slow-growing, hyperplastic epidermal lesions
- Most commonly due to human papillomavirus
- Raised, piled-on growth of variable size; located on skin or mucus membranes, most commonly on hands
- Different clinical presentations based on serotype of infecting HPV and location of lesion
  - Anogenital: HPV 6, 11 (16 and 18 cause cervical cancer)
  - Nongenital: HPV 1–4 cause skin warts

Epidemiology

- Most common viral infection of the skin
- Most common during teen years
- Incubation period of 2 months to 2 years

Differential Dx

- Squamous cell carcinoma
- Secondary syphilis
- Verrucous nevi
- Molluscum contagiosum
- Seborrheic keratosis
- Actinic keratosis
- Lichen planus
- Callus
- Corn

Signs/Symptoms

- Common warts (verruca vulgaris) occur on hands; asymptomatic; single or multiple; most disappear within 2 yrs
- Flat warts (verruca plana) occur on face, hands, legs; multiple—possibly hundreds; flat-topped papules
- Plantar warts (verruca plantaris) are located on the plantar surface of the foot; usually single; often tender; classically these lesion demonstrate pinpoint bleeding when removed; may coalesce into large pustules forming mosaic warts
- Anogenital or venereal warts (condyloma acuminatum) appear as "cauliflower-like" growths on penis, vulva, vagina, cervix, perianal region; cervical lesions are often premalignant

Diagnosis

- Diagnosis is based on clinical examination
- Biopsy confirms the diagnosis; may also determine the serotype of HPV involved
- Distinguish condyloma accuminatum (HPV skin wart) from condyloma lata (skin wart in secondary syphilis)

Treatment

- Most warts are self-limited; tend to disappear within 2 years
- Surgical excision is the treatment of choice
  - Excise if the diagnosis is unclear as lesions may be malignant
- CO_2 laser therapy
- Liquid nitrogen cryotherapy
- Keratolytic agents: Combinations of salicylic acid, lactic acid, podophyllin, and cantharidin
- 5-Fluorouracil cream for flat warts and vaginal warts
- Tretinoin cream for flat warts
- Anogenital lesions must be considered for malignant potential

Prognosis/Clinical Course

- HPV infection is associated with frequent recurrences and spontaneous remission
- Explosive verrucae may be the first indication of HIV infection

198. Viral Exanthems

Etiology

- Rubeola (measles): Paramyxovirus; spread via respiratory droplets
- Rubella (German measles): Spread by respiratory droplets
- Varicella (chickenpox): Due to varicella-zoster virus; spread by respiratory droplets or vesicular fluid
- Erythema infectiosum (fifth disease): B19 parvovirus

Epidemiology

- Rubeola: Affects children > age 10; older adults may be susceptible due to waning immunity
- Rubella: Affects older children/young adults; occurs in springtime
- Varicella: Affects any age; occurs in late winter-spring; increased incidence in immunocompromised hosts
- Erythema infectiosum: Mostly children; female > male; springtime

Differential Dx

- Enterovirus infection
- Herpes simplex
- Erythema multiforme
- Urticaria
- Toxic shock syndrome
- Kawasaki disease
- Rocky Mountain spotted fever
- Dengue
- Infectious mononucleosis
- Scarlet fever
- Roseola infantum
- Other viral diseases
- Insect bites
- Drug reaction
- Dermatitis

Signs/Symptoms

- Rubeola: *Prodrome*—cough, coryza, conjunctivitis; fever; *Rash*—Koplik spots (blue/gray macules) on buccal mucosa; nonpruritic maculopapular rash spreads from head to trunk to extremities
- Rubella: *Prodrome*—URI symptoms, HA; *Rash*—maculopapular; begins on forehead and spreads to face, trunk, and extremities; petechiae on soft palate; postauricular lymphadenopathy
- Varicella: *Prodrome*—fever, HA, malaise for 24 hours; *Rash*—pruritic, "dew drop on rose petal" vesicles on torso, head/face, sclera
- Erythema infectiosum: Maculopapular, reddish rash on cheeks ("slapped cheek") with perioral pallor, arthritis

Diagnosis

- Clinical diagnosis for all exanthems
- Laboratory tests may be helpful
  - Rubeola: Leukopenia, thrombocytopenia, antimeasles IgM and IgG; lymphoid biopsy shows giant cells
  - Rubella: Leukopenia, thrombocytopenia, anti-IgM and IgG
  - Varicella: Tzanck smear, thrombocytopenia, CXR if significant respiratory symptoms
  - Erythema infectiosum: Eosinophilia may be present, IgM levels
- Lack of previous immunization for rubeola, rubella, and varicella may help with diagnosis

Treatment

- All exanthems are self-limited; supportive care is most common
- Rubeola and rubella: Antipyretics, analgesics, hydration, vitamin A supplementation in patients with severe disease
- Varicella
  - Baths, lotions, cool compresses
  - Antihistamines, acetaminophen (*do not* use aspirin—Reye's syndrome may result)
  - Antivirals: Acyclovir, valacyclovir, famciclovir
- Erythema infectiosum: Supportive treatment only

Prognosis/Clinical Course

- Rubeola: 1–2 wk incubation; rash lasts 1 wk; highly contagious throughout; complications include pneumonia, encephalitis, otitis media
- Rubella: 2–3 wk incubation; rash lasts 2–3 days; highly contagious throughout and even after rash disappears; complications include arthritis, encephalitis; congenital rubella syndrome if transmitted in utero
- Varicella: 2–3 wk incubation; 3–5 day eruptions; very contagious several days before eruptions until lesions crust; complications include bacterial superinfection, pneumonia (pregnancy), encephalitis; hepatitis in immunocompromised
- Erythema infectiosum: 2-week incubation; mildly contagious only before rash appears; avoid exposure of pregnant women

199. Herpes Zoster

Etiology

- Zoster (shingles) is due to reactivation of latent varicella-zoster virus from dorsal root sensory neurons; occurs when patient is immunocompromised (e.g., from cancer, trauma, stress, fatigue, illness, or steroid use)
- Opportunistic infection in HIV patients

Differential Dx

- Differential diagnosis depends on area affected
- Angina
- GERD
- Herpes simplex
- Insect bites
- Viral exanthem

Epidemiology

- Increased incidence with age
- Increased incidence in HIV and underlying malignancy

Signs/Symptoms

- Affects trunk, face, and neck along dermatomes
- Unilateral dermatomal distribution
- Rash appears as erythema, then becomes vesicular blisters
- Pain may precede lesions (may be confused with angina, GERD, or ulcer)
- Lymphadenopathy

Diagnosis

- Tzanck smear, direct fluorescent antibody, culture of vesicle fluid; biopsy rarely needed
- Herpes zoster ophthalmicus: Involving the ophthalmic branch of the fifth cranial nerve (in or near the eye, or on the side or tip of the nose); may result in invasive eye disease

Treatment

- Zoster
  - Antivirals: Acyclovir, valcyclovir, famciclovir
  - Antihistamines
  - Analgesics (narcotics)
  - Steroids (especially in elderly) may prevent post-herpetic neuralgia
  - Soothing creams and soaks
- Herpes zoster ophthalmicus requires immediate referral to an ophthalmologist for treatment

Prognosis/Clinical Course

- Pain may precede rash; lasts 2–6 weeks (often increasing duration with age); rarely contagious; complications include ophthalmic zoster, disseminated disease, post-herpetic neuralgia
- Post-herpetic neuralgia: Debilitating pain may persist for months to years after resolution of rash

Rheumatologic & Immunologic Disease

CAROLYN O'CONNOR, MD
KAREN CARPENCY, MD

200. Avascular Necrosis

Etiology

- Infarction and necrosis of bone marrow, trabecular bone, and subchondral bone due to compromised blood supply (in later stages, the articular cartilage is affected and subchondral bone collapses)
- Common etiologies include trauma, corticosteroid use, alcohol abuse, sickle cell anemia, radiation therapy, Gaucher's disease, decompression injury (deep-sea diving), pancreatitis, hyperlipidemia, and thrombosis
- Any joint may be affected, but most commonly occurs in the femoral head

Differential Dx

- Rheumatoid arthritis
- Osteoarthritis
- Spondyloarthropathy
- Septic arthritis
- SLE

Epidemiology

Signs/Symptoms

- Early in the course of AVN, the patient may be asymptomatic
- Later, the patient develops severe pain, a limited and painful range of motion, and a limp (if lower extremity involved)
- Decreased pain with rest
- Noninflammatory joint effusion

Diagnosis

- History and physical examination
- MRI
- Bone scan
- X-ray shows irregular contour of joint articulation; however, may take several months to show evidence of disease

Treatment

- Prevention is most important: Avoid prolonged corticosteroid use; prevent decompression injury; rapid reduction of joint dislocations
- Early stages can be treated with limited weight bearing and analgesics
- Surgical options
    - Core decompression
    - Osteotomy and bone grafting to prevent bone collapse
    - Total joint replacement
    - Joint fusion

Prognosis/Clinical Course

- Disease is usually bilateral, even though the opposite side may be asymptomatic early on
- Small lesions may resolve spontaneously
- Patients with larger lesions tend to progress to subchondral collapse and usually require some type of surgical intervention

201. Gout

Etiology

- A syndrome in which hyperuricemia leads to precipitation of monosodium urate crystals, resulting in inflammation, tissue injury, tophi, and arthritis
- Most cases due to decreased excretion of uric acid (chronic renal disease, low-volume states, diuretics); other cases due to excess production of uric acid (enzyme deficiency/defect, increased cell turnover as in leukemias, psoriasis, and hemoglobinopathies)

Epidemiology

- Middle-aged men are most affected
- Rare in premenopausal women
- High risk in transplant patients on cyclosporine

Differential Dx

- Septic arthritis
- Pseudogout (precipitation of calcium pyrophosphate crystals)
- Other crystal deposition disorders (i.e., calcium hydroxyapatite or calcium oxalate)
- Rheumatoid arthritis
- Osteoarthritis
- Cellulitis
- Trauma
- Stress fracture

Signs/Symptoms

- Acute gouty arthritis
  - Repeated attacks of severe joint pain, swelling, and erythema
  - First MTP joint is most commonly affected (podagra)
  - Also commonly involved are ankle, intertarsal joints, knee, wrist
  - Fever
- Chronic tophaceous gout
  - Palpable tophi develop as crystals are deposited in subcutaneous tissues, periarticular areas, or bone

Diagnosis

- Aspiration of synovial fluid or tophi is diagnositic
  - Negatively birefringent, needle-shaped crystals; up to 60,000 cells/mm^3; >70% PMNs
  - Aspirate of tophi show urate crystals (versus rheumatoid nodules)
- X-ray: "Punched-out" lytic areas with overhanging bony edges (Martel's sign)
- Serum: Leukocytosis, elevated ESR, and elevated uric acid may or may not be present
- 24-hour urine uric acid collection may help distinguish overproducers of uric acid from underexcreters: >800 mg of uric acid in urine indicates overproduction of uric acid rather than decreased excretion

Treatment

- Acute attacks
  - Indomethacin and other NSAIDs
  - Oral colchicine
  - Corticosteroids (intra-articular/oral/IM/IV) in severe disease or contraindications to NSAIDs/colchicine
  - Avoid hypouricemic treatment (i.e., allopurinol) or diuretics during acute attacks
  - Ice
- Prophylaxis
  - Allopurinol: Inhibits xanthine oxidase to decrease production of uric acid; used in overproducers, tophaceous gout, nephrolithiasis, creatinine clearance <50 cc/mL
  - Low-dose colchicine
  - Uricosuric drugs decrease renal reabsorption of uric acid: Probenicid, sulfapyrazone

Prognosis/Clinical Course

- Acute attacks are often triggered by trauma, stress, surgery, illness, alcohol, diet, and changes in uric acid levels
- Avoid alcohol
- Chronic destructive arthropathy may result if not properly diagnosed and treated

202. Low Back Pain

Etiology

- LBP can be loosely categorized into 4 groups
  - Arthritic: OA/DJD, RA, spondyloarthropathies
  - Mechanical: Spondylolisthesis, muscular, fracture, disk/facet disease
  - Postural: Osteoporosis/poor posture → excessive demands of back musculature to support weight → lactic acid buildup → crampy pain
  - Myofascial: Due to muscle co-contraction → lactic acid buildup → crampy pain
- Additional serious causes include malignancy, infection, and referred pain

Epidemiology

- 50% of population will experience LBP by age 20
- 80% by age 60
- Second most common cause of doctor visits (#1 is cold)
- At any given time, up to 20% of the population is experiencing LBP

Differential Dx

- Osteoarthritis/DJD
- Ankylosing spondylitis
- Psoriatic arthritis
- Degenerative disk disease
- Spondylolisthesis
- Compression fracture
- 1° or 2° malignancy (mets from prostate, breast, lung; myeloma)
- Osteomyelitis
- Disk space infection
- Osteoporosis
- Scoliosis
- Fibromyalgia
- Referred pain from AAA, pancreatitis, PUD, renal colic, endocarditis, etc

Signs/Symptoms

- Arthritic
  - OA: Stiffness and soreness after activity; relieved by rest; soreness upon waking
  - Spondyloarthropathies: Early age of onset; pain with rest; improves with activity; decreased mobility of spine
- Mechanical: Pain with movement; possible radiation to leg; better with rest
- Postural: Progressive pain when up and about; increased pain as day progresses, relief with lying down
- Myofascial: Aching, stiffness, and soreness with inactivity; better when active; worse as day progresses; worse with tension and stress; not relieved by rest; pain elicited with palpation
- See "red flags" below

Diagnosis

- History and physical examination are the most important diagnostic tools
- Imaging studies indicated if "red flags" are present, if pain or limited function is refractory to treatment, or if trauma has occurred
  - X-ray: To diagnose osteomyelitis, cancer, fractures, ankylosing spondylitis, segmental instability
  - CT/MRI: To diagnose disk herniation, stenosis, cauda equina tumors, epidural masses
  - Bone scan: To diagnose osteomyelitis, metastases
  - Discography if necessary
  - EMG/nerve conduction studies: To diagnose peripheral nerve injuries

Treatment

- In absence of red flag symptoms:
  - Return to activity as soon as possible; rest has not been shown to improve recovery
  - Acetaminophen, NSAIDs, opioids, muscle relaxants for pain
  - Epidural corticosteroid injections
  - Patient education: Proper back biomechanics and ergonomics
  - Physical therapy: Pain relief modalities (ice, heat, ultrasound), stretching, strengthening, aerobic conditioning, relaxation
  - Surgery in refractory disease, large neurologic deficits, unbearable pain or limitations
- In presence of red flags, workup is necessary based on the underlying symptoms

Prognosis/Clinical Course

- All patients with LBP must be screened for "red flag" symptoms, which may indicate serious disease:
  - Fever
  - Trauma
  - Age >50 or <20
  - Drug abuse
  - Refractory to treatment
  - History of cancer
  - Incontinence
  - Progressive neurologic deficits
  - Weight loss
  - Night pain
  - Impotence
- Precise diagnosis often not pinpointed
- Most patients (those without red flag symptoms) improve within one month without any specific treatment
- Remember myotomes and dermatomes to pinpoint areas of deficits

203. Osteoarthritis

Etiology

- Also known as degenerative joint disease, a noninflammatory "wear-and-tear" disease of the articular surface
- Idiopathic versus secondary OA
  - Idiopathic OA has strong association with family history of OA; may be related to hereditary defects in collagen biochemistry
  - OA may occur secondary to acute or repetitive trauma, joint hypermobility, congenital hip dysplasia, Legg-Calves-Perthes disease, or prior meniscus injury

Epidemiology

- By age 40, 90% of the population has X-ray evidence of osteoarthritic changes, even if they are asymptomatic
- Affects more males than females under age 45; affects more females than males after age 55
- Obesity predisposes to OA of the knees and ankles

Differential Dx

- Avascular necrosis
- Rheumatoid arthritis
- Gouty arthritis
- Calcium pyrophosphate arthropathy
- Spondyloarthropathies
- Osteonecrosis
- Neuropathic joint related to endocrine disease
- Septic arthritis
- Reiter's syndrome
- Tendonitis/bursitis
- SLE
- Polymyalgia rheumatica
- Hemochromatosis

Signs/Symptoms

- Deep, gnawing joint pain that increases with activity
- Morning stiffness <30 minutes
- Pain often subsides with rest
- Joints most involved: Hip, knee, DIP, PIP, first MTP, first CMC, AC joint, disks and facets of spine
- Joint swelling
- Joint deformities may be present, especially in hands: Heberden's nodes (DIP) and Bouchard's nodes (PIP)
- Bony enlargement
- Decreased and painful range of motion
- Crepitus
- Tenderness to palpation

Diagnosis

- History and physical examination
  - History of trauma to joint, sports participation (wear-and-tear), obesity, poor conditioning, meniscal tear
  - Physical findings of crepitus, decreased range of motion, bony enlargement
- X-ray: Joint space narrowing, subchondral sclerosis, osteophyte formation, subchondral cysts
- Synovial fluid analysis: Few WBCs, <25% PMNs, no crystals, normal viscosity
- Arthroscopic evidence
- Normal ESR

Treatment

- NSAIDs or acetaminophen for pain; intra-articular steroid injections for severe pain
- Physical therapy and regular exercise
- Supplements (glucosamine and chondroitin sulfate) may be effective in treating pain
- Viscosupplementation (Synvisc or Hyalgan injections): These hyaluronic acid injections may preserve and/or replenish articular cartilage, and have been shown to decrease pain for 6 months
- Ligamentous reconstruction tendinous interposition at the carpometacarpal joint of the thumb
- Total or partial joint replacement surgery

Prognosis/Clinical Course

- Insidious onset with chronic, sometimes debilitating sequelae
- Symptoms can be treated, but the progression of the disease is unaffected
- Ultimately, many patients with advanced disease will require surgical treatment
- The results of surgical intervention are usually very good, as it allows patients to return to all or most activities of daily living

204. Poly/Dermatomyositis

Etiology

- Idiopathic inflammatory myopathy
- It is postulated that viral infection by Coxsackie B virus or *Toxoplasma gondii* results in an autoimmune process that attacks muscle cells
- Proximal, bilateral muscle weakness ensues

Differential Dx

- Muscle weakness with normal muscle enzymes
    - Motor neuron disease (ALS)
    - Myasthenia gravis
    - Muscular dystrophy
    - Inherited myopathies
    - Steroids
- Weakness with ↑ enzymes
    - Hypothyroidism
    - Sarcoidosis
    - Inclusion body myositis
    - Amyloidosis
    - Trauma
    - Infections
    - Drugs (penicillamine, statins, cocaine, alcohol)

Epidemiology

- Most common acquired cause of muscle weakness
- May be associated with mixed connective tissue diseases and other autoimmune diseases (e.g., scleroderma, RA, SLE)
- Affects more females than males (2:1)

Signs/Symptoms

- Initial presentation of muscle weakness
    - Proximal
    - Bilateral and symmetrical
    - Difficulty combing hair, rising from prone or seated position, and so on
- No ocular muscle involvement
- Dermatomyositis is often preceded by heliotropic upper eyelid rash and periorbital edema, macular facial rash, and rash on knuckles (Gottron's rash)
- Fever, malaise
- Arthralgias
- Weight loss
- Dysphagia may occur (due to involvement of striated muscle in upper third of esophagus)

Diagnosis

- Diagnosis is established by abnormal muscle biopsy
- EMG may show diagnostic pattern
- Elevated enzymes: Creatine kinase (may be up to 50 × normal), myoglobin, aldolase, LDH, glutamate, pyruvate
- Dermatomyositis may be diagnosed by characteristic rash without muscle findings
- Positive ANA in 80% of cases

Treatment

- Treatment is aimed at increasing muscle strength
- Prednisone
    - Discontinue if strength does not improve in 3 months—3/4 of patients fail to improve with steroids
    - DM is more responsive than PM
- Immunosuppressive agents may be used to decrease steroid dosages: Azathioprine, methotrexate
- Some patients respond temporarily to IVIG
- Topical corticosteroids
- Physical therapy
- Avoid sun exposure

Prognosis/Clinical Course

- Symptoms progress over weeks to months
- Dermatomyositis has the better prognosis—80% 5-year survival
- Most deaths occur from pulmonary or cardiac complications, including conduction defects, arrythmias, dilated cardiomyopathy, interstitial lung disease, and pulmonary dysfunction
- Other complications include joint contractures and subcutaneous calcifications
- Increased incidence of neoplasia—breast, ovarian, colon, and melanoma
- Milder disease occurs in patients with coexisting RA, SLE, scleroderma, or Sjögren's syndrome

205. Paget's Disease (Osteitis Deformans)

Etiology

- A disease of excessive bone destruction and disorganized remodeling
- The disease begins with a period of osteoclastic bone resorption, followed by a period of bone formation, which leads to a net gain in bone mass
- New bone is made in a haphazard, disorganized fashion and is therefore architecturally unstable, resulting in bone deformities and frequent fractures
- Cause is unknown but may be due to a paramyxovirus infection

Differential Dx

- Multiple myeloma
- Osteogenic sarcoma
- Osteitis fibrosa cystica
- Metastatic bone cancer
- Fibrogenesis imperfecta ossium
- Hyperparathyroidism

Epidemiology

- Most commonly occurs in middle-aged and elderly patients
- Genetic factors: Up to 25% of family members of affected patients will develop the disease
- Monostotic lesions (disease of only one bone) are fairly common; polyostotic lesions (true Paget's disease) are rare

Signs/Symptoms

- Most cases are mild and/or asymptomatic, often discovered as an incidental finding
- Pain is usually the presenting symptom and the most common complaint; it is generally localized to the affected bone(s)
- Skull, femur, tibia, pelvis, and humerus are the most common sites of involvement
- Can present with DJD, fracture, or neurologic encroachment
- Skull: Bone overgrowth (frontal bossing); may lead to large head and headaches
- May see anterior bowing of the femur and/or tibia; kyphosis
- Deafness, tinnitus, vertigo, and cranial nerve palsies may occur (due to nerve compression by enlarged bone)

Diagnosis

- X-ray: Often diagnostic; shows dense, coarsened trabeculae, multiple fractures, and remodeled cortices
- Bone scan is the most sensitive test to identify bone lesions; may show lesions even before the disease is clinically or radiologically apparent
- Bone biopsy may help to distinguish Paget's disease from metastatic bone disease
- Histology: Irregular broad trabeculae, reversal of cement lines, osteoclastic activity, and fibrous vascular tissue between trabeculae
- Increased serum alkaline phosphatase level
- Increased urinary hydroxyproline excretion
- Generally normal serum calcium and phosphate

Treatment

- The primary goal of treatment is pain relief; thus, many asymptomatic patients are not treated
- Treatment is aimed at slowing the activity of osteoclasts
  - Bisphosphonates (etidronate, pamidronate, alendronate, tiludronate, and risedronate)
  - Subcutaneous or nasal calcitonin
  - Gallium nitrate
- NSAIDs and acetaminophen
- Surgery: Joint replacement, fixation of pathologic fractures, osteotomy
- Care should be taken to adequately treat the patient for increased risk of bleeding before any surgery (such as arthroplasty) as the hypervascularized bone tends to bleed profusely

Prognosis/Clinical Course

- The majority of cases are mild
- Arthritis often presents in joints of involved bones
- Bone tumors are much more common in patients with Paget's disease
  - Osteosarcomas are the most common types of tumors to develop
  - Most frequently occur in pelvis, humerus, femur, and skull
  - Present as abrupt onset of severe bone pain, swelling, and elevated alkaline phosphatase
  - Sarcomas have a poor prognosis—less than 20% long-term survival

206. Primary Amyloidosis

Etiology

- Systemic disorder with irreversible accumulation of amyloid proteins
- Amyloid protein is derived from a fragment of the light-chain immunoglobulin → these fibrils infiltrate and are deposited in various tissues (e.g., heart, muscle, tongue, kidney), replacing normally functioning tissue → results in enlargement and decreased function of the involved tissues
- No apparent cause, but sometimes associated with plasma cell disorders (Multiple myeloma, Waldenstrom's macroglobulinemia)

Differential Dx

- 2° amyloidosis
- Other amyloid-like protein depositions
- Sarcoidosis
- Hemochromatosis
- Multiple myeloma
- Waldenstrom's macroglobulinemia
- Rheumatoid arthritis
- Malignancy

Epidemiology

- Affects middle-aged and elderly individuals

Signs/Symptoms

- Fatigue and weight loss
- Orthostatic hypotension
- Bradycardia
- Organ-specific presentation
  - Heart: Restrictive cardiomyopathy, conduction abnormality, arrhythmias
  - Kidney: Renal tubular acidosis, nephrotic syndrome
  - Musculoskeletal: Arthritis, carpal tunnel syndrome, "shoulder pad" sign
  - GI: Macroglossia, malabsorption (due to small bowel infiltration), hepatosplenomegaly with normal liver function
  - Neurological: Autonomic neuropathy, peripheral neuropathy

Diagnosis

- Biopsy of involved tissue(s) is diagnostic
  - Congo red staining results in green birefringence under polarized light
  - Aspiration and examination of abdominal fat are easiest
- Monoclonal spike in urine or serum
- Specific testing based on involved organ(s): EKG, echocardiogram, U/A, LFTs, EMG

Treatment

- No cure exists
- Prednisone, melphalan, and/or colchicine may be effective
- Stem cell transplantation is under investigation
- Supportive care and organ-specific treatment
- Dialysis/kidney transplantation in renal failure
- Avoid digitalis and calcium-channel blockers

Prognosis/Clinical Course

- Poor prognosis—depends on organ(s) involved and associated diseases
- Patients with multiple myeloma often die within 1 year
- Cardiac involvement may lead to life-threatening arrhythmias and heart failure

207. Rheumatoid Arthritis

Etiology

- A chronic inflammatory state of unknown etiology characterized by synovial proliferation, cartilage destruction, and bony erosion
- Juvenile forms also occur

Epidemiology

- Affects about 1% of population; 3–5% of Native Americans
- Affects more females than males
- Peak onset ages 20–50
- Higher risk in close family members

Differential Dx

- Articular SLE
- Sjögren's syndrome
- Sarcoidosis
- Hepatitis C
- Polymyalgia rheumatica
- Lyme disease
- Gout
- Felty's syndrome (RA, splenomegaly, neutropenia)

Signs/Symptoms

- Early morning stiffness that lasts >1 hour
- Symmetrical joint pain and swelling
  - Worse with motion
  - Relieved by rest
- Fever, malaise
- Swan-neck deformity: Extended PIP joint, flexed DIP joint
- Boutonniere deformity: Flexed PIP, extended DIP
- Subcutaneous nodules
- Extra-articular manifestations
  - Eye: Keratoconjunctivitis, scleromalacia perforans
  - Pleuropericarditis
  - Pulmonary nodules

Diagnosis

- Joint fluid aspiration is diagnostic: >2000 WBCs/μL; >75% PMNs; absence of crystals
- 4 of 7 diagnostic criteria
  - Morning stiffness lasting more than 1 hour, experienced for more than 6 weeks
  - Symmetrical joint swelling for more than 6 weeks
  - Must involve PIP, MCP, or wrist joint
  - More than 3 joints affected for more than 6 weeks
  - Subcutaneous nodules
  - Positive rheumatoid factor (IgM antibody to IgG)
  - X-ray evidence of joint erosion or osteopenia of hand or wrist
- Anemia of chronic disease
- Elevated ESR
- In endemic areas, *Borrelia burgdorferi* infection should be excluded by ELISA testing and Western blot

Treatment

- Nonpharmacologic treatment includes rest, hot baths, paraffin wax, and physiotherapy
- Pain relief with NSAIDs and aspirin
- Aggressive early intervention with multiple medications
  - Methotrexate
  - Hydroxychloroquine
  - Sulfasalazine
  - Minocycline
  - Gold salts
  - Low-dose prednisone
  - Intra-articular steroids
- New biologic agents probably prevent bone erosions: Etanercept and infliximab (TNF-α receptor antibodies) and anakinra (IL-1 receptor antibody)
- Reconstructive surgery in patients who develop destructive arthropathy

Prognosis/Clinical Course

- Goals of therapy: Prevent joint destruction, relieve pain/inflammation, maintain ROM
- There are different patterns of progression: Some patients have a slow onset with multiple remissions and relapses; others have an acute, rapid onset
- Half of patients are disabled within 10 years
- Reconstructive surgery often significantly improves quality of life
- Decreased life expectancy by 3–7 years
- Poor prognosis in white females, rheumatoid factor positive, >20 joints affected, elevated ESR, rheumatoid nodules, joint changes on X-ray
- Complications: Permanent joint deformities, carpal tunnel syndrome, vasculitis, pericardial effusion, atlantoaxial subluxation

208. Sjögren's Syndrome

Etiology

- Chronic inflammatory disease of unknown etiology characterized by lymphocytic infiltration and destruction of exocrine glands
- Destruction of exocrine glands → absence of physiologic secretions → dryness of mucus membranes and conjunctiva → keratoconjunctivitis sicca, xerostomia, and other manifestations

Epidemiology

- Affects 0.5–1% of the population
- 90% of patients are female
- Patients with RA, SLE, or scleroderma have >25% chance of secondary Sjögren's syndrome
- HLA associations

Differential Dx

- Salivary gland enlargement
  - Sarcoidosis
  - HIV
  - Lymphoma
  - Tuberculosis
  - Hemochromatosis
  - Amyloidosis
  - Mumps
  - Alcoholism
  - Graft-versus-host disease
- Dry eyes
  - Vitamin A deficiency
  - Mebomian gland dysfunction
  - Drugs (e.g., anticholinergic)

Signs/Symptoms

- Initially presents with mucosal dryness
- Eyes: Dry, burning, red eyes; photosensitivity
- Mouth: Dysphagia, enlarged salivary glands, cavities
- Systemic: Raynaud's phenomenon, lung infections, fibrosis, renal disease, pancreatitis, thyroiditis, arthralgias, myositis

Diagnosis

- Diagnosis likely if 3 criteria are met, definite if 4 + criteria are present
  - Dry eyes every day for >3 months
  - Dry mouth every day for >3 months
  - Positive Schirmer test: Measures degree of tear wetting
  - Positive salivary gland biopsy
  - Decreased salivary flow
  - Antibodies to protein Ro (SS-A), protein La (SS-B), ANA, or rheumatoid factor
- Lip biopsy showing lymphocytic infiltration is diagnostic
- Keratoconjunctivitis on slit lamp exam
- Elevated ESR

Treatment

- No specific cure
- Treat dry eyes with ophthalmic drops PRN
- Emergent referral for patients with corneal ulceration
- Dry mouth: Pilocarpine; maintain excellent oral hygiene to avoid cavities
- Treat arthralgias with hydroxychloroquine
- May need steroids for systemic symptoms

Prognosis/Clinical Course

- Full disease progresses over 8–10 years
- With an earlier onset, anti-Ro or anti-La antibodies tend to signify more severe disease
- Complications include corneal ulceration, dental caries, and increased risk of lymphoma
- Systemic manifestations in 1/3 of patients

209. Spondyloarthropathies

Etiology

- A group of inflammatory polyarthropathies characterized by sacroiliitis and the presence of HLA-B27
  - Ankylosing spondylitis (AS): Sacroiliitis in young men (this illness is the paradigm for spondyloarthropathies)
  - Reiter's syndrome: Urethritis, conjunctivitis, and lower limb polyarthritis
  - Reactive arthritis: Reiter's syndrome following infectious diarrhea and *Chlamydia* infection
  - Psoriatic arthritis
  - Inflammatory bowel disease-associated arthropathy

Epidemiology

- AS: Young men
- Psoriatic arthritis: 10% of psoriasis patients
- High incidence of HLA-B27

Differential Dx

- Rheumatoid arthritis
- Infectious arthritis
- SLE
- Polymyalgia rheumatica
- Gout/pseudogout
- Amyloidosis
- Fracture
- Hemarthrosis
- Osteoarthritis
- Neoplasia

Signs/Symptoms

- Low back pain
  - Worse in morning
  - Improved as the day goes on and by exercise
- Limited motion of spine
- Limited chest expansion
- Sacroiliitis; tender SI joints
- Enthesopathy: Inflammation of tendon and ligaments at their insertion to bone
- Extra-articular involvement: Iritis, keratoderma blenorrhagicum, aortic insufficiency

Diagnosis

- X-ray
  - Bilateral sacroiliitis in AS
  - Unilateral sacroiliitis in Reiter's syndrome, psoriatic arthritis, and IBD-associated arthropathy
  - Later stages may show a "bamboo spine"
- Elevated ESR and serum IgA levels may also be observed

Treatment

- No curative treatment
- NSAIDs for pain control and suppression of inflammation; intra-articular corticosteroid injections into acutely inflamed joints
- Azulfidine and methotrexate
- Physical therapy and daily exercise emphasizing extension exercises
- Hip arthroplasty and surgical correction of deformities
- Preliminary evidence shows that TNF receptor inhibitors are effective in refractory cases

Prognosis/Clinical Course

- Highly variable prognosis; spontaneous remissions and exacerbations, particularly in early stages of the disease
- Morbidity is related to fused joints in the spine
- Complications include severe hip arthritis requiring arthroplasty, spinal fractures, secondary amyloidosis, apical pulmonary fibrosis, and complications secondary to NSAIDs

210. Systemic Lupus Erythematosis

Etiology

- Chronic inflammatory disease of uncertain etiology characterized by B-cell hyperreactivity, activation of complement, and T-cell defects

Differential Dx

- Rheumatoid arthritis
- Vasculitis
- Lymphoma
- HIV
- Drug-induced SLE (procainamide, isoniazid, hydralazine)
- Poly/dermatomyositis
- Sjögren's syndrome

Epidemiology

- 90% of patients are female
- Blacks have the greatest incidence
- Peak onset in teens and middle-aged individuals
- HLA associations; increased incidence in close relatives
- Flare-ups often occur with pregnancy

Signs/Symptoms

- Malar ("butterfly") or discoid (red, raised, scaly) rash
- Fatigue
- Myalgias and arthralgias
- Arthritis—symmetrical and migratory; especially in fingers, hands, wrists, and knees
- Photosensitivity
- Seizures
- Cognitive dysfunction
- Fever
- Alopecia
- Lymphadenopathy
- Edema secondary to renal disease

Diagnosis

- American College of Rheumatology suggests 4 of 11 criteria should be present for diagnosis (all at once or separately)
  – Malar rash
  – Discoid rash
  – Photosensitivity
  – Painless mouth ulcers
  – Arthritis in more than 2 joints
  – Pleural or pericardial effusion/inflammation
  – Proteinuria (at least 3+ or >0.5 g/day)
  – Seizure activity not attributable to other causes
  – Anemia, leukopenia, or thrombocytopenia
  – Anti-DNA, anti-Smith, or antiphospholipid antibodies or false-positive VRDL
  – Antinuclear antibodies (98% of patients have positive ANA)

Treatment

- Avoid sun exposure
- NSAIDs for arthralgias, myalgias, and fever
- Hydroxychloroquine for skin rashes
- Severe disease with complications
  – Glucocorticoids
  – Cytotoxic drugs: Cyclophosphamide, azathioprine, mycophenolate, methotrexate
- Warfarin for anticoagulation in cases of antiphospholipid antibody syndrome
- IVIG for acute thrombocytopenia, hemolytic anemia
- Screen for and treat osteoporosis

Prognosis/Clinical Course

- Chronic course with exacerbations and remissions
- Complications include Jacoud's arthropathy (tendon disease and rupture), avascular necrosis of hip and other joints (due to chronic steroid use), thrombosis, vasculitis, glomerulonephritis, pericarditis, pleural effusions, pneumonitis
- >90% are alive 2 years after diagnosis; 70% are alive 20 years after diagnosis
- Indicators of poor prognosis: HTN, nephritic syndrome, creatinine >1.4, anemia, antiphospholipid antibody
- Most common causes of death in the initial decade after diagnosis are infections and renal failure; thromboembolic events are the most common cause of death thereafter

211. Systemic Sclerosis (Scleroderma)

Etiology

- Autoimmune disease characterized by vascular injury to skin, lungs, GI tract, and kidneys → leads to vasoconstriction, ischemia, collagen deposition, and fibrosis (sclerosis) of skin and internal organs
- Exposure to silica, polyvinyl chloride, benzene, and toluene may predispose to scleroderma
- Variants include visceral involvement without skin involvement, rapid skin and organ damage, and CREST syndrome (calcinosis, Raynaud's phenomenon, esophageal dysmotility, sclerodactyly, telangiectasias)

Differential Dx

- Limited cutaneous sclerosis
- Diffuse systemic sclerosis
- Systemic sclerosis sine scleroderma
- Mixed connective tissue disease
- Eosinophilic fasciitis
- Overlap syndromes
- Amyloidosis
- Drug-induced sclerosing diseases (bleomycin, pentazocine, toxic oil)

Epidemiology

- Affects more females than males (3:1)
- Associated with HLA-DR529 (lung fibrosis)
- Prevalent worldwide in all races

Signs/Symptoms

- Raynaud's phenomenon: Digital vasospasm upon exposure to cold (cold hands and feet)
- Tight, hidebound skin
- Extension/flexion contractures and ulcerations of fingers
- Arthralgias, polyarthritis
- Reflux esophagitis, dysphagia
- Bloating, abdominal pain
- Dyspnea on exertion, cough
- Dry eyes and mouth
- "Skin softening" may occur later in the disease

Diagnosis

- Presence of sclerodermatous skin fingers on both hands plus involvement of any of the following: Hands proximal to MCP joint, extremity, face, neck, chest, or abdomen
- Any two of the following: Sclerodactyly, pitting scars/loss of finger pads, or bilateral pulmonary fibrosis
- Skin biopsy may be helpful
- Anti-topoisomerase antibodies
- Anti-centromere antibodies in 60% of CREST syndrome cases

Treatment

- Treatment is based on which manifestations present
  - Skin sclerosis may improve with D-penicillamine
  - Screen for and treat reflux esophagitis
  - Treat pulmonary hypertension
  - Pulmonary inflammation: Cyclophosphamide and steroids
  - Renal disease: ACE inhibitors
  - Raynaud's phenomenon: Calcium-channel blockers, nitrates, sildenafil

Prognosis/Clinical Course

- 75% 10-year survival
- Limited disease has better prognosis: Sclerosis restricted to hands and feet; CREST syndrome (see Etiology); pulmonary hypertension
- Diffuse disease: Extensive skin involvement with greater risk of renal, pulmonary, and cardiac disease
- Digital gangrene occurs in smokers

Index

231

Acute tubular necrosis, as differential diagnosis for nephritic syndrome (glomerulonephritis), 104

Acute tubular necrosis (ATN), as differential diagnosis for diabetes insipidus, 125

Acute valvular dysfunction of non-infectious etiology, as differential diagnosis for infectious endocarditis, 8

Addison's disease, 130

Adenitis, as differential diagnosis for Hodgkin's disease, 170

Adenoma, as differential diagnosis for thyroid cancer, 129

Adenomatous polyp, as differential diagnosis for gastric carcinoma, 69

Adenomyosis, as differential diagnosis for leiomyoma (fibroids), 183

Adhesions, as differential diagnosis for bowel obstruction, 93

Adrenal adenoma, as differential diagnosis for hyperaldosteronism, 132

Adrenal cancer, as differential diagnosis for hyperaldosteronism, 132

Adrenal crisis, as differential diagnosis for shock, 30

Adrenal deficiency, as differential diagnosis for SIADH, 124

Adrenal hyperplasia, acquired or congenital, as differential diagnosis for polycystic ovarian syndrome (PCOS), 187

Adrenal hyperplasia, as differential diagnosis
for Cushing's syndrome, 131
for hyperaldosteronism, 132

Adrenal hyperplasia, congenital, as differential diagnosis for pituitary disorders, 137

Adrenal neoplasm, as differential diagnosis for Cushing's syndrome, 131

Adrenal tumor, isolated, as differential diagnosis for multiple endocrine neoplasia (MEN), 135

Adrenoleukodystrophy, as differential diagnosis for Addison's disease, 130

Adult polycystic kidney disease (PKD), 108

Afibrinogenemia, as differential diagnosis for von Willebrand's disease, 166

Airway foreign body, as differential diagnosis for chronic cough, 37

Albinism, 208

Albright's syndrome, as differential diagnosis for neurofibromatosis, 157

Alcohol use, as differential diagnosis
for erectile dysfunction, 194
for secondary hypertension, 26

Alcohol withdrawal, as differential diagnosis for status epilepticus, 153

Alcoholic hepatitis, as differential diagnosis
for alcoholic liver disease, 80
for α_1-Antitrypsin deficiency, 81
for autoimmune hepatitis, 79
for hepatitis A, 74
for hepatitis B, 75
for hepatitis C, 76
for hepatitis D, 77
for hepatitis E, 78

Alcoholic liver disease, 80

Alcoholic liver disease, as differential diagnosis for Wilson's disease, 83

Alcoholism, as differential diagnosis for Sjogren's syndrome, 226

Aleukemic acute leukemia, as differential diagnosis for hemolytic anemia, 175

Aleukemic leukemia, as differential diagnosis for myeloproliferative disorders, 176

Allergic contact dermatitis, 205

Allergic vaginitis, as differential diagnosis for vaginal discharge, 188

Alport syndrome, as differential diagnosis for hematuria, 191

Alveolar hemorrhage, diffuse, as differential diagnosis for ARDS, 34

Alveolar proteinosis
as cause of interstitial lung diseases, 44
as differential diagnosis for idiopathic pulmonary fibrosis (IPF), 47

Alzheimer's dementia, as differential diagnosis for normal-pressure hydrocephalus, 143

Alzheimer's disease, 140

Alzheimer's disease, as differential diagnosis for Huntington's chorea, 144

Amebic abscess, as differential diagnosis for liver abscess, 88

Amenorrhea, as differential diagnosis for endometriosis, 185

Amiodarone-induced epididymitis, as differential diagnosis for epididymitis, 193

Amphetamines, as differential diagnosis for secondary hypertension, 26

Amyloid-like protein depositions, as differential diagnosis for primary amyloidosis, 224

Amyloidosis, as differential diagnosis
for Addison's disease, 130
for diabetes insipidus, 125
for gastric carcinoma, 69
for hypothyroidism, 128
for pituitary disorders, 137
for poly/dermatomyositis, 222
for Sjogren's syndrome, 226
for solitary pulmonary nodule, 56
for spondyloarthropathies, 227
for systemic sclerosis (scleroderma), 229

Amyloidosis as cause of interstitial lung diseases, 44

Amyotrophic lateral sclerosis (ALS), 149

Amyotrophic lateral sclerosis (ALS), as differential diagnosis
for Guillain-Barré syndrome, 148
for Myasthenia gravis, 146

Analgesic nephropathy, as differential diagnosis for hematuria, 191

Anaphylaxis, as differential diagnosis for shock, 30

Anaplastic carcinoma, as differential diagnosis for thyroid cancer, 129

Androgen-producing tumors of ovary or adrenal gland, as differential diagnosis for polycystic ovarian syndrome (PCOS), 187

Anemia, as differential diagnosis
for congestive heart failure (CHF), 4
for syncope, 151

Pancreatic tumors, as differential diagnosis for diabetes mellitus (DM), 126

Pancreatitis, as differential diagnosis
  for abdominal aortic aneurysm (AAA), 27
  for acute myocardial infarction (MI), 3
  for aortic dissection, 28
  for cholecystitis, 91
  for coronary artery disease (CAD), 2
  for diabetes mellitus (DM), 126
  for exudative pleural effusion, 55
  for gastritis, 67
  for gastroesophageal reflux disease (GERD), 66
  for low back pain, 220
  for megaloblastic anemia, 161
  for nephrolithiasis, 109
  for pancreatic cancer, 72
  for peptic ulcer disease (PUD), 68

Papillary breast cancer, 182

Papillary carcinoma, as differential diagnosis for thyroid cancer, 129

Papillary necrosis, as differential diagnosis for nephrolithiasis, 109

Paraneoplastic syndromes, as differential diagnosis for myeloproliferative disorders, 176

Parasitic infections, as differential diagnosis
  for Hodgkin's disease, 170
  for non-Hodgkin's lymphoma, 171

Parasitic infections, cutaneous, 204

Parathyroid growth, as differential diagnosis for thyroid cancer, 129

Parathyroid tumor, isolated, as differential diagnosis for multiple endocrine neoplasia (MEN), 135

Parkinson's disease, 145

Parkinson's disease, as differential diagnosis
  for Alzheimer's disease, 140
  for normal-pressure hydrocephalus, 143

Paroxysmal nocturnal hemoglobinuria (PNH), as differential diagnosis
  for hemolytic anemia, 162
  for myelodysplastic syndromes, 175

Pasteurella
  in osteomyelitis, 118
  in septic arthritis, 119

PCP. *See* Pneumocystis (PCP)

Pelvic cancer, as differential diagnosis
  for colon cancer, 99
  for diverticular disease, 98

Pelvic inflammatory disease (PID), as differential diagnosis
  for appendicitis, 95
  for colon cancer, 99
  for diverticular disease, 98
  for endometriosis, 185
  for leiomyoma (fibroids), 183
  for STD, 178
  for urinary tract infection (UTI), 192

Pelvic kidney, as differential diagnosis for ovarian cysts and tumors, 186

Pelvic mass, as differential diagnosis for prostate cancer, 197

Pelvic surgery, as differential diagnosis for erectile dysfunction, 194

Pelvic trauma, as differential diagnosis for incontinence, 190

Pemphigus vulgaris, 201

Peptic ulcer disease (PUD), 68

Peptic ulcer disease (PUD), as differential diagnosis
  for acute pancreatitis, 70
  for cholecystitis, 91
  for chronic pancreatitis, 71
  for esophagitis, 63
  for gastric carcinoma, 69
  for gastritis, 67
  for gastroesophageal reflux disease (GERD), 66
  for hiatal hernia, 62
  for low back pain, 220

Perforated peptic ulcer, as differential diagnosis for appendicitis, 95

Perforated ulcer, as differential diagnosis
  for abdominal aortic aneurysm (AAA), 27
  for pancreatic cancer, 72

Perforated viscous, as differential diagnosis for acute pancreatitis, 70

Pericardial disease, 10

Pericardial effusion, as differential diagnosis for pericardial disease, 10

Pericarditis, as differential diagnosis
  for acute myocardial infarction (MI), 3
  for aortic dissection, 28
  for Budd-Chiari syndrome, 87
  for coronary artery disease (CAD), 2
  for exudative pleural effusion, 55
  for pneumothorax (PTX), 54

Pericarditis/tamponade, as differential diagnosis for pulmonary embolism (PE), 53

Perineal surgery, as differential diagnosis for erectile dysfunction, 194

Peripheral vascular disease (PVD), 29

Peripheral vascular disease (PVD), as differential diagnosis for syphilis, 180

Perirectal abscess, as differential diagnosis for prostatitis, 196

Peritoneal dialysis, as differential diagnosis for transudative pleural effusion, 55

Peutz-Jeghers syndrome, as differential diagnosis for gastric carcinoma, 69

Phenylephrine, as differential diagnosis for hypertension (HTN), 25

Pheochromocytoma, 136

Pheochromocytoma, as differential diagnosis
  for hypertension (HTN), 25
  for myeloproliferative disorders, 176
  for secondary hypertension, 26

Photodermatitis, as differential diagnosis for dermatitis, 205

Pick's disease, as differential diagnosis
  for Alzheimer's disease, 140
  for Huntington's chorea, 144

Pickwickian syndrome, as differential diagnosis for sleep apnea, 58

Piebaldism, as differential diagnosis for hypopigmentary disorders, 208

Pigmented epithelioma, as differential diagnosis for skin cancer, 210

for dysfunctional uterine bleeding
(DUB), 184
for gonorrhea, 179
for hypercoagulable states, 169
for leiomyoma (fibroids), 183
for megaloblastic anemia, 161
for urinary tract infection (UTI), 192
Pregnancy-induced hypertension, as differential
diagnosis for hypertension (HTN), 25
Premature atrial beats, as differential diagnosis for
atrial fibrillation, 13
Premature ventricular beats, as differential diagnosis
for atrial fibrillation, 13
Primary aldosteronism, 132
Primary aldosteronism, as differential diagnosis
for hypertension (HTN), 25
Primary alveolar hypoventilation, as differential
diagnosis for sleep apnea, 58
Primary amyloidosis, 224
Primary biliary cirrhosis, as differential diagnosis
for portal hypertension, 85
for Wilson's disease, 83
Primary biliary cirrhosis (PBC), 90
Primary bone tumor, as differential diagnosis for
osteomyelitis, 118
Primary lateral sclerosis, as differential diagnosis for
amyotrophic lateral sclerosis (ALS), 149
Primary lung cancer, as differential diagnosis for
solitary pulmonary nodule, 56
Primary malignancy, as differential diagnosis for low
back pain, 220
Primary muscle dysfunction, as differential diagnosis
for achalasia, 60
Primary pulmonary HTN, as differential diagnosis in
HIV-related lung diseases, 43
Primary sclerosing cholangitis (PSC), 89
Prior urologic/gynecologic surgery, as differential
diagnosis for incontinence, 190
Progressive spinal muscular atrophy, as differential
diagnosis for amyotrophic lateral sclerosis
(ALS), 149
Prolactinemia, as differential diagnosis for polycystic
ovarian syndrome (PCOS), 187
Prolactinoma, as differential diagnosis for polycystic
ovarian syndrome (PCOS), 187
Prolonged exogenous ACTH use, as differential
diagnosis for Cushing's syndrome, 131
Prolymphocytic leukemia, as differential diagnosis
for chronic lymphocytic leukemia (CLL), 173
Propionbacterum acne, in acne vulgaris, 200
Prostate cancer, 197
Prostate cancer, as differential diagnosis
for benign prostatic hypertrophy (BPH), 195
for hematuria, 191
for incontinence, 190
for prostatitis, 196
Prostate disorders, 195–197
Prostatic swelling after alcohol consumption, as
differential diagnosis for benign prostatic
hypertrophy (BPH), 195
Prostatitis, 196
Prostatitis, as differential diagnosis
for benign prostatic hypertrophy (BPH), 195
for epididymitis, 193

for hematuria, 191
for incontinence, 190
for prostate cancer, 197
for urinary tract infection (UTI), 192
Prostatodynia, as differential diagnosis for
prostatitis, 196
Proteus, in urinary tract infection (UTI), 192
Proteus mirabilis, in prostatitis, 196
"Pseudoclaudication," as differential diagnosis
for peripheral vascular disease
(PVD), 29
Pseudocushing's, as differential diagnosis for
Cushing's syndrome, 131
Pseudo-dementia, as differential diagnosis for
Alzheimer's disease, 140
Pseudoepitheliomatous hyperplasia, as differential
diagnosis for skin cancer, 210
Pseudofolliculitis, as differential diagnosis for
folliculitis, 206
Pseudogout, as differential diagnosis
for gout, 219
for septic arthritis, 119
for spondyloarthropathies, 227
Pseudohyperparathyroidism, as differential diagnosis
for hyperparathyroidism, 133
Pseudohypoparathyroidism, as differential diagnosis
for hypocalcemia, 134
Pseudomonas
in folliculitis, 206
in HIV-related lung diseases, 43
infection in burns, 202
infections in cystic fibrosis (CF), 39
in neutropenic fever, 117
in osteomyelitis, 118
in pneumonia, 40
in sepsis, 112
in septic arthritis, 119
in urinary tract infection (UTI), 192
Pseudomonas aeruginosa, in prostatitis, 196
Psoriasis, 209
Psoriasis, as differential diagnosis
for cutaneous fungal infections, 203
for folliculitis, 206
for hyperpigmentary disorders, 207
Psoriatic arthritis, 227
as differential diagnosis for low back
pain, 220
Psychiatric disturbance, as differential diagnosis for
coma, 156
Psychiatric disturbances, as differential diagnosis for
normal-pressure hydrocephalus, 143
Psychogenic coma, 156
Psychogenic cough, as differential diagnosis for
chronic cough, 37
Psychogenic stroke, as differential diagnosis for
stroke, 141
Pulmonary alveolar proteinosis, as differential
diagnosis for BOOP, 48
Pulmonary anthrax, 121
Pulmonary diseases, 34–58
Pulmonary edema, as differential diagnosis
for asthma, 35
for hemoptysis, 50
for pneumoconioses, 46

Wegener's granulomatosis, as differential diagnosis
    for Goodpasture's Syndrome, 51
    for sarcoidosis, 49
Whipple's disease, as differential diagnosis for
    infectious diarrhea, 114
"White coat hypertension," as differential diagnosis
    for hypertension (HTN), 25
Wilson's disease, 83
Wilson's disease, as differential diagnosis
    for alcoholic liver disease, 80
    for Alzheimer's disease, 140
    for α_1-Antitrypsin deficiency, 81
    for autoimmune hepatitis, 79
    for hemochromatosis, 82
    for Parkinson's disease, 145

Wolf-Parkinson-White Syndrome, as differential
    diagnosis
    for supraventricular tachycardia, 15
    for ventricular tachycardia, 16

Xanthoma, 211

Yersinia, in infectious diarrhea, 114

Zollinger-Ellison syndrome, as differential diagnosis
    for megaloblastic anemia, 161
Zoster. *See* Herpes zoster